PHLEBOTOMY

ESSENTIALS

Fourth Edition

Ruth E. McCall
Retired Program Director and Instructor
Central New Mexico Community College
Albuquerque, New Mexico

Cathee M. Tankersley, MT(ASCP)
Retired Program Director
Faculty, Emeritus
Phoenix College
Phoenix, Arizona

 Wolters Kluwer | Lippincott Williams & Wilkins

Philadelphia · Baltimore · New York · London
Buenos Aires · Hong Kong · Sydney · Tokyo

Acquisitions Editor: Peter Sabatini
Managing Editor: Andrea M. Klingler
Marketing Manager: Allison M. Noplock
Production Editor: Julie Montalbano
Designer: Doug Smock
Compositor: Nesbitt Graphics, Inc.

Printed in China

First Edition, 1993
Second Edition, 1998
Third Edition, 2003

Library of Congress Cataloging-in-Publication Data

McCall, Ruth E.
    Phlebotomy essentials/Ruth E. McCall, Cathee M. Tankersley.--4th ed.
      p.; cm.
    Includes bibliographical references and index.
    ISBN 978-0-7817-6138-3
    1. Phlebotomy. I. Tankersley, Cathee M. II. Title.
    [DNLM: 1. Phlebotomy. WB 381 M478p 2008]
RB45.15.M33 2008
616.07'561--dc22

                                                                2006039356

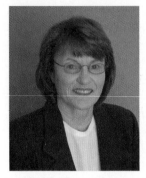

Ruth McCall received her bachelor's degree from the University of Iowa and her medical technology certificate after a year's internship at Saint Joseph's School of Medical Technology in Phoenix, Arizona, and has worked or taught in the area of Clinical Laboratory Sciences and Health Care Education since 1969. Ruth recently retired as Director of the Phlebotomy and Clinical Laboratory Assistant Programs after 18 years of teaching in the Health, Wellness and Public Safety Department at Central New Mexico (CNM) Community College (formerly TVI Community College). While at CNM Ruth proposed creation of the Clinical Laboratory Assistant Program, was instrumental in its development, and was responsible for it becoming one of the first programs at CNM offered entirely through distance education. Ruth participated with science instructors from a local high school in a program that introduced the students to health careers and was the first CNM phlebotomy instructor to teach phlebotomy to high school students through concurrent enrollment. She has lectured on phlebotomy at conferences throughout the United States, served as an expert witness in phlebotomy injury cases, and especially enjoyed participating in a medical technology exchange trip to China. Most recently Ruth had the privilege of being a member of the CLSI Working Group on Venipuncture charged with the 6th revision of the H3 Venipuncture Standard.

Ruth loves the outdoors. She enjoys hiking in the beautiful southwest and downhill skiing in the mountains of Colorado and New Mexico. She has even tried her hand at paragliding. She has been married for 40 years to her husband, John, and has two sons, Christopher and Scott. Christopher and his wife Tracy are parents of her adorable grandchildren, Katie and Ryan.

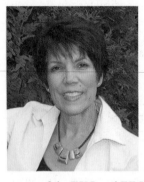

Cathee Tankersley recently retired as Faculty Emeritus after 27 years of teaching at Phoenix College in the Health Enhancement Department. She has worked or taught in the area of Clinical Laboratory Sciences and Health Care Education since graduating from New Mexico State University in Medical Technology in 1964. As an instructor, she has found her 30 graduate hours in Computer Applications to be very worthwhile. Cathee has been active in many professional organizations since she became a medical technologist. She has served on many committees at the state and national level. While at St. Joseph's Hospital and Medical Center, she was the Director of the Medical Technology Program during her last two years at that facility. Her tenure at Phoenix College has been as Clinical Coordinator for the MLT Program, Director of the EKG and EEG Programs, and as the Phlebotomy Program Director since the spring of 1982. While at PC, she established the first and only college-based Law Enforcement Phlebotomy Program in the United States.

She served on the initial NCA Phlebotomy Certification Committee as chair from 1983 to 1985. She was one of the original six members of the NAACLS Approval Committee for Phlebotomy Programs in 1985. She went on to serve as the chair of that committee from 1993 to 1995. Since 1997 when she established her company, NuHealth Educators, LLC, she has been a health care educator and consultant for several organizations. She has served as an expert witness in the area of phlebotomy techniques and has lectured at numerous conferences across the United States.

Cathee moves into active retirement this fall, teaching only 49%, giving her time to enjoy her husband of 41 years, Earl, their two children, Todd and Jaime, and their spouses, Chris and Darin. Most of her spare time will be devoted to the two very special people in her life right now, her grandsons, Trevor and Connor.

Phlebotomy Essentials, 4th edition, was written for all who want to correctly and safely practice phlebotomy. The authors have over 70 years of combined experience in laboratory sciences, phlebotomy program direction, and teaching many different levels and diverse populations of phlebotomy students. As with previous editions, the goal of *Phlebotomy Essentials*, 4th edition, is to provide accurate, up-to-date, and practical information and instruction in phlebotomy procedures and techniques, along with a comprehensive background in phlebotomy theory and principles. It is appropriate for use as an instructional text or as a reference for those who wish to update skills or study for national certification.

ORGANIZATION

Much care has been taken to present the material in a clear and concise manner that encourages learning and promotes comprehension. A good deal of time was spent organizing and formatting the information into a logical and student-friendly reading style in an order that allows the reader to build on information from previous chapters.

The book is divided into four units. Unit I, The Healthcare Setting, presents a basic description of the healthcare system and the role of the phlebotomist within it. Major topics include communication skills, healthcare financing and delivery with an emphasis on clinical laboratory services, quality assurance and legal issues and their relationship to the standard of care, and comprehensive instruction in infection control and safety.

Unit II, Overview of the Human Body, provides a foundation in medical terminology and a basic understanding of each of the body systems, including associated disorders and diagnostic tests. An entire chapter is devoted to the circulatory system, with special emphasis on the vascular system, including blood vessel structure, vascular anatomy of the arm, and blood composition.

Unit III, Blood Collection Procedures, describes phlebotomy equipment (including the latest safety equipment and order of draw) and proper procedures and techniques for collecting venipuncture and capillary specimens based upon the latest CLSI standards. Also included is an extensive explanation of preanalytical variables, complications, and procedural errors associated with blood collection.

Unit IV, Special Procedures, offers information and instruction on how to handle special blood and nonblood specimen collections and point-of care-tests. A separate chapter on arterial puncture is included for those who anticipate advancing beyond venous collection. The last chapter gives good insight into how the LIS works, since it is such an important part of the laboratory process and is used by the phlebotomist in specimen collection. The unit ends with instruction in routine and special handling and processing of specimens, with an emphasis on safety.

FEATURES

This new edition includes various features meant to help the reader learn and retain the information in *Phlebotomy Essentials*.

- **Key Terms** and **Objectives** open each chapter and help students recognize important terms and concepts they will come across while reading the chapter.
- Consistently organized step-by-step **Procedures** with an explanation or rationale for each step assist the student in learning and understanding phlebotomy techniques.
- **Cautions** highlight critical information to help students identify and avoid dangerous practices.
- **FYIs** are interesting notes and fun facts that will enhance practical application of the information.
- **Memory Joggers** offer a proven way to aid some students in remembering important information.
- **Study & Review Questions** at the end of each chapter provide a review of content covered in the chapter.
- A **video-camera icon** is placed throughout the text (usually in Procedures) to indicate where there is supplemental information included on an accompanying CD.
- The **Student Resource CD** includes video clips of skills and procedures, critical thinking questions, games, a glossary with audio pronunciations, and electronic flashcards.
- An optional **student workbook**—*Phlebotomy Essentials Fourth Edition Workbook*—provides additional study questions and case studies, along with a variety of exercises that enhance the learning process, and may be included in this package as well.
- The text is supported by an **Instructor's Resource CD.** This very important guide includes lesson plans, PowerPoint presentations, image and test banks, procedure evaluation forms, and activity log and signature paper samples. It is a valuable tool for first-time instructors and provides an opportunity for seasoned instructors to enhance or update their curriculum.

The content in this new edition of *Phlebotomy Essentials* was designed in accordance with applicable National Accrediting Agency for Clinical Laboratory Science (NAACLS) competencies. Procedures have been written to conform to the latest OSHA safety regulations and, wherever applicable, standards developed by the Clinical and Laboratory Standards Institute (CLSI).

RUTH E. MCCALL
CATHEE M. TANKERSLEY

USER'S GUIDE

This User's Guide shows you how to put the features of *Phlebotomy Essentials* to work for you.

CHAPTER OPENING ELEMENTS

Each chapter begins with the following elements, which will help orient you to the material:

KEY TERMS are listed in the beginning of each chapter and defined in the glossary.

OBJECTIVES provide a quick overview of content to be covered.

PHLEBOTOMY CHAPTER
*Past and Present and the
Healthcare Setting*

1

key·terms

AHCCS	HIPAA	phlebotomy
APC	HMOs	polycythemia
certification	ICD-9-CM	PPOs
CLIA '88	IDS	PPS
communication barriers	kinesic slip	primary care
continuum of care	kinesics	proxemics
CPT	MCOs	reference laboratories
DRGs	Medicaid	secondary care
exsanguinate	Medicare	tertiary care
gatekeeper	PHI	third-party payer

objectives

Upon successful completion of this chapter, the reader should be able to:

1. Define the key terms and abbreviations listed at the beginning of this chapter.
2. Describe the evolution of phlebotomy and the role of the phlebotomist in today's healthcare setting.
3. Describe the traits that form the professional image and identify national organizations that support professional recognition of phlebotomists.
4. Describe the basic concepts of communication as they relate to healthcare and how appearance and nonverbal messages affect the communication process.
5. Describe proper telephone protocol in a laboratory or other healthcare setting.
6. Demonstrate an awareness of the different types of healthcare settings.
7. Compare types of third-party payers, coverage, and methods of payment to the patient, provider, and institutions.
8. Describe traditional hospital organization and identify the healthcare providers in the inpatient facility.
9. List the clinical analysis areas of the laboratory and the types of laboratory procedures performed in the different areas.
10. Describe the different levels of personnel found in the clinical laboratory and how Clinical Laboratory Improvement Amendment regulations affect their job descriptions.

3

SPECIAL FEATURES

Unique chapter features will aid readers' comprehension and retention of information—and spark interest in students and faculty:

> **caution** IA discard tube must be drawn to protect the critical 9:1 blood-to-additive ratio of a coagulation tube that is the first or only tube collected using a butterfly, because air in the tubing displaces blood in the tube.

CAUTION BOXES alert students to potential mistakes and problems before they occur.

Microbial Contamination

Blood cultures detect microorganisms in the blood and require special site-cleaning measures prior to collection to prevent contamination of the specimen by microorganisms normally found on the skin. Blood culture tubes or bottles are sterile and are collected first in the order of draw to ensure that they are collected when sterility of the site is optimal and to prevent microbial contamination of the needle from the unsterile tops of tubes used to collect other tests. Blood cultures do not often factor into the sequence of collection because they are typically drawn separately.

> **key • point** Contamination of blood culture bottles can lead to false positive results and inappropriate or delayed care for the patient.

CLSI Order of Draw

To minimize the chance of specimen contamination, the CLSI recommends the following order of draw for both ETS collection and when filling tubes from a syringe:

1. Sterile tube (blood culture)
2. Blue-top coagulation tube
3. Serum tube with or without clot activator, with or without gel
4. Heparin tube with or without gel plasma separator
5. EDTA tube
6. Glycolytic inhibitor tube

MEMORY JOGGERS reinforce memorization.

memory • jogger For the order of draw:

Stop	Light	Red.	Stay	Put.	Green	Light	Go
(Sterile)	(Lt. Blue)	(Red)	(SST)	(PST)	(Green)	(Lavender)	(Gray)

VIDEO ICONS direct you to informative videos on the CD-ROM that bring material to life.

TABLES outline important information in an easy-to-understand format.

Today, healthcare organizations are downsizing, reorganizing, and shifting the responsibilities for all healthcare providers in an effort to better serve the patient. The development of teams and the sharing of tasks have become necessary as healthcare organizations attempt to find the balance between cost-effective treatment and quality care. Advances in laboratory technology are making point-of-care testing (POCT) more common, centralized laboratory services are giving way to decentralized activities, and other health professionals are being cross-trained to perform venipunctures.

Official Recognition

CERTIFICATION

Certification is evidence that an individual has mastered fundamental competencies in a particular technical area. Certification is a process that indicates the completion of defined academic and training requirements and the attainment of a satisfactory score on an examination. This is verified by the awarding of a title, signified by initials that a phlebotomist is allowed to display after his or her name. National agencies that certify phlebotomists along with the title and corresponding initials awarded are listed in Table 1-1.

LICENSURE AND REGISTRATION

A license is a document or permit granted by the state indicating that permission has been granted for a person to perform a certain service after having met the education and experience requirements and successfully completing an examination. A health professional who has successfully passed a national certification examination or a state licensure examination will be put on a list called a registry. This listing is maintained as long as the health professional pays the registration fee annually (e.g., to the American Society of Clinical Pathology [ASCP] Board of Registry).

Culturally aware healthcare providers enhance the potential for more rewarding interpersonal experiences. This can lead to increased job satisfaction for them and increased patient satisfaction with the healthcare services they provide.

TABLE 1-1 Phlebotomist Certification Agencies and Title, and Initials Awarded

Certification Agency	Certification Title	Certification Initials
American Society for Clinical Pathology (ASCP)	Phlebotomy Technician	PBT (ASCP)
American Society for Phlebotomy Technicians (ASPT)	Certified Phlebotomy Technician	CPT (ASPT)
National Credentialing Agency (NCA) for Medical Laboratory Personnel	Clinical Laboratory Phlebotomist	CLPlb (NCA)
National Phlebotomy Association (NPA)	Certified Phlebotomy Technician	CPT (NPA)
American Medical Technologists (AMT)	Registered Phlebotomy Technician	RPT (AMT)

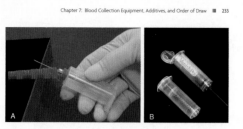

FIGURE 7-13
Safety tube holders. **A.** Venipuncture Needle-Pro with needle resheathing device. **B.** Vanishpoint tube holder with needle-retracting device (Courtesy Retractible Technologies, Little Elm, TX.)

Vacuum   Evacuated tubes fill with blood automatically because there is a **vacuum** (negative pressure, or artificially created absence of air) in them. The vacuum is premeasured by the manufacturer so that the tube will draw the precise volume of blood indicated. To reach its stated volume, a tube must be allowed to fill with blood until the normal vacuum is exhausted. A tube that has prematurely lost all or part of its vacuum will fail to properly fill with blood.

🔑 key • point   Tubes do not fill with blood all the way to the stopper. When filled properly, there is always a consistent amount of headspace between the level of blood in the tube and the tube stopper.

KEY POINTS help to identify and retain important concepts.

Premature loss of vacuum can occur from improper storage, opening the tube, dropping the tube, advancing the tube too far onto the needle before venipuncture, or pulling the needle bevel partially out of the skin during venipuncture. Premature loss of vacuum, removing the tube before the vacuum is exhausted, or stoppage of blood flow during the blood draw can result in an underfilled tube called a partial draw or **"short draw"**. Some manufacturers offer special **"short draw" tubes** designed to partially fill without compromising test results. These tubes are used in situations in which it is difficult or inadvisable to draw larger quantities of blood.

fyi   Manufacturer partial draw tubes are often the same size as standard-volume tubes but do not fill to the same level and may fill more slowly.

FYI BOXES present you with interesting and relevant information.

PROCEDURE 1–2

Performing Venipuncture Below An IV

Purpose: To obtain a blood specimen by venipuncture below an IV.
Equipment: Applicable ETS or Syringe system supplies and equipment.

Steps	Explanation/Rationale
1. Ask the patient's nurse to turn off the IV for at least two minutes prior to collection.	A phlebotomist is not qualified to make IV adjustments. Turning off the IV for two minutes allows IV fluids to dissipate from the area.
2. Apply the tourniquet distal to the IV.	Avoids disturbing the IV.
3. Select a venipuncture site distal to the IV	Venous blood flows up the arm towards the heart. Drawing below an IV affords the best chance of obtaining blood that is free of IV fluid contamination.
4. Perform the venipuncture in a different vein than the one with the IV if possible.	IV fluids can be present below an IV due to backflow and may still be there after the IV is shut off due to poor venous circulation.
5. Ask the nurse to restart the IV after the specimen has been collected.	IV flow rates must be precise and starting or adjusting them is not part of a phlebotomist's scope of practice.
6. Document that the specimen was collected below an IV, indicate the type of fluid in the IV, and identify which arm.	This aids laboratory personnel and the patient's physician in the event test results are questioned.

PROCEDURES are presented in easy-to-follow steps with explanations.

CONFIDENTIALITY

Patient confidentiality is seen by many as the ethical cornerstone of professional behavior in the healthcare field. It serves to protect both the patient and the practitioner. As a professional, the healthcare provider should recognize that all patient information is absolutely private and confidential. Information, such as a patient's test results, treatment, or condition, is not to be discussed any place where the information might be overheard. In addition, patient information should not be released to unauthorized people. Any questions relating to patient information, such as inquiries from a reporter in the case of a celebrity, should be referred to the proper person in administration. Unauthorized release of information concerning a patient is considered invasion of privacy. Information should only be given out with the written consent of the patient.

CHAPTER CLOSING ELEMENTS

Each chapter closes with the following elements, which will help aid in further study:

CASE STUDIES bring concepts to life and enhance critical thinking skills.

> 16 ■ Chapter 1: Phlebotomy: Past and Present and the Healthcare Setting
>
> ## CASE · STUDY
>
> ### An Accident Waiting to Happen
>
> A female phlebotomist works alone in an outpatient clinic. It is almost time to close for lunch when a patient arrives for a blood test. The phlebotomist is flustered because she has a special date for lunch. she is dressed up for the occassion, wearing a nice dress and high heels. She looks nice except for a large scratch on her left wrist that she got while playing with her cat this morning. she quickly draws the patient's blood. As she turns to put the specimen in the rack, she slips and falls. One of the tubes breaks. She does not get cut, but blood splashes everywhere, including her left wrist.
>
> QUESTIONS:
> 1. What is the first thing the phlebotomist should do?
> 2. How did the phlebotomist's actions contribute to this accident?
> 3. What should she have done that might have prevented the exposure, despite the tube breaking?
> 4. What type of exposure did she receive?

> Chapter 1: Phlebotomy: Past and Present and the Healthcare Setting ■
>
> ## STUDY & REVIEW QUESTIONS
>
> 1. Early equipment used for blood-letting includes all of the following *except* the
>   a. hemostat.   c. fleam.
>   b. lancet.   d. leech.
>
> 2. A factor that contributes to the phlebotomist's professional image is
>   a. personal hygiene.   c. a pleasant smile and a positive attitude.
>   b. national certification.   d. all of the above.
>
> 3. The initials for the title granted after successful completion of the National Credentialing Agency phlebotomy examination are
>   a. CLPlb.   c. CPT.
>   b. CLT.   d. PBT.
>
> 4. The principles of right and wrong conduct as they apply to professional problems are called
>   a. certification.   c. esteem.
>   b. ethics.   d. tort.
>
> 5. An example of a third-party payer is
>   a. Medicare.   c. OSHA.
>   b. DRG.   d. CPT.
>
> 6. Which of the following is a duty of a phlebotomist?
>   a. Chart patient results   c. Analyze specimens for hematology
>   b. Obtain blood pressures and temperatures of patients   d. Perform laboratory computer operations
>
> 7. Which of the following is an example of proxemics?
>   a. Eye contact   c. Facial expressions
>   b. Zone of comfort   d. Personal hygiene
>
> 8. Which of the following is proper telephone technique?
>   a. Wait for the phone to ring three or four times so as not to appear anxious.
>   b. Do not identify yourself in case there are problems later.
>   c. Be careful of the tone of voice used and keep answers simple.
>   d. Listen carefully; do not take notes because it takes too much time.

STUDY & REVIEW QUESTIONS provoke thought and help test your comprehension of each chapter's major concepts.

ADDITIONAL LEARNING RESOURCE

This powerful learning tool also includes:

> Student Resource CD-ROM to Accompany
>
> PHLEBOTOMY
> *Essentials*
> FOURTH EDITION
>
> To Run Program:
> Insert the CD-ROM. The program should run automatically. If it does not:
> 1. Double-click on the 'My Computer' icon on your desktop.
> 2. Double-click on your CD-ROM drive.
> 3. Double-click on 'Start' or 'Start.exe'.
>
> Ruth McCall
> Cathee Tankersley
>
> LWW Technical Support:
> 1-800-638-3030
> technicalsupport3@wolterskluwer.com
>
> Copyright © 2007
>
> ● Wolters Kluwer | Lippincott Williams & Wilkins

STUDENT CD-ROM with animations, electronic flashcards, exercises and games, clinical procedures videos, and a glossary with audio pronunciations. Materials are also available on a companion website: **http://thepoint.lww.com/mccall4e.**

ACKNOWLEDGMENTS

Many individuals gave of their time, talent, and expertise to make this edition of *Phlebotomy Essentials* and the accompanying student and instructor CDs possible. The authors sincerely wish to express their gratitude to all including Nancy Ackerman, Judy Arbique, Blanca Bujanda, Glenda Hiddessen, Bruce Knaphus, Monica Lewis, Dorothy "Mimi" Roush, and graduates of the Phoenix College program, Rebecca Bautista, Kaylin A. Oddo, Zhengyun "Sophie" Qiao, Timothy L. Slim, and Debra A. Waffle. Others we wish to thank include videographer Michael Norde; ancillary editor Molly Ward; Shannon Conley, Phlebotomy Supervisor at John C. Lincoln Hospital in Phoenix; Judi Armstrong from Beckman Coulter; and all the manufacturers who allowed us to illustrate their products. In addition, we are grateful for the support and dedication of the staff at LWW, especially those with whom we worked most closely, Acquisitions Editor Pete Sabatini, Managing Editor Andrea Klingler, Production Editor Julie Montalbano, and Associate Marketing Manager, Allison Noplock.

CONTENTS

The Healthcare Setting

PHLEBOTOMY

CHAPTER

Past and Present and the Healthcare Setting

1

key•terms

AHCCCS	HIPAA	phlebotomy
APC	HMOs	polycythemia
certification	ICD-9-CM	PPOs
CLIA '88	IDS	PPS
communication barriers	kinesic slip	primary care
continuum of care	kinesics	proxemics
CPT	MCOs	reference laboratories
DRGs	Medicaid	secondary care
exsanguinate	Medicare	tertiary care
gatekeeper	PHI	third-party payer

objectives

Upon successful completion of this chapter, the reader should be able to:

1. Define the key terms and abbreviations listed at the beginning of this chapter.
2. Describe the evolution of phlebotomy and the role of the phlebotomist in today's healthcare setting.
3. Describe the traits that form the professional image and identify national organizations that support professional recognition of phlebotomists.
4. Describe the basic concepts of communication as they relate to healthcare and how appearance and nonverbal messages affect the communication process.
5. Describe proper telephone protocol in a laboratory or other healthcare setting.
6. Demonstrate an awareness of the different types of healthcare settings.
7. Compare types of third-party payers, coverage, and methods of payment to the patient, provider, and institutions.
8. Describe traditional hospital organization and identify the healthcare providers in the inpatient facility.
9. List the clinical analysis areas of the laboratory and the types of laboratory procedures performed in the different areas.
10. Describe the different levels of personnel found in the clinical laboratory and how Clinical Laboratory Improvement Amendment regulations affect their job descriptions.

Healthcare, today, has evolved into an integrated delivery system offering a full range of services to ensure that the patient gets what is needed at the right time and in the right way. In addition to physicians, nurses, and patient support personnel, allied health professionals such as clinical laboratory personnel play a role in the delivery of patient care. The clinical laboratory provides physicians with some of medicine's most powerful diagnostic tests. Before patient test results can be reported to the physician, specimens must be collected and analyzed. The phlebotomist has been a key player in this process for some time. In addition to blood collection skills, successful specimen collection requires the phlebotomist to demonstrate competence, professionalism, good communication and public relations skills, thorough knowledge of the healthcare delivery system, and familiarity with clinical laboratory services. An understanding of phlebotomy from an historical perspective helps the phlebotomist appreciate the significance of his or her role in healthcare today.

PHLEBOTOMY: AN HISTORICAL PERSPECTIVE

Since very early times, man has been fascinated by blood and has believed in some connection between the blood racing through his veins and his well-being. From this belief, certain medical principles and procedures dealing with blood evolved, some surviving to the present day.

An early medical theory developed by Hippocrates (460–377 BC) stated that disease was the result of excess substance, such as blood, phlegm, black bile, and yellow bile, within the body. It was thought that removal of the excess would restore balance. The process of removal and extraction became the treatment and could be done either by expelling disease materials through the use of drugs or by direct removal during surgery. One important surgical technique was **phlebotomy**—the process of bloodletting. Bloodletting involved cutting into a vein with a sharp instrument and releasing blood in an effort to rid the body of evil spirits, cleanse the body of impurities, or as in Hippocrates' time, bring the body into proper balance. Literal translation of the word phlebotomy comes from the Greek words *phlebos*, meaning veins, and *tome*, meaning incision.

Some authorities believe phlebotomy dates back to the last period of the Stone Age, when crude tools were used to puncture vessels to allow excess blood to drain out of the body. A painting in a tomb showing the application of a leech to a patient evidences bloodletting in Egypt in about 1400 BC. Early in the Middle Ages, barber-surgeons flourished. By 1210, the Guild of Barber-Surgeons was formed and divided the surgeons into Surgeons of the Long Robe and Surgeons of the Short Robe. Soon the Short Robe surgeons were forbidden by law to do any surgery except bloodletting, wound surgery, cupping, leeching, shaving, tooth extraction, and enema administration.

To distinguish their profession from that of the Long Robe surgeon, barber–surgeons placed a striped pole from which a bleeding bowl was suspended outside their doors. The pole represented the rod squeezed by the patient to promote bleeding and the white stripe on the pole corresponded to the bandages, which were also used as tourniquets. Soon, handsomely decorated ceramic bleeding bowls (Fig. 1-1) came into fashion and were passed down from one generation to the next. These bowls, which often doubled as shaving bowls, usually had a semicircular area cut out on one side to facilitate placing the bowl under the chin.

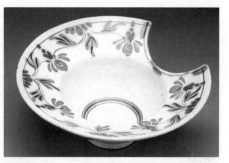

FIGURE 1-1
Bleeding bowl.

During the 17th and early 18th centuries, phlebotomy was considered a major therapeutic (treatment) process, and anyone willing to claim medical training could perform phlebotomy. The lancet, a tool used for cutting the vein during a procedure called venesection, was perhaps the most prevalent medical instrument of the times. The usual amount of blood withdrawn was approximately 10 mL, but excessive phlebotomy was common.

fyi   Excessive phlebotomy was thought to have contributed to George Washington's death in 1799, when he was diagnosed with a throat infection and the physician bled him four times in 2 days. It was because of Washington's request to be allowed to die without further medical intervention that the physician did not completely **exsanguinate** or remove all blood from him.

During this same period, phlebotomy was also accomplished by cupping and leeching. The art of cupping required a great deal of practice to maintain the high degree of dexterity necessary so as not to appear clumsy and frighten the patient away. Cupping involved the application of a heated suction apparatus, called the "cup," to the skin to draw the blood to the surface before severing the capillaries in that area by making a series of parallel incisions with a lancet or fleam. The typical fleam was a wide double-edged blade at right angles to the handle. Eventually, multiple fleams (Fig. 1-2) were attached and folded into a

FIGURE 1-2
Typical fleams.

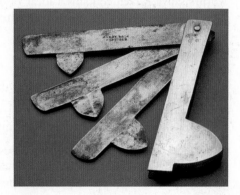

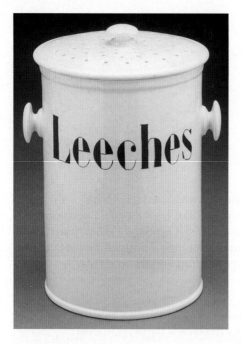

FIGURE 1-3
Leech jar.

brass case for easy carrying. The blades were wiped clean with only a rag and readily transmitted a host of bloodborne infections from patient to patient.

Fleams were used for general phlebotomy to open an artery or, more commonly, a vein to remove large amounts of blood. For more localized bloodletting, leeches were used. This procedure involved enticing the *Hirudo medicinalis*, a European medicinal leech, to the spot needing bloodletting with a drop of milk or blood on the patient's skin. After the leech was engorged with blood, which took about an hour, it was allowed to drop off by itself. By the mid-18th century, leeching was widely practiced in Europe, especially in France. Leeches were kept in special vessels that were filled with water and had perforated tops so that the leeches could breathe. Early leech jars were glass, and later ones ceramic (Fig. 1-3). Within the last decade, leeches have made a comeback as defenders from the complications of microsurgical replantation (Fig. 1-4). The value of leech therapy lies in the components of the worm's saliva, which contains a local vasodilator (substance that increases the diameter of blood vessels), a local anesthetic, and hirudin, an anticoagulant (substance that prevents clotting).

PHLEBOTOMY TODAY

The practice of phlebotomy continues to this day; however, principles and methods have improved dramatically. Today, phlebotomy is performed to

- Obtain blood for diagnostic purposes and monitoring of prescribed treatment
- Remove blood for transfusions at a donor center
- Remove blood for therapeutic purposes such as treatment for **polycythemia**, a disorder involving overproduction of red blood cells

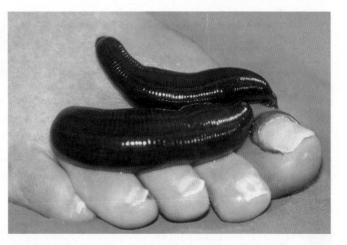

FIGURE 1-4
Toe with leech.

Phlebotomy is primarily accomplished by one of two procedures:

- Venipuncture, which involves collecting blood by penetrating a vein with a needle and syringe or other collection apparatus
- Capillary puncture, which involves collecting blood after puncturing the skin with a lancet

The Role of the Phlebotomist in a Changing Healthcare Environment

The term phlebotomist is applied to a person who has been trained in various techniques to perform phlebotomy procedures. It is the responsibility of a phlebotomist to collect blood for laboratory analysis that is necessary for the diagnosis and care of a patient. A well-prepared phlebotomist must have good manual dexterity, special communication skills, good organizational skills, and a thorough knowledge of laboratory test requirements and departmental policies. The most common duties and responsibilities of a phlebotomist are listed in Box 1-1.

Today, healthcare organizations are reorganizing, merging, and integrating healthcare delivery due to increased pressure to contain costs and improve quality. By focusing on a holistic, coordinated system of healthcare services called a **continuum of care**, they are shifting the responsibilities for all healthcare providers in an effort to better serve the patient, now often referred to as the customer. The development of teams and the sharing of tasks have become necessary as healthcare organizations attempt to find the balance between cost-effective treatment and high-quality care. Advances in laboratory technology are making point-of-care testing (POCT) more common, and services that were once unique to the laboratory can now be provided at other locations. As a result, many health professionals are being cross-trained to perform phlebotomy (or blood collection procedures.) Consequently, the term "phlebotomist" is being applied to anyone who has been trained to collect blood specimens.

During this time of transition, the profession of phlebotomy maintains a standardized educational curriculum with a recognized body of knowledge. Structured programs exist in

BOX • 1-1   Duties and Responsibilities of a Phlebotomist

- Prepare patients for collection procedures associated with laboratory samples
- Collect routine skin puncture and venous specimens for testing as required
- Prepare specimens for transport to ensure stability of sample
- Maintain patient confidentiality
- Perform quality control checks while carrying out clerical, clinical, and technical duties
- Transport specimens to the laboratory
- Comply with all procedures instituted in the procedure manual
- Promote good public relations with patients and hospital personnel
- Assist in collecting and documenting monthly workload and recording data
- Maintain safe working conditions
- Perform laboratory computer operations
- Participate in continuing education programs
- Collect and perform point-of-care testing (POCT)
- Perform quality control checks on POCT instruments
- Perform skin tests
- Process specimens and perform basic laboratory tests
- Collect urine drug screen specimens
- Perform electrocardiography
- Perform front office duties, current procedural terminology coding, and paperwork

hospitals, vocational schools, and colleges that incorporate classroom instruction and clinical practice to prepare the student for national certification.

Official Recognition

CERTIFICATION

Certification is evidence that an individual has mastered fundamental competencies in a particular technical area. Certification indicates the completion of defined academic and training requirements and the attainment of a satisfactory score on an examination. This is verified by the awarding of a title, signified by initials that a phlebotomist is allowed to display after his or her name. Examples of national agencies that certify phlebotomists along with the title and corresponding initials awarded are listed in Table 1-1.

TABLE 1-1 Phlebotomist Title and Initials Awarded by Certification Agency		
Certification Agency	**Certification Title**	**Certification Initials**
American Medical Technologists	Registered Phlebotomy Technician	RPT(AMT)
American Certification Agency	Certified Phlebotomy Technician	CPT(ACA)
American Society for Clinical Pathology	Phlebotomy Technician	PBT(ASCP)
National Center for Competency Testing	National Certified Phlebotomy Technician	NCPT(NCCT)
National Credentialing Agency	Clinical Laboratory Phlebotomist	CLPlb(NCA)
National Health Career Association	Certified Phlebotomy Technician	CPT(NHA)

Mailing and email addresses and telephone numbers can be found in McCall, R. Phlebotomy exam review (2nd ed).

LICENSURE AND REGISTRATION

A license is a document or permit granted by the state indicating permission for a person to perform a certain service after having met the education and experience requirements and successfully completing an examination. A health professional who has successfully passed a national certification examination or a state licensure examination will be awarded credentials and put on a list called a registry. These credentials indicate competency only at the time of examination. Recertification is a mechanism used to demonstrate continued competency through either reexamination or continuing education.

CONTINUING EDUCATION

It is important for phlebotomists to participate in continuing education to keep their knowledge base and skills up-to-date. Many organizations sponsor workshops, seminars, and self-study programs that award continuing education units (CEUs) to those who participate. Most certifying and licensing agencies require CEUs or other proof of continuing education for renewal of credentials. Employers may offer in-service education or provide funds for employees to attend offsite programs offered by organizations such as the American Society for Clinical Laboratory Sciences (ASCLS) and the American Medical Technologists (AMT).

Public Relations and Client Interaction

As a member of the clinical laboratory team, the phlebotomist plays an important role in public relations for the laboratory. Positive public relations involves promoting good will and a harmonious relationship with staff, visitors, and especially patients. The phlebotomist is often the only real contact the patient has with the laboratory. In many cases, patients equate this encounter with the caliber of care they receive while in the hospital. A confident phlebotomist with a professional manner and a neat appearance helps to put the patient at ease and helps establish a positive relationship.

RECOGNIZING DIVERSITY

Despite similarities, fundamental differences among people arise from nationality, ethnicity, and culture, as well as from family background, life experiences, and individual challenges. These differences affect the health beliefs and behaviors of both patients and providers.

Culturally aware healthcare providers enhance the potential for more rewarding interpersonal experiences. This can lead to increased job satisfaction for them and increased patient satisfaction with the healthcare services they provide.

Critical factors in the provision of healthcare services that meet the needs of diverse populations include understanding the:

* Beliefs and values that shape a person's approach to health and illness
* Health-related needs of patients and their families according to the environments in which they live
* Knowledge of customs and traditions related to health and healing
* Attitudes toward seeking help from healthcare providers

key • point By recognizing diversity the phlebotomist promotes good will and harmonious relationships that directly improve health outcomes, the quality of services, and public relations.

PROFESSIONALISM

Professionalism is defined as the conduct and qualities that characterize a professional person. As part of a service-oriented industry, persons performing phlebotomy must practice professionalism.

The overall impression conveyed by a person creates an image. The professional image is the way in which an occupation or a member of that profession is perceived. This image is formed from several characteristics or traits. The first characteristic deals with the superficial aspects of a person, for example, the way a person dresses or his or her manner of speaking. In fact, general appearance and grooming reflect directly on whether the phlebotomist is perceived as a professional. Conservative clothing, proper personal hygiene, and physical well-being contribute to a professional appearance. Institutional policies for attire are influenced by a federal standard that requires employers to provide protective clothing for laboratory workers, including phlebotomists.

Professionalism also involves personal behaviors or characteristics, including the following.

Integrity Professional standards of integrity or honesty require a person to do what is right regardless of the circumstances. For example, a phlebotomist often functions independently and may be tempted to take procedural shortcuts when pressed for time. A phlebotomist with integrity understands that following the rules for collection is essential to the quality of test results—and respects those rules.

Compassion A phlebotomist may show compassion and still remain professional. Compassion simply means being sensitive to a patient's or customer's needs and being willing to offer reassurance in a caring and interested way.

Motivation   Phlebotomists with motivation find the workplace a challenge no matter what their tasks entail. Motivation is a direct reflection of a person's attitude about life. If phlebotomists have a positive attitude and a willingness to perform at their peak every day, the healthcare environment will consistently offer adventure and growth, especially during this exciting time of changing roles and responsibilities.

Dependability   Dependability and work ethic go hand-in-hand. An individual who is dependable and who takes personal responsibility for his or her actions is extremely refreshing in today's environment and is a very desirable candidate for job opportunities in the healthcare setting or anywhere.

Diplomacy/Ethical Behavior   A phlebotomist should demonstrate diplomacy and ethical behavior at all times. Diplomacy means that the phlebotomist uses effective communication skills and tact while dealing with the patient, even in stressful situations. Ethical behavior entails conforming to a standard of right and wrong conduct to avoid harming the patient in any way. Based on a system of principles called ethics, the professional can identify conduct that is morally desirable. A code of ethics, although not enforceable by law, leads to uniformity and defined expectation by the members of that profession. Professional organizations, such as ASCLS, have developed codes of ethics for healthcare professionals. As stated in the Hippocratic oath, "primum non nocere," or "first do not harm," the primary objective in any healthcare professional's code of ethics must always be the patient's welfare. A guide to working with that principle in mind is a document of accepted quality-care principles developed by the American Hospital Association, and related to patient rights.

PATIENT RIGHTS

The phlebotomist, like any other member of the healthcare team, must recognize the rights and privileges a patient has while in a hospital or other healthcare facility. These rights have been clearly defined in a document first adopted in 1973 by the American Hospital Association, called **A Patient's Bill of Rights**. This document, although not legally binding nor federally mandated, is an accepted statement of principle that encourages and guides healthcare institutions to customize this document to ensure that patients and their families understand their rights and responsibilities.

The latest revision approved by the AHA Board in 2003 is entitled **"The Patient Care Partnership"**. This easy-to-read brochure replaces the AHA's Patients' Bill of Rights and is designed to help patients understand their expectations during their hospital stay with regard to their rights and responsibilities. It states that the first priority of all healthcare professionals, including phlebotomists, is to provide high-quality patient care in a clean and safe environment, while also maintaining the patient's personal rights and dignity by being sensitive to cultural, racial, religious, gender, age, and other differences. Expectations listed in the brochure are summarized in Box 1-2.

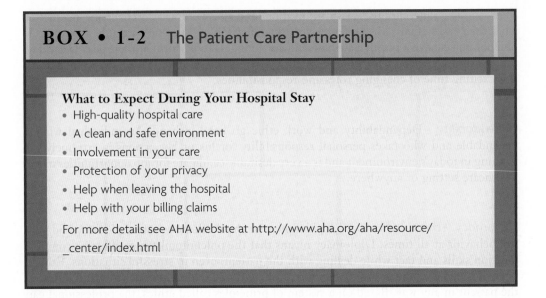

BOX • 1-2 The Patient Care Partnership

What to Expect During Your Hospital Stay
- High-quality hospital care
- A clean and safe environment
- Involvement in your care
- Protection of your privacy
- Help when leaving the hospital
- Help with your billing claims

For more details see AHA website at http://www.aha.org/aha/resource/
_center/index.html

CONFIDENTIALITY

Patient confidentiality is seen by many as the ethical cornerstone of professional behavior in the healthcare field. It serves to protect both the patient and the practitioner. As a professional, the healthcare provider should recognize that all patient information is absolutely private and confidential.

key • point Maintaining confidentiality is such an important issue in testing for HIV that the patient must sign a consent form before the specimen for the test can be collected.

Any questions relating to patient information should be referred to the proper authority. Unauthorized release of information concerning a patient is considered invasion of privacy. In 1996, a federal law was passed requiring all healthcare providers to obtain a patient's consent in writing before disclosing medical information such as a patient's test results, treatment, or condition to any unauthorized person. That law is the **Health Insurance Portability and Accountability Act** (HIPAA) of 1996.

HIPAA As a person's health information has become more easily transferred from one facility or entity to the next through electronic exchange, a growing problem with a person's rights and confidentiality has arisen. The HIPAA law, which became effective in 2003, was enacted in order to more closely secure this information and regulate patient privacy. The law established national standards for the electronic exchange of **protected health information** (PHI). Penalties for HIPAA violations include disciplinary action, fines, and possible jail time.

The law states that patients must be given information on their rights concerning the release of PHI and how it will be used. **Healthcare workers** (HCWs) must obtain the patient's written authorization for any use or disclosure of PHI unless the use or disclosure is for treatment, payment, or healthcare operations. To avoid litigation in this area, all HCWs and students must sign a confidentiality and nondisclosure agreement affirming that they understand HIPAA and will keep all patients' information confidential.

Communication Skills

Phlebotomy is both a technical and a people-oriented profession. Many different types of people or customers interact with phlebotomists. Often, the customer's perception of the healthcare facility is derived from the employees they deal with on a one-to-one basis, such as a phlebotomist. Customers expect high-quality service. A phlebotomist who lacks a good bedside manner (the ability to communicate empathically with the patient) increases the chances of becoming part of a legal action should any difficulty arise while obtaining the specimen. Favorable impressions result when professionals respond properly to patient needs, and this occurs when there is good communication between the healthcare provider and the patient.

COMMUNICATION DEFINED

Communication is a skill. Defined as the means by which information is exchanged or transmitted, communication is one of the most important processes that takes place in the healthcare system. This dynamic or constantly changing process involves three components: verbal skills, nonverbal skills, and the ability to listen.

COMMUNICATION COMPONENTS

Verbal Communication Expression through the spoken word is the most obvious form of communication. Effective healthcare communication should be an interaction in which both participants are affected. It involves a *sender* (speaker), a *receiver* (listener), and, when complete, a process called *feedback*, creating what is referred to as the *communication feedback loop* (Fig. 1-5). Accurate verbal exchange depends upon feedback, as it is through feedback that the listener or receiver is given the chance to correct miscommunication.

Normal human behavior sets up many **communication barriers** (biases or personalized filters) that are major obstructions to hearing and understanding what has been said and a frequent cause of miscommunication. Examples of communication barriers are language limitations, culture diversity, emotions, age, and physical disabilities such as hearing loss.

To encourage good verbal communication, the phlebotomist should use a vocabulary that is easily understood by clients. To avoid creating suspicion and distrust in individuals from other countries, the phlebotomist should be aware of cultural differences and avoid clichés and nonverbal cues that could be misunderstood.

Nonverbal Communication It has been stated that 80% of language is unspoken. Unlike verbal communication, formed from words that are one-dimensional, nonverbal communication is multidimensional and involves the following elements.

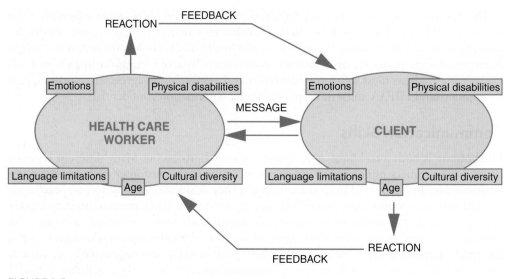

FIGURE 1-5

Verbal communication feedback loop.

Kinesics

The study of nonverbal communication is also called **kinesics** and includes characteristics of body motion and language such as facial expression, gestures, and eye contact. Figure 1-6 illustrates an exaggerated and simplified form of the six emotions that are most easily read by nonverbal facial cues. Body language, which most often is unintentional, plays a major role in communication because it is continuous and more reliable than verbal communication. In fact, if the verbal and nonverbal messages do not match, it is called a **kinesic slip**. When this happens, people tend to trust what they see rather than what they hear.

As health professionals, the phlebotomist can learn much about patients' feelings by observing nonverbal communication, which seldom lies. The patient's face often tells the health professional what the patient will not reveal verbally. For instance, when a patient is anxious, nonverbal signs may include tight eyebrows, an intense frown, narrowed eyes, or a downcast mouth (Fig. 1-6). Researchers have found that certain facial appearances, such as a smile, are universal expressions of emotion. Worldwide, we all recognize the meaning of a smile; however, strong cultural customs often dictate when it is used.

key • point To communicate effectively with someone, it is important to establish good eye contact. A patient or client may be made to feel unimportant and more like an object rather than a human being if no eye contact is established.

Proxemics

Proxemics is the study of an individual's concept and use of space. This subtle but powerful part of nonverbal communication plays a major role in patient relations. Every

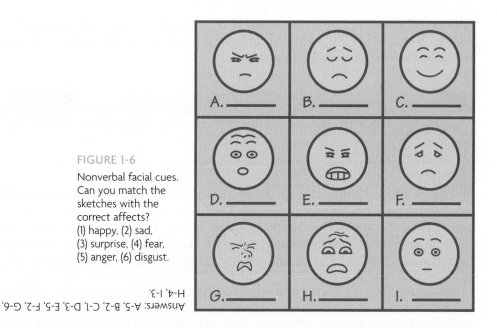

FIGURE 1-6

Nonverbal facial cues. Can you match the sketches with the correct affects? (1) happy, (2) sad, (3) surprise, (4) fear, (5) anger, (6) disgust.

Answers: A-5, B-2, C-1, D-3, E-5, F-2, G-6, H-4, I-3.

individual is surrounded by an invisible "bubble" of personal territory in which he or she feels most comfortable. The size of the bubble or territorial "zone of comfort" depends on the individual's needs at the time. Four categories of naturally occurring territorial zones and the radius of each are listed in Table 1-2. These zones are very obvious in human interaction. Entering personal or intimate zones is often necessary in the health-care setting, and if not carefully handled, the patient may feel threatened, insecure, or out of control.

Appearance

Most healthcare facilities have dress codes because it is understood that appearance makes a statement. The impression the phlebotomist makes as he or she approaches the patient sets the stage for future interaction. The right image portrays a trustworthy professional. A phlebotomist's physical appearance should communicate cleanliness and confidence. Lab coats, when worn, should completely cover the clothing underneath and should be clean and pressed. Shoes should be conservative and polished. Close attention should be paid to personal hygiene. Bathing and deodorant use should be a daily routine. Strong perfumes or colognes should be avoided. Hair and nails should be clean and look natural. Hair, if long,

TABLE 1-2 Territorial Zones and Corresponding Radii	
Territorial Zone	**Zone Radius**
Intimate	1 to 18 inches
Personal	$1\frac{1}{2}$ to 4 feet
Social	4 to 12 feet
Public	More than 12 feet

must be pulled back and fingernails should be short for safety's sake. In October 2002, CDC released new hand hygiene guidelines stating that healthcare workers with direct care contact cannot wear artificial nails or extenders.

key • point Phlebotomists will find that when dealing with patients who are ill or irritable a confident and professional appearance will be most helpful to doing their job.

Touch

Touching can take a variety of forms and convey many different meanings. For example, accidental touching may happen in a crowded elevator. Social touching takes place when a person grabs the arm of another while giving advice. Today, therapeutic touch that is designed to aid in healing has found a new place in medical practice. This special type of nonverbal communication is very important to the well-being of humans and even more so to diseased (dis-eased) humans.

Because medicine is a contact profession, touching privileges are granted to and expected of healthcare workers under certain circumstances. Whether a patient or healthcare provider is comfortable with touching is based on his or her cultural background. Because touch is a necessary part of the phlebotomy procedure, it is important to realize that, as a phlebotomist, patients are often much more aware of your touch than you are of theirs; there may even be a risk of the patient questioning the appropriateness of touching. Generally speaking, patients respond favorably when touch portrays a thoughtful expression of caring.

Active Listening   It is more difficult to communicate than just to speak because effective communication requires that the listener participate. It is always a two-way process. The ordinary person can absorb verbal messages at about 500 to 600 words per minute, and the average speaking rate is only 125 to 150 words per minute. Therefore, to avoid distraction, the listener must use the extra time for active listening. Active listening means taking positive steps through feedback to ensure that the listener is interpreting what the speaker is saying exactly as the speaker intended. Listening forms the foundation for good interpersonal communication and is particularly valuable in building rapport with patients.

EFFECTIVE COMMUNICATION IN HEALTHCARE

It is not easy for the patient or the health professional to face disease and suffering every day. For many patients, being ill is a terrifying experience; having their blood drawn only contributes to their anxiety. Patients reach out for comfort and reassurance through conversation. Consequently, a phlebotomist must understand the unusual aspects of healthcare communication and its importance in comforting the patient.

Communication between the health professional and patient is more complicated than normal interaction. Not only is it often emotionally charged, but it also involves, in many instances, other people who are very close to the patient and who may tend to be very critical of the way the patient is handled. Recognizing some of the elements in healthcare communication, such as empathy, control, trust, and confirmation, will aid the phlebotomist in successfully interacting with the patient.

Elements in Healthcare Communication
Empathy

Defined as identifying with the feelings or thoughts of another person, empathy is an essential factor in interpersonal relations. It involves putting yourself in the place of another and attempting to feel like that person. Thoughtful and sensitive people generally have a high degree of empathy. Empathic health professionals help patients handle the stress of being in a healthcare institution. A health professional who recognizes the needs of the patient and allows the patient to express his or her emotions helps to validate the patient's feelings and gives the patient a very necessary sense of control.

Control

An important element relating to communication in the healthcare setting is control. Feeling in control is essential to an individual's sense of well-being. People like to think that they can influence the way things happen in their lives. A hospital is one of the few places where individuals give up control over most of the personal tasks they normally perform. Many patients perceive themselves as unable to cope physically or mentally with events in a hospital because they feel fearful and powerless because of this loss of control. Consequently, the typical response of the patient is to act angry, which characterizes him or her as a "bad patient," or to act extremely codependent and agreeable, which characterizes him or her as a "good patient."

If a patient refuses to have blood drawn, the phlebotomist should allow that statement of control to be expressed and even agree with the patient. Patients who are allowed to exert that right will often change their minds and agree to the procedure, because then it is their decision. Sharing control with the patient may be difficult and often time-consuming, but awareness of the patient's need is important.

Confirmation

Too often, busy healthcare workers resort to labeling patients when communicating with coworkers and even with patients themselves. They may say, for example, "oh, you're the one with no veins" or "you're the bleeder, right?" Such communication is dehumanizing and is a subtle way of "disconfirming" patients. Each patient needs to be accepted as a unique individual with special needs. An example of initiating a confirming exchange with the patient in the first example could be, "Mrs. Jones, I seem to remember that we had a hard time finding a suitable vein last time we drew your blood." Or in the second case, "Mr. Smith, wasn't there a problem getting the site to stop bleeding after the draw last time?"

Trust

Another variable in the process of communication is trust. Trust, as defined in the healthcare setting, is the unquestioning belief by the patient that health professionals are performing their job responsibilities as well as they possibly can. As is true with most professionals, healthcare providers tend to emphasize their technical expertise while sometimes completely ignoring the elements of interpersonal communication that are essential in a trusting relationship with the patient. Having blood drawn is just one of the situations in which the consumer must trust the health professional. Developing trust takes time, and phlebotomists spend very little time with each patient. Consequently, during this limited interaction, the phlebotomist must do everything possible to win the patient's confidence by consistently appearing knowledgeable, honest, and sincere.

In summary, by recognizing the elements of empathy, control, trust, and confirmation, the phlebotomist can enhance communication with patients and assist in their recovery. Understanding these communication elements will help when used with other means of communication, such as the telephone.

Telephone Communication   The telephone is presently a fundamental part of communication. It is used 24 hours a day in the laboratory. To phlebotomists or laboratory clerks, it becomes just another source of stress, bringing additional work and uninvited demands on their time. The constant ringing and the interruption to the workflow often cause laboratory personnel to overlook the effect their style of telephone communication has on the caller. To maintain a professional image, every person given the responsibility of answering the phone should review proper protocol. Each one should be taught how to answer, put someone on hold, and transfer calls properly. To promote good communication, proper telephone etiquette (see Table 1-3) should be followed.

THE HEALTHCARE SETTING

Virtually everyone in the United States becomes a healthcare consumer at some time in his or her life. For many, working through the bureaucracy involved in receiving healthcare can be confusing. Healthcare personnel who understand how healthcare is organized and financed and their role in the system can help consumers successfully negotiate the process with minimal frustration.

Healthcare Delivery

Two general categories of facilities, inpatient (nonambulatory) and outpatient (ambulatory), support all three (**primary, secondary,** and **tertiary**) levels of healthcare presently offered in the United States. See Box 1-3 for a listing of services and practitioners associated with the two categories.

AMBULATORY CARE AND HOMEBOUND SERVICES

Changes in healthcare practices that have significantly decreased the amount of time a patient spends in the hospital have led to innovative ways to serve healthcare, including offering a wide range of ambulatory services. These services meet the needs of patients who may still require healthcare provisions such as nursing care, lab tests, or other follow-up procedures after being discharged from the hospital. In addition, new health services are being developed for the fastest growing segment of the population, the elderly. Many homebound elderly require nursing care and physical therapy to be given and specimens for

TABLE 1-3 Proper Telephone Etiquette

Proper Etiquette	Communication Tips	Rationale
Answer promptly		• If the phone is allowed to ring too many times, the caller may assume that the people working in the laboratory are inefficient or insensitive
State your name and department		• The caller has a right to know to whom they are speaking
Be helpful	Ask how you can be of help to assist the caller and facilitate the conversation Keep your statements and answers simple and to the point to avoid confusion	• When a phone rings, it is because someone needs something. Because of the nature of the healthcare business, the caller may be emotional and need a calm, pleasant voice on the other end to respond to the request
Prioritize calls	Inform callers if they are interrupting another call Always ask callers if they can be put on hold in case it is an emergency that must be handled immediately	• Coordinating several calls takes an organized person • Callers should be informed if they are interrupting another call
Transfer and put on hold properly	Tell callers when you are going to transfer or put them on hold and learn how to do this properly **Note:** Do not leave the line open	• Disconnecting callers while transferring or putting them on hold irritates them • Leaving the line open so that conversations be heard by the one on hold is discourteous and can compromise confidentiality
Be prepared to record information	Have a pencil and paper close to the phone Listen carefully, which means clarifying, restating, and summarizing the information received	• Documentation is necessary when answering the phone at work to ensure that accurate information is transmitted to the necessary person
Know the laboratory policies	Make answers consistent by learning laboratory polices	• People who answer the telephone need to know the laboratory policies to avoid misinformation • Consistent answers help establish the laboratory's credibility, because a caller's perception of the lab involves more than accurate test results
Diffuse hostile situations	When a caller is hostile you might say "I can see why you are upset. Let me see what I can do."	• Some callers are angry because of lost results or errors in billing • Validating a hostile caller's feelings will often diffuse the situation • After the caller has been calmed down, the issue can be addressed
Try to assist everyone	Refer the caller to someone who can address the caller's issue if you are uncertain Remind yourself to keep your attention on one person at a time	• It is possible to assist callers and show concern even if you are not actually answering their questions • Validate callers' requests by giving a response that tells them something can be done • Sincere interest in the caller will enhance communication and contribute to the good reputation of the laboratory

BOX • 1-3 Two Categories of Healthcare Facilities

Outpatient	Inpatient
• Principal source of healthcare services for most people	• The key resource and center of the American healthcare system
• Offer routine care in physician's office to specialized care in a freestanding and ambulatory setting	• Offer specialized instrumentation and technology to assist in unusual diagnosis treatment
• Serve the **primary care** physician who assumes ongoing responsibility for maintaining patients' health	• Serve the **tertiary care** (highly complex services and therapy) level practitioners. Usually require that patients stay overnight or longer
• Serve a **secondary care** level physician (specialist) who performs routine surgery, emergency treatments, therapeutic radiology, and so on in same-day service centers	• Examples are acute care hospitals, nursing homes, extended care facilities, hospice, and rehabilitation centers

laboratory tests to be collected where they reside, either in their homes or in long-term care facilities. A number of agencies employ nurses, respiratory therapists, phlebotomists, and other healthcare workers to provide these services.

PUBLIC HEALTH SERVICE

One of the principal units under the Department of Health and Human Services is the Public Health Service (PHS). PHS agencies at the local or state level offer defense against infectious diseases that might spread among the populace. These agencies are constantly monitoring, screening, protecting, and educating the public (see Table 1-4 for examples of services provided by local health departments). Public health departments provide their services for little or no charge to the entire population of a region, with no distinction between rich or poor, simple or sophisticated, interested or disinterested. Public health facilities offer ambulatory care services through clinics, much as with those in hospital outpatient areas, military bases, and Veterans Administration and Indian Health Service facilities.

TABLE 1-4 Examples of Services Provided by Local Health Departments

Vital statistics collection	Tuberculosis screening
Health education	Immunization and vaccination
Cancer, hypertension, and diabetes screening	Operation of health centers
Public health nursing services	Venereal disease clinics

As the country moves into managed care, integration between primary prevention and primary/ambulatory care is necessary. Because containment of healthcare costs is the driving force behind managed care, proactive public health programs can significantly contribute to reducing overall healthcare costs.

Healthcare Financing

Healthcare is expensive and the cost continues to escalate. The consumer must make choices based on financial considerations as well as medical need and can no longer afford to be passive in the process. The healthcare provider, such as the phlebotomist, in addition to being a consumer is also an employee of an institution that relies on third-party payers (health insurers) for a major portion of his or her income.

THIRD-PARTY PAYERS

A **third-party payer** can be an insurance company or government program that pays for healthcare services on behalf of a patient. Third-party payers have greatly influenced the direction of medicine. In the past decade, major changes have come about in healthcare payments and third-party reimbursements. Table 1-5 shows methods of payments and coding that have been used to standardize healthcare expenses.

DIAGNOSIS AND BILLING CODES

Managed care systems face major challenges in remaining fiscally strong in the coming years. For that reason, it is imperative that all services be billed correctly and as quickly as possible, but with the advent of new technologies and electronic transfer of data, billing has become even more challenging. The lack of standardization and confusion in the diagnostic and

TABLE 1-5 Methods of Payment and Diagnosis Coding		
Method of Payment	**Abbreviation**	**Description**
Prospective payment system	PPS	Begun in 1983 to limit and standardize the Medicare/Medicaid payments made to hospitals
Diagnosis-related groups	DRGs	Originally designed by the American Hospital Association, hospitals are reimbursed a set amount for each patient procedure using established disease categories
Ambulatory patient classification	APC	A new classification system implemented in 2000 for determining payment to hospitals for outpatient service
Diagnosis Codes	**Abbreviation**	**Description**
International Classification of Diseases, Ninth Revision, Clinical Modification	ICD-9-CM	For coding of diagnoses, all major payers use this coding system that groups together similar diseases and operations for reimbursement

procedural coding led to the passage in 1996 of HIPAA. This bill was designed to improve the efficiency of the healthcare system by establishing standards for electronic data exchange including coding systems. The goal of HIPAA regulations is to move to one universal procedural coding system as the future standard. The Center for Medicare and Medicaid Services (CMS) is in the process of developing the latest version of the ICD coding system. It will be called *International Classification of Diseases–Tenth Revision, Clinical Modification* or ICD-10-CM.

The **current procedural terminology** (CPT) codes were originally developed in the 1960s by the American Medical Association to provide a terminology and coding system for physician billing. Physician offices have continued to use it to report their services. Now all types of healthcare providers use CPT to classify, report, and bill for a variety of healthcare services. Currently, ICD-9-CM procedure codes are used for inpatients and CPT procedure codes are used for patients seen in the ambulatory setting and for professional services in the inpatient setting.

REIMBURSEMENT

The history of institutional reimbursement is tied to **entitlement programs** such as Medicare and public welfare in the form of Medicaid. Before 1983, hospitals were paid retrospectively and reimbursed for all services performed on Medicare and Medicaid patients. A comparison of Medicare and Medicaid Programs is listed in Box 1-4.

Arizona is the only state that has devised its own system outside of Medicaid, called **Arizona Healthcare Cost Containment System** (AHCCCS). It differs in that the providers (private physician groups) must bid annually for contracts to serve this population and patients are able to choose their healthcare provider through annual open enrollment.

BOX • 1-4   Medicare and Medicaid Program Comparison

Medicare	Medicaid
First enacted in 1965	First enacted in 1965
Federally funded program for providing healthcare to persons over the age of 65, regardless of their financial status, and to the disabled	Federal and state program that provides medical assistance for low-income Americans
An entitlement program because it is a right earned by individuals through employment	No entitlement feature; recipients must prove their eligibility
Financed through Social Security payroll deductions and copayments	Funds come from federal grants and state and local governments and are administered by the state
Benefits divided into two categories; Part A, called hospital services, and Part B, called supplementary medical insurance (SMI), which is optional	Benefits cover inpatient care, outpatient and diagnostic services, skilled nursing facilities, and home health and physician services

The Changing Healthcare System

Healthcare systems are currently undergoing major revisions. The driving force behind these changes is the perceived need to control the cost of healthcare. Government social programs and other managed healthcare plans continually negotiate discounts on the amount they will reimburse the healthcare facilities, forcing them to cut costs and downsize operations. It has become the goal of all healthcare organizations to deliver high-quality, cost-effective care in the most appropriate setting, or in other words strictly manage care.

MANAGED CARE

Managed care is a generic term for a payment system that attempts to manage cost, quality, and access to healthcare by

- Detecting illnesses or risk factors early in the disease process
- Putting into practice various financial incentives for providers
- Offering patient education
- Encouraging healthy lifestyles

Most managed care systems do not provide the healthcare to enrollees; instead, they enter into contracts with healthcare facilities, physicians, and other healthcare providers who supply medical services to the enrollees/clients in the plan.

Benefits or payments paid to the provider are made according to a set fee schedule, and enrollees must comply with managed care policies such as preauthorization for certain medical procedures and approved referral to specialists for claims to be paid. Because the association of provider, payer, and consumer is the foundation of managed care systems, several concepts have been developed to control this relationship, including gatekeepers and large services networks.

Primary Care Gatekeepers   One of the most important concepts in managed care is that of the primary care physician filling the role of **gatekeeper**. As the patient's advocate, this person has the responsibility to advise the patient on healthcare needs and coordinate responses to those needs. Gatekeeper responsibilities also include providing early detection and treatment for disease, which should reduce the total cost of care.

Network Service Systems   Today's large **managed care organizations** (MCOs) evolved from prepaid healthcare plans such as **health maintenance organizations** (HMOs) and **preferred provider organizations** (PPOs). HMOs are group practices reimbursed on a prepaid, negotiated, and discounted basis of admission. PPOs are independent groups of physicians or hospitals that offer services to employers at discounted rates in exchange for a steady supply of patients. MCOs contract with local providers to establish a complete network of services. Providers are reimbursed on the basis of the number of enrollees served— not on the number of services delivered. The goal of the MCO is to reduce the total cost of care while maintaining patient satisfaction; and this can best be done if the patient can get the right care from the right provider at the right time. To accomplish this, **Integrated healthcare delivery systems** (IDSs) have been developed. An IDS is a healthcare provider made up of a number of associated medical facilities that furnish coordinated healthcare services from prebirth to death. Some of the institutions through which the services are offered along this continuum of care are acute care hospitals, subacute care facilities, ambulatory surgery centers, physician office practices, outpatient clinics, and skilled nursing facilities (SNFs). The focus of an IDS arrangement is holistic, coordinated care rather than fragmented care performed by many medical specialists.

Medical Specialties   In managed care, the primary physician is most often a family practitioner, a pediatrician, or an internist. As gatekeeper, he or she is expected to refer to the appropriate specialist as needed. Some of the many healthcare areas in which a doctor of medicine (MD) or doctor of osteopathy (DO) can specialize are listed in Table 1-6.

TABLE 1-6 Medical Specialties		
Specialty	**Area of Interest**	**Specialist Title**
Anesthesiology	Partial or complete loss of sensation usually by injection or inhalation	Anesthesiologist
Cardiology	Diseases of the heart and blood vessels and cardiovascular surgery, a subspecialty of internal medicine	Cardiologist
Dermatology	Diseases and injuries of the skin more recently, concerned with skin cancer prevention	Dermatologist
Endocrinology	Disorders of the endocrine glands, such as, sterility, diabetes, and thyroid problems	Endocrinologist
Gastroenterology	Digestive tract and related structure diseases, a subspecialty of internal medicine	Gastroenterologist
Gerontology	Effects of aging and age-related disorders	Gerontologist
Hematology	Disorders of the blood and blood-forming organs	Hematologist
Internal Medicine	Diseases of internal organs and general medical condition, uses nonsurgical therapy	Internist
Nephrology	Diseases related to structure and function of the kidney	Nephrologist
Neurology	Disorders of the brain, spinal cord, and nerves	Neurologist
Obstetrics and Gynecology	Women through pregnancy, childbirth, disorders of the reproductive system, and menopause	Gynecologist
Oncology	Tumors, including benign and malignant conditions	Oncologist
Ophthalmology	Eye examinations, eye diseases, and surgery	Ophthalmologist
Orthopedics	Disorders of the musculoskeletal system, including preventing disorders and restoring function	Orthopedist
Otorhinolaryngology	Disorders of the eye, ear, nose, and throat	Otorhinolaryngologist
Pediatrics	Diseases of children from birth to adolescence; does wellness checks and gives vaccinations	Pediatrician
Psychiatry	Mental illness, clinical depression, and other behavioral and emotional disorders	Psychiatrist
Pulmonary Medicine	Function and disorders of the lungs and respiratory system	Pulmonologist
Rheumatology	Rheumatic diseases (acute and chronic conditions characterized by inflammation and joint disease)	Rheumatologist
Urology	Urinary tract disease and male reproductive organ disorders	Urologist

Departments Within the Hospital Setting

Hospitals are often large organizations with a complex internal structure. The healthcare delivery system in hospitals has traditionally been arranged by departments or medical specialties. People who do similar tasks are grouped into departments, the goal being to perform each task as efficiently and accurately as possible. This style of management segregates the departments and their processes (See Fig. 1-7 for a typical hospital organization flow chart). Consequently, it is difficult to look at an institution-wide final outcome and judge patient satisfaction.

Managed care has led to a reduction in the number of healthcare personnel, whereas the number of services remains the same. This has resulted in the formation of teams of cross-trained personnel and the consolidation of services. Such reengineering, as it is called, is designed to make the healthcare delivery system more process-oriented by combining related groups of tasks into a system that is customer-focused. This management of process is reflected in a new type of hospital organization that blends former distinct departments into service or process areas. The intent is to create a "gentle handoff" for patients between service areas, instead of the abrupt "toss and catch" approach that can occur in traditional settings

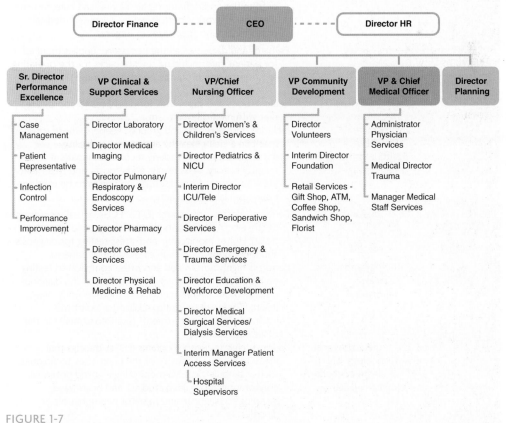

FIGURE 1-7

Example of a hospital organizational chart.

TABLE 1-7 Essential Service Areas of a Hospital

Service Area	Departments Within Area	Services Performed
PATIENT CARE SERVICES	Nursing Care	Direct patient care, Includes careful observation to assess conditions, administering medications and treatments prescribed by a physician, evaluation of patient care, and documentation in the health record that reflects this. Staffed by many types of nursing personnel including registered nurses (RNs), licensed practical nurses (LPNs), and certified nursing assistants (CNAs)
	Emergency Services	Around-the-clock service designed to handle medical emergencies that call for immediate assessment and management of injured or acutely ill patients. Staffed by specialists such as emergency medical technicians (EMTs) and MDs who specialize in emergency medicine
	Intensive Care Units (ICUs)	Designed for increased bedside care of patients in fragile condition. Found in many areas of the hospital and named for the type of patient care they provide (e.g., trauma ICU, pediatric ICU, medical ICU)
	Surgery	Concerned with operative procedures to correct deformities and defects, repair injuries, and cure certain diseases. All work is performed by a licensed medical practitioner who specializes in surgery
SUPPORT SERVICES	Central Supply	Prepares and dispenses all the necessary supplies required for patient care, including surgical packs for the operating room, intravenous pumps, bandages, syringes, and other inventory controlled by computer for close accounting
	Dietary Services	Selects foods and supervises food services to coordinate diet with medical treatment
	Environmental Services	Includes housekeeping and grounds keepers whose services maintain a clean, healthy and attractive facility
	Health Information Technology	Maintains accurate and orderly records for inpatient medical history, tests results and reports, and treatment plans and notes from doctors and nurses to be used for insurance claims, legal actions, and utilization reviews
PROFESSIONAL SERVICES	Cardiodiagnostics (EKG or ECG)	Performs electrocardiograms (EKGs/ECGs, actual recordings of the electrical currents that are detectable from the heart), Holter monitoring, and stress testing for diagnosis and monitoring therapy in cardiovascular patients
	Pathology and Clinical Laboratory	Performs highly automated and often complicated testing on blood and other body fluids to detect and diagnose disease, monitor treatments, and, more recently, assess health. There are several specialized areas of the laboratory called departments (see Departments in the Clinical Laboratory)
	Electroneurodiagnostic Technology (ENT) or electroencephalography (EEG)	Performs electroencephalograms (EEGs), tracings that measure electrical activity of the brain. Uses techniques, such as ambulatory EEG monitoring, evoked potential, polysomnography (sleep studies), and brain wave mapping to diagnose and monitor neurophysiologic disorders

continued

Service Area	Departments Within Area	Services Performed
PROFESSIONAL SERVICES, *continued*	Occupational Therapy (OT)	Uses techniques designed to develop or assist mentally, physically, or emotionally disabled patients to maintain daily living skills
	Pharmacy	Prepares and dispenses drugs ordered by physicians; advises the medical staff on selection and harmful side effects of drugs, therapeutic drug monitoring, and drug use evaluation
	Physical Therapy (PT)	Diagnoses physical impairment to determine the extent of disability and provides therapy to restore mobility through individually designed treatment plans
	Respiratory Therapy (RT)	Diagnoses, treats, and manages patient's lung deficiencies (e.g., analyzes arterial blood gases [ABGs], tests capacity of the lungs, administers oxygen therapy)
	Diagnostic Radiology Services	Diagnoses medical conditions by taking x-ray films of various parts of the body. Uses latest procedures including powerful forms of imaging that do not involve radiation hazards, such as ultrasound machines, magnetic resonance (MR) scanners, and positron emission tomography (PET) scanners

TABLE 1-7 *(continued)*

with distinct and separate departments. Although the lines between former departments are becoming blurred, Table 1-7 shows the services areas that are identified as essential.

Clinical Laboratory Services

Clinical laboratory (lab) services perform tests on patient specimens. Results of testing are primarily used by physicians to confirm health or aid in the diagnosis, evaluation, and monitoring of patient medical conditions. Clinical labs are typically located in hospitals, outpatient clinics, physicians' offices, and large reference laboratories.

TRADITIONAL LABORATORIES

There are two major divisions in the clinical laboratory, the clinical analysis area and the anatomic and surgical pathology area. All laboratory testing is associated with one of these two areas (see Box 1-5).

Clinical Analysis Areas
Hematology

The hematology department performs laboratory tests that identify diseases associated with blood and the blood-forming tissues. The most commonly ordered hematology test is the complete blood count (CBC). The CBC is performed using automated instruments, such as the Coulter counter (Fig. 1-8), that electronically count the cells and calculate results.

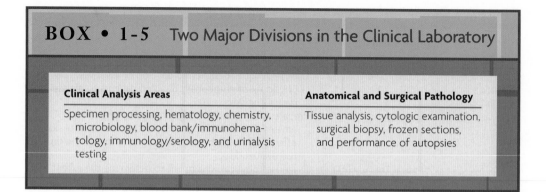

BOX • 1-5   Two Major Divisions in the Clinical Laboratory

Clinical Analysis Areas	Anatomical and Surgical Pathology
Specimen processing, hematology, chemistry, microbiology, blood bank/immunohematology, immunology/serology, and urinalysis testing	Tissue analysis, cytologic examination, surgical biopsy, frozen sections, and performance of autopsies

A CBC is actually a multipart assay that is reported on a form called a hemogram (Tables 1-8 and 1-9).

Coagulation

Coagulation is the study of the ability of blood to form and dissolve clots. Coagulation tests are closely related to hematology tests, and the department is often housed in the hematology area. Coagulation tests are used to discover, identify, and monitor defects in the blood-clotting mechanism. They are also used to monitor patients who are taking medications called anticoagulants (chemicals that inhibit blood clotting) or "blood thinners." The two most common coagulation tests are the prothrombin time, used to monitor warfarin therapy, and the activated partial thromboplastin time for evaluating heparin therapy (Table 1-10).

Chemistry

The chemistry department performs most laboratory tests. This department often has subsections such as toxicology and radioimmunoassay. Computerized instruments (Fig. 1-9)

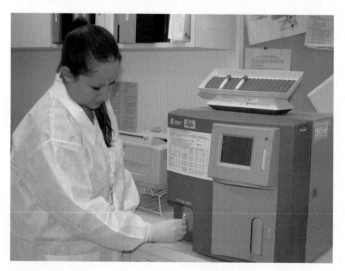

FIGURE 1-8

Coulter A^c Tdiff 2 automated hematology analyzer.

TABLE 1-8 Hemogram for Complete Blood Count (CBC) Assay

Name of Test	Abbreviation	Examples of Clinical Significance
Hematocrit	Hct	Values correspond to the red cell count and hemoglobin level; when decreased, indicate anemic conditions
Hemoglobin	Hgb	Decreased values indicate anemic conditions; values normally differ with age, sex, altitude, and hydration
Red blood cell count	RBC	Measure of erythropoietic activity; decrease in numbers related to anemic condition
White blood cell count	WBC	Abnormal leukocyte response indicative of various conditions, such as infections and malignancies; when accompanied by WBC, differential test becomes more specific
Platelet count	Plt Ct	Decreased number indicative of hemorrhagic diseases; values may be used to monitor chemotherapy or radiation treatments
Differential white count	Diff	Changes in appearance or number of specific cell type signifies specific disease conditions; values also used to monitor chemotherapy or radiation treatments
Indices		Changes in RBC size, weight, and Hgb content indicate certain types of anemias
Mean corpuscular hemoglobin	MCH	Reveals the weight of the hemoglobin in the cell, regardless of the size. Decreased hemoglobin content indicative of iron deficiency anemia, increased hemoglobin content found in macrocytic anemia
Mean corpuscular volume	MCV	Reveals the size of the cell. Decreased MCV associated with thalassemia and iron deficiency anemia; increased MCV because of folic acid or vitamin B12 deficiency and chronic emphysema
Mean corpuscular hemoglobin concentration	MCHC	Reveals the hemoglobin concentration per unit volume of RBCs. Below-normal range means red cells are deficient in hemoglobin as in thalassemia, overhydration, or iron deficiency anemia; above-normal range will be seen in severe burns, prolonged dehydration, and hereditary spherocytosis
Red blood cell distribution width	RDW	Reveals the size differences of the RBCs. An early predictor of anemia before other signs and symptoms

used in this area are capable of performing discrete (individualized) tests or metabolic panels (multiple tests) from a single sample. Examples of panels frequently ordered to evaluate a single organ or specific body system are given in Table 1-11.

The most common chemistry specimen is serum; however, other types of specimens tested include plasma, whole blood, urine, and various other body fluids. Examples of tests normally performed in the automated clinical laboratory section are provided in Table 1-12.

Serology or Immunology

Serology literally means the study of serum. Serology tests deal with the body's response to the presence of bacterial, viral, fungal, or parasitic diseases that stimulate antigen–antibody reactions that can easily be demonstrated in the laboratory (Table 1-13). Autoimmune reactions, in which autoantibodies produced by B lymphocytes attack normal cells, are

TABLE 1-9 Other Common Hematology Tests

Test	Examples of Clinical Significance
Bone marrow	Detects abnormal blood cells and evaluates blood cell formation and function
Cerebrospinal (CSF) and other body fluids	Presence or absence, number and type of cells Hematocrit on fluid indirectly measures fluid volume
Eosinophil count	Increased numbers in direct count indicate parasitic infections and allergies
Erythrocyte sedimentation rate (ESR)	Increased rate at which red blood cells settle out is indicative of inflammatory conditions or necrosis of tissue
Lupus erythematosus (LE prep)	Presence of typical LE cells is diagnostic of systemic LE
Osmotic fragility	Increased red cell fragility is indicative of hemolytic and autoimmune anemias, decreased fragility is indicative of sickle cell and thalassemia
Reticulocyte count (retic count)	Increased number of retics in circulating blood attest to bone marrow hyperactivity
Sickle cell	Sickling of red cells indicates presence of abnormal hemoglobin variant, Hgb S

TABLE 1-10 Common Coagulation Tests

Test	Examples of Clinical Significance
Activated partial thromboplastin time	Prolonged times may indicate stage one defects; values reflect adequacy of heparin therapy
Bleeding time (BT)	Increased BT indicates hemorrhagic disorders associated with decreased platelet activity and lack of elasticity of capillary walls
D dimer test	Evaluates thrombin and plasmin activity and is very useful in testing for disseminated intravascular coagulation (DIC) and used in monitoring thrombolytic therapy
Fibrin degradation products (FDP)	High levels result in FDP fragments that interfere with platelet function and clotting
Fibrinogen	Fibrinogen deficiency suggests hemorrhagic disorders and is used most frequently in obstetrics
Prothrombin time (PT)	Prolonged times may indicate stage two and three defects; values used to monitor warfarin therapy

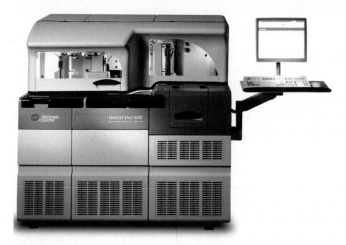

FIGURE 1-9

Automated chemistry analyzer, DXC600 Pro. (Courtesy of Beckman Coulter, Fullerton, CA.)

TABLE 1-11 Disease- and Organ-Specific Chemistry Panels (CMS Approved)

Panel Grouping	Battery of Selected Diagnostic Tests
Basic metabolic panel (BMP)	Glucose, BUN, creatinine, sodium, potassium, chloride, CO_2, calcium
Comprehensive metabolic panel (CMP)	Glucose, BUN, creatinine, sodium, potassium, chloride, CO_2, AST, ALT, alkaline phosphatase total protein, albumin, total bilirubin, calcium
Hepatic function panel A	AST, ALT, alkaline phosphatase, total protein, albumin, total bilirubin, direct bilirubin
Renal function panel	Glucose, BUN, creatinine, sodium, potassium, chloride, CO_2, calcium, albumin, phosphorus

ALT, alanine aminotransferase; AST, aspartate aminotransferase; BUN, blood urea nitrogen; CO_2, carbon dioxide.

TABLE 1-12 Common Chemistry Tests

Test	Associated Body System	Examples of Clinical Significance
Alanine amino-transferase (ALT)	Liver	Marked elevations point to liver disease; used for monitoring liver treatment
Alpha-fetoprotein (AFP)	Liver	Increased values in hepatic carcinoma; elevation of AFP in prenatal screening indicates neural tube disorder
Alkaline phosphatase (ALP)	Liver or bone	Elevated ALP levels because of biliary obstruction and bone disease
Ammonia	Liver	Increased blood levels indicate cirrhosis and hepatitis
Amylase	Pancreas and liver	Increased levels of this enzyme diagnostic of acute pancreatitis; decreased values associated with liver disease, cholecystitis, and advanced cystic fibrosis
Aspartate amino-transferase (AST)	Liver or heart	Increase in enzyme indicative of liver dysfunction; significant increase following myocardial infarction
Bilirubin	Liver	Increased levels in the blood stream point to red cell destruction and liver dysfunction
Blood gases (ABG)	Kidneys, lungs	Measures pH, partial pressure of carbon dioxide (Pco_2), partial pressure of oxygen (Po_2) to evaluate the acid-base balance
Blood urea nitrogen (BUN)	Kidney	Elevated values because of impaired renal function from toxins, inflammation, or obstruction
Carcinoembryonic antigen (CEA)	Nonspecific	Increased in the cases of malignancy, effective in the early detection of colorectal cancer
Calcium	Bone	Increased levels associated with diseases of the bone; used in monitoring effects of renal failure
Cholesterol (total)	Heart	Indicative of high risk for cardiovascular disease
Cortisol	Adrenals	Elevated levels signify adrenal hyperfunction (Cushing syndrome); decreased levels indicate adrenal hypofunction (Addison's disease)
Creatine kinase (CK)	Heart or muscle	Elevated values point to muscle damage (i.e., myocardial infarction, muscular dystrophy, or strenuous exercise)
Creatinine	Kidney	Increased levels indicate renal impairment; decreased levels associated with muscular dystrophy

continued

TABLE 1-12 *(continued)*

Test	Associated Body System	Examples of Clinical Significance
Drug analysis		Values monitored to maintain therapeutic range and avoid toxic levels for drugs such as barbiturates, digoxin, gentamicin, lithium, primidone, phenytoin, salicylates, theophylline, or tobramycin
Electrolytes (sodium, potassium, chloride, CO_2)	Kidney, adrenals, heart	Sodium values, increased in disorders of the kidney and adrenals; decreased values of potassium seen in irregular heartbeat; chloride values are increased in kidney and adrenal disorders and decreased in diarrhea
Glucose	Pancreas	Elevated levels signify diabetic problems; decreased values support liver disease and malnutrition
Glycosylated hemoglobin	Pancreas	Glycohemoglobin level shows what type of diabetic control has occurred over the past several months
Gamma-glutamyl transferase (GGT)	Liver	Elevated values assist in the diagnosis of liver problems, specific for hepatobiliary problems
Lactate dehydrogenase (LD)	Heart, lungs, liver	Elevated levels confirm acute myocardial infarction; chronic lung, kidney, and liver dysfunction
Lipase	Pancreas	Increased levels in acute pancreatitis, pancreatic carcinoma, and obstruction
Prostate specific antigen (PSA)	Prostate	Performed to screen patients for the presence of prostate cancer, monitor progression of disease and the response of the patient to treatment
Total protein	Liver or kidney	Low levels point to liver and kidney disorders; elevated levels may occur with multiple myeloma and dehydration
Triglycerides	Heart	Increased values indicate lipid metabolism disorders and serve as an index for evaluating atherosclerosis possibilities
Uric acid	Kidney	Elevated values found in renal disorders and gout
Vitamin B_{12} and folate	Liver	Decreased levels indicate anemias and disease of the small intestine

becoming more prevalent and can be detected by serologic tests. Testing is done by enzyme immunoassay (EIA), agglutination, complement fixation, or precipitation to determine the antibody or antigen present and to assess its concentration or titer.

Urinalysis

The urinalysis (UA) department may be housed in the hematology or chemistry area or may be a completely separate section. Urine specimens may be analyzed manually or using automated instruments. UA is a routine urine test that includes physical, chemical, and microscopic evaluations (Table 1-14). The physical examination assesses the color, clarity, and specific gravity of the specimen. The chemical evaluation, performed using chemical reagent strips, screens for substances such as sugar and protein. A microscopic examination establishes the presence or absence of blood cells, bacteria, crystals, and other substances.

TABLE 1-13 Common Serology and Immunology Tests

Test	Examples of Clinical Significance
Bacterial Studies	
Antinuclear antibody (ANA)	Positive results in autoimmune disorders, specifically systemic lupus erythematosus
Antistreptolysin O (ASO) titer	To demonstrate infection from streptococcus bacteria
Cold agglutinins	Present in cases of atypical pneumonia
Febrile agglutinins	Presence of antibodies to specific organisms indicates disease condition (i.e., tularemia)
FTA-ABS	Fluorescent treponemal antibody absorption test, confirmatory test for syphilis
Rapid plasma reagin (RPR)	Positive screen indicates syphilis; positives need to be confirmed
Rheumatoid factor (RF)	Presence of antibody indicates rheumatoid arthritis
Viral Studies	
Anti-HIV	Human immunodeficiency virus is screened
Cytomegalovirus antibody (CMV)	Confirmation test
Epstein-Barr virus (EBV)	Presence of this heterophil antibody indicates infectious mononucleosis
Hepatitis B surface antigen (HBsAg)	Demonstrates the presence of hepatitis antigen on the surface of the red cells
General Studies	
C-reactive protein (CRP)	Increased levels in inflammatory conditions
Human chorionic gonadotropin (HCG)	Present in pregnancy (serum and urine)

TABLE 1-14 Common Urinalysis Tests

Test	Examples of Clinical Significance
Physical Evaluation	
Color	Abnormal colors that are clinically significant result from blood melanin, bilirubin, or urobilin in the sample
Clarity	Turbidity may be the result of chyle, fat, bacteria, RBCs, WBCs, or precipitated crystals
Specific gravity	Variation in this indicator of dissolved solids in the urine is normal; inconsistencies suggest renal tubule involvement or ADH deficiency
Chemical Evaluation	
Blood	Hematuria may be the result of hemorrhage, infection, or trauma
Bilirubin	Aids in differentiating obstructive jaundice from hemolytic jaundice, which will not cause increased bilirubin in the urine
Glucose	Glucosuria could be the result of diabetes mellitus, renal impairment, or ingestion of a large amount of carbohydrates
Ketones	Occurs in uncontrolled diabetes mellitus and starvation
Leukocyte esterase	Certain white cells (neutrophils) in abundance indicate urinary tract infection
pH	Variations in pH indicate changes in acid—base balance, which is normal; loss of ability to vary pH is indicative of tissue breakdown
Protein	Proteinuria is indicator of renal disorder, such as injury and renal tube dysfunction
Nitrite	Positive result suggests bacterial infection but is only significant on first-morning specimen or urine incubated in bladder for at least 4 hours
Urobilinogen	Occurs in increased amounts when patient has hepatic problems or hemolytic disorders
Microscopic Evaluation	Analysis of urinary sediment reveals status of the urinary tract, hematuria pyuria, and presence of casts and tissue cells are pathologic indicators

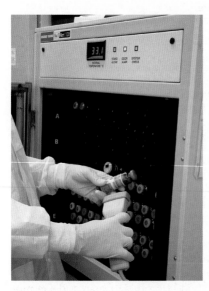

FIGURE 1-10

Microbiologist reviews blood cultures processed by the BactALERT 3D.

Microbiology

The microbiology department analyzes body fluids and tissues for the presence of microorganisms, primarily by means of culture and sensitivity (C & S) testing (Fig. 1-10). Results of a C & S tell the physician the type of organisms present and the particular antibiotics that would be most effective for treatment. Collecting and transporting microbiology specimens properly is very important in the identification of microorganisms. Subsections of microbiology are bacteriology (study of bacteria), parasitology (study of parasites), mycology (study of fungi), and virology (study of viruses) (Table 1-15).

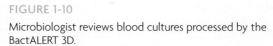

Test	Examples of Clinical Significance
Acid fast bacilli (AFB)	Positive stain means pulmonary tuberculosis; used to monitor the treatment for TB
Blood culture	Positive culture results (bacterial growth in media) indicate bacteremia or septicemia
CLOtest	Presence of *Helicobacter pylori*
Culture & sensitivity (C & S)	Growth of a pathogenic microorganism indicates infection (culture); in vitro inhibition by an antibiotic (sensitivity) allows the physician to select the correct treatment
Fungus culture and identification	Positive culture detects the presence of fungi and determines the type
Gram stain	Positive stain for specific types of pathogenic microorganisms permits antimicrobial therapy to begin before culture results are known
Occult blood	Positive test indicates blood in the stool, which is associated with gastrointestinal bleeding from carcinoma
Ova and parasites	Microscopic examination of stool sample showing ova and parasites solves many "etiology unknown" intestinal disorders

TABLE 1-15   Common Microbiology Tests

Blood Bank or Immunohematology

The blood bank or immunohematology department of the laboratory prepares blood products to be used for patient transfusions. Blood components dispensed include whole blood, platelets, packed cells, fresh frozen plasma, and cryoprecipitates. Blood samples from all donors and the recipient must be carefully tested before transfusions can be administered so that incompatibility and transfusion reactions can be avoided (Table 1-16). Transfusion services offered by the blood bank department, collect, prepare, and store units of blood from donors or patients who wish to donate their own units for autologous transfusion, if necessary.

Anatomic and Surgical Pathology
Histology

Histology is literally defined as the study of the microscopic structure of tissues. In this department, pathologists evaluate samples of tissue from surgeries and autopsies under a microscope to determine if they are normal or pathologic (diseased). Histologic techniques include two of the most diagnostic tools found in the laboratory (1) biopsy, obtaining samples by removal of a plug (small piece) of tissue from an organ and examining it microscopically, and (2) frozen sections, obtaining tissue from surgery and freezing and examining it immediately to determine whether more extensive surgery is needed. Before tissues can be evaluated, they must be processed and stained. This is the role of a person called an histologist.

Cytology

Cytology and histology are often confused. Whereas histology tests are concerned with the structure of tissue, cytology tests are concerned with the structure of cells. In this department, cells in body tissues and fluids are identified, counted, and studied to diagnose malignant and premalignant conditions. Histologists often process and prepare the specimens for evaluation by a pathologist or cytotechnologist. The Pap smear, a test for early detection of cancer cells, primarily of the cervix and vagina, is one of the most common examinations performed by this department.

TABLE 1-16 Common Blood Bank and Immunohematology Tests

Test	Examples of Clinical Significance
Antibody (Ab) screen	Agglutination indicates abnormal antibodies present in patient's blood
Direct antihuman globulin test (DAT)	Positive results point to autoimmune hemolytic anemia, hemolytic disease of the newborn (HDN), and transfusion incompability
Type and Rh	Determination of blood group (ABO) and type (Rh) by identifying agglutinins present or absent
Type and crossmatch	Determination of blood group and general screening for antibodies of recipient's blood and then recipient and donor blood are checked against each other for compatibility
Compatibility testing	Detection of unsuspected antibodies and antigens in recipient's and donor's blood that could cause severe reaction if transfused

Cytogenetics

An area found in larger labs is cytogenetics. In this section, samples are examined for chromosomal deficiencies that relate to genetic disease. Specimens used for chromosomal studies include tissue, blood, and amniotic fluid. The DNA histogram is the latest in tests for genetic and malignant disorders. DNA fingerprinting and molecular genotyping have become the form of scientific testing for forensic medicine.

STAT LABS

In today's healthcare environment, laboratory services in many tertiary care facilities exist as STAT labs only. STAT means immediately. Consequently, tests performed are primarily those needed to respond to medical emergencies, along with some of the more frequently ordered tests. Specimens for all other laboratory tests are collected, processed, and sent to an offsite location or reference laboratory. This efficient way of performing lab work allows hospital laboratories to produce immediately needed test results without having to maintain the equipment and reagents necessary to do all routine testing.

Reference Laboratories   **Reference laboratories** are large, independent laboratories that receive specimens from many different facilities located in the same city, other cities in the same state, or even out of state. They provide routine and more specialized analysis of blood, urine, tissue, and other patient specimens. These laboratories offer fast **turnaround time** (TAT) and reduced costs because of the high volume of tests they perform. Specimens sent to offsite laboratories must be carefully packaged in special containers designed to protect the specimens and meet federal safety regulations for transportation of human specimens.

Clinical Laboratory Personnel

LABORATORY DIRECTOR/PATHOLOGIST

The pathologist is a physician who specializes in diagnosing disease, through the use of laboratory tests results, in tissues removed at operations and from postmortem examinations. It is his or her duty to direct laboratory services so they benefit the physician and patient. The laboratory director may be a pathologist or a clinical laboratory scientist with a doctorate. The laboratory director and the laboratory administrator share responsibilities for managing the laboratory.

LABORATORY ADMINISTRATOR/LABORATORY MANAGER

The lab administrator is usually a technologist with an advanced degree and several years of experience. Duties of the administrator include overseeing all operations involving physician and patient services. Today, the laboratory administrator may supervise several ancillary services, such as radiology and respiratory therapy, or all the laboratory functions in a healthcare system consisting of separate lab facilities across a large geographic area.

TECHNICAL SUPERVISORS

For each laboratory section or subsection, there is a technical supervisor who is responsible for the administration of the area and who reports to the laboratory administrator. This person usually has additional education and experience in one or more of the clinical laboratory areas.

MEDICAL TECHNOLOGIST/CLINICAL LABORATORY SCIENTIST

The medical technologist (MT) or clinical laboratory scientist (CLS) generally has a bachelor's degree in chemistry or biology, with study in an MT program for 1 year or more. Some states require licensing for this level of personnel. The responsibilities of the MTs include performing all levels of testing in any area of the laboratory procedures, reporting results, performing quality control, evaluating new procedures, and conducting preventive maintenance and troubleshooting on instruments.

MEDICAL LABORATORY TECHNICIANS/CLINICAL LABORATORY TECHNICIANS

The medical laboratory technician (MLT) or clinical laboratory technician (CLT) is most often an individual with an associate degree from a 2-year program or certification from a military or proprietary (private) school. As with MTs, some states may require licensing for medical/clinical laboratory technicians. The technician is responsible for performing routine testing, operating all equipment, performing basic instrument maintenance and recognizing instrument problems, and assisting in problem solving.

CLINICAL LABORATORY ASSISTANT

Before the arrival of computerized instrumentation in the laboratory, the clinical laboratory assistant (CLA) was a recognized position. Today, because of reduction in the laboratory staff, this category of personnel has been revived. A clinical laboratory assistant is a person with phlebotomy experience who has skills in specimen processing and basic laboratory testing. Clinical laboratory assistants are generalists, responsible for assisting the MT or MLT with the workload in any area.

PHLEBOTOMIST

The phlebotomist is trained to collect blood for laboratory tests that are necessary for diagnosis and care of patients. A number of facilities use phlebotomists as laboratory assistants or specimen processors (see Box 1-1 for duties). Formal phlebotomy programs in colleges and private schools usually require a high school diploma or the equivalent to enroll. After completing the program or acquiring 1 year of work experience, a phlebotomist can become certified by passing a national examination. A few states require licensing for this level of personnel.

OTHER LABORATORY PERSONNEL

Other laboratory personnel include programmers and laboratory information systems (LIS) operators, quality assurance managers, and point-of-care coordinators. Computer programmers and LIS operators are often laboratorians who, through additional training, have become experts in laboratory computer software. Quality assurance (QA) managers are detail-oriented MTs who collect statistics for QA purposes. Point-of-care coordinators are MTs who work closely with the nursing staff to ensure the quality of point-of-care testing results. In some hospital settings, maintenance and QA checks on the POCT instruments have become the responsibility of the phlebotomy staff.

Clinical Laboratory Improvement Act

The **Clinical Laboratory Improvement Amendments of 1988** (CLIA '88) were signed into law on October 31, 1988, and became effective in 1992. This public law mandates that all laboratories must be regulated using the same standards regardless of the location, type, or size. The law requires that every clinical laboratory facility in the country obtain a certificate from the federal government assuring the customers that laboratory testing performed at that facility is reliable and accurate. Laboratories that fall under the CLIA regulations include those in hospitals, clinics, government facilities, independent laboratories, HMOs, and physician office laboratories. The regulations put in force by this law deal with, among other things, laboratory standards. The standards are designed for two types of laboratory facilities. The lab type is determined by the complexity of testing done at that facility; for example, moderately complex or highly complex. Personnel qualifications for each of the types are stated in the regulations.

STUDY & REVIEW QUESTIONS

1. Early equipment used for bloodletting includes all of the following *except* the
   - a. Fleam
   - b. Hemostat
   - c. Lancet
   - d. Leech

2. A factor that contributes to the phlebotomist's professional image is
   - a. A pleasant smile and a positive attitude
   - b. National certification
   - c. Personal hygiene
   - d. All of the above

3. The initials for the title granted after successful completion of the National Credentialing Agency phlebotomy examination are
   - a. CLPlb
   - b. CLT
   - c. CPT
   - d. PBT

4. The principles of right and wrong conduct as they apply to professional problems are called
   - a. Certification
   - b. Esteem
   - c. Ethics
   - d. Torts

5. The law that established national standards for the electronic exchange of protected health information is
   - a. CLIA
   - b. HIPAA
   - c. OSHA
   - d. PHS

6. Which of the following is a duty of a phlebotomist?
   - a. Analyze specimens for hematology
   - b. Chart patient results
   - c. Obtain blood pressures and temperatures of patients
   - d. Perform laboratory computer operations

7. Which of the following is an example of proxemics?
   - a. Eye contact
   - b. Facial expressions
   - c. Personal hygiene
   - d. Zone of comfort

8. Which of the following is proper telephone technique?
   - a. Be careful of the tone of voice used and keep answers simple
   - b. Do not identify yourself in case there are problems later
   - c. Listen carefully; do not take notes because it takes too much time
   - d. Wait for the phone to ring three or four times so as not to appear anxious

9. **An institution that provides inpatient services is a**
   a. Clinic
   b. Day-surgery
   c. Doctor's office
   d. Hospital

10. **State and federally funded insurance is called**
    a. ASCP
    b. HIPPA
    c. Medicaid
    d. PPO

11. **The specialty that treats disorders of old age is called**
    a. Cardiology
    b. Gerontology
    c. Pathology
    d. Psychiatry

12. **The department in the hospital that records brain waves for diagnosis is**
    a. Electroneurodiagnostics
    b. Occupational therapy
    c. Physical therapy
    d. Radiology

13. **The microbiology department in the laboratory performs**
    a. Compatibility testing
    b. Culture and sensitivity testing
    c. Electrolyte monitoring
    d. Enzyme-linked immunoassay

14. **The abbreviation for the routine hematology test that includes hemoglobin, hematocrit, red blood count, and white blood count determinations is called**
    a. CBC
    b. CDC
    c. CPK
    d. CRP

15. **Which of the following laboratory professionals is specified by CLIA'88 as responsible for administration of a clinical area?**
    a. Clinical laboratory scientist
    b. Clinical laboratory technician
    c. Laboratory manager
    d. Technical supervisor

CASE · STUDY · 1-1

Telephone Etiquette and Irate Caller

Sally is a new phlebotomist working for a small hospital in the suburbs of Chicago. As she finds out right away, her coworkers have many different job responsibilities and are required to cover for one another. Today it is Sally's turn to cover the reception area of the lab while the regular person takes a few days off. This is Sally's first time, and she is rather hesitant to answer the first call because she is afraid that she does not know enough to answer all inquiries. Consequently, she lets it ring more than 10 times. She finally answers the phone. The caller, a nurse, sounds irritated. He has been very anxious to obtain some results on a patient. He tells Sally that they were to be faxed 2 days ago and he has not yet received them. Sally tells him she will transfer him to the technician in the back. Being unfamiliar with this phone, she loses his call in the process. The nurse calls back in a few minutes and wants to speak to "someone who knows what they are doing." The other line starts ringing. This time rather than lose him she keeps the line open, puts the phone down on the counter, and calls out "someone please take this call. I have a call on the other line."

Questions

1. Name three telephone etiquette errors Sally made.
2. Which error creates the chance for a HIPAA violation to occur? Explain why.
3. What should Sally have done differently that would have prevented all three errors?
4. What responsibility does the laboratory administrator have?

Bibliography and Suggested Readings

Johns, M. L. (2006). Health information management technology—an applied approach (2nd ed.). Chicago: American Health Information Management Association.

CLIA '88. (1992). Final standard is published. Clinical Chemistry News, March.

Cmiel, P. (1990). Postoperative management of the replant patient: monitoring, complications, and education. Critical Care Nursing Quarterly 1990;13(1):47.

Davis, A., & Appel, T. (1979). Bloodletting instruments in the National Museum of History and Technology. Washington, DC: Smithsonian Institution Press.

Fischbach, F. (2003). A manual of laboratory and diagnostic tests (7th ed.). Philadelphia: Lippincott Williams & Wilkins.

Henry, J. B. (2001). Clinical diagnosis and management by laboratory methods (20th ed.). Philadelphia: W. B. Saunders.

Mitchell, J., & Haroun, L. (2002). Introduction to health care. Albany, NY: Delmar Publishers.

National Center for Cultural Competence. Policy Brief 1, Rationale for culture competence in primary healthcare. Washington, DC: Georgetown University Child Development Center.

Williams, S. J. (2005). Essentials of health services. New York: Delmar Publishers.

QUALITY ASSURANCE AND LEGAL ISSUES

key•terms

assault	discovery	QI
battery	due care	QC
breach of confidentiality	fraud	QSE
civil actions	GLPs	quality indicators
CLSI	informed consent	respondeat superior
CMS	invasion of privacy	standard of care
competencies	malpractice	statute of limitations
defendant	negligence	threshold values
delta check	plaintiff	tort
deposition	QA	vicarious liability

objectives

Upon successful completion of this chapter, the reader should be able to:

1. Define the key terms and abbreviations listed at the beginning of this chapter.
2. Identify national organizations, agencies, and regulations that support quality assurance in healthcare.
3. Define quality and performance improvement measurements as they relate to phlebotomy.
4. List and describe the components of a quality assurance (QA) program and identify areas in phlebotomy subject to quality control (QC).
5. List areas in phlebotomy subject to QC and identify QC procedures associated with each.
6. Demonstrate knowledge of the legal aspects associated with phlebotomy procedures by defining legal terminology and describing situations that may have legal ramifications.

QUALITY ASSURANCE IN HEALTHCARE

Consumer awareness has increased lawsuits in all areas of society. This is especially true in the healthcare industry. Healthcare institutions search for ways to guarantee quality patient care by identifying and minimizing situations that pose risks to patients and employees. Guidelines are developed for all processes used and all personnel involved, and when formally adopted, they become the institution's **quality improvement** (QI) program. Measurement of performance and quality improvement projects are now part of the accreditation requirements for all types of healthcare facilities and are found in every aspect of healthcare, including phlebotomy. One of the ways to improve quality is through compliance with and use of national standards and regulations.

National Standard and Regulatory Agencies

JOINT COMMISSION ON ACCREDITATION OF HEALTH CARE ORGANIZATIONS

One of the key players in bringing quality assessment review techniques to healthcare is the **Joint Commission on Accreditation of Health Care Organizations** (JCAHO). JCAHO, now referred to as the Joint Commission, is a voluntary, nongovernmental agency charged with, among other things, establishing standards for the operation of hospitals and other health-related facilities and services. Presently, it is the largest healthcare standards-setting body in the world, accrediting more than 15,000 healthcare organizations. Current Joint Commission standards stress performance improvement by requiring the facility to be directly accountable to their customer. This means that all departments of a healthcare facility are required to have ongoing evaluations of their activities and customer expectations. To evaluate and track complaints about healthcare organizations relating to quality of care, the Office of Quality Monitoring was created. The office has a toll-free line that can assist people in registering their complaints. Information and concerns often come from patients, their families, and healthcare employees. A complaint may be submitted by using the *Online Complaint Submission Form* that will go directly to the Joint Commission over the internet or by summarizing the issue in a letter of no more than two pages and providing the name, street address, city and state of the accredited healthcare organization. When a report is submitted, the Joint Commission reviews any past reports and the organization's most recent accreditation decision. Depending on the nature of the reported concern, the Joint Commission will

- Request from the organization a written response to the reported concern
- Incorporate the concern into the performance improvement database that is used to identify trends or patterns in performance
- Conduct an on-site, unannounced assessment of the organization if the report raises serious concerns about a continuing threat to patient safety or a continuing failure to comply with standards
- Review the reported concern and compliance at the organization's next accreditation survey

COLLEGE OF AMERICAN PATHOLOGISTS

Another agency that influences quality improvement in phlebotomy through standards is the **College of American Pathologists** (CAP). This national organization is an outgrowth of the **American Society for Clinical Pathology** (ASCP), a not-for-profit organization for professionals in the field of laboratory medicine. The membership in this specialty organization is composed entirely of board-certified pathologists. CAP offers **proficiency testing** and a continuous form of laboratory inspection by a team made up of pathologists and laboratory managers. The CAP Inspection and Accreditation Program does not compete with the Joint Commission accreditation for healthcare facilities because CAP is designed for pathology/laboratory services only. A CAP-certified laboratory also meets Medicare/Medicaid standards because Joint Commission grants reciprocity to CAP in the area of laboratory inspection.

CLINICAL LABORATORY IMPROVEMENT AMENDMENTS OF 1988

The **Clinical Laboratory Improvement Amendments of 1988** (CLIA '88) are federal regulations passed by Congress and administered by the **Centers for Medicare and Medicaid Services** (CMS), an agency that manages federal healthcare programs of Medicare and Medicaid. These regulations establish quality standards that apply to all facilities, including clinics and physicians' office laboratories that test human specimens for the purpose of providing information used to diagnose, prevent, or treat disease or to assess health status. The aim of the standards is to ensure the accuracy, reliability, and timeliness of patient test results, regardless of the location, type, or size of the laboratory. The standards address quality assurance, quality control, proficiency testing, laboratory records, and personnel qualifications.

All laboratory facilities subject to CLIA'88 regulations are required to obtain a certificate from the CMS according to the complexity of testing performed there. Three categories of testing are recognized: waived (simple with a low risk of error), moderate (which includes provider-performed microscopy), and high complexity. Complexity of testing is based on the difficulty involved in performing the test and the degree of risk of harm to a patient if the test is performed incorrectly. CLIA requirements are more stringent for labs that perform moderate- and high-complexity testing than waived testing, and their facilities are subject to routine inspections. Specimen collection is an important part of CLIA inspections, and laboratories that are moderate or high complexity are required to have written protocols for patient preparation, and specimen collection, labeling, preservation, and transportation.

As of April 2002, CMS began on-site visits to approximately 2% of **Certificate of Waiver** (COW) labs across the country as a result of study findings indicating significant gaps in the quality of their testing practices. The on-site visits are known in advance and are for education and gathering information. In addition, the **Clinical Laboratory Improvement Advisory Committee** (CLIAC) has developed ten QA recommendations for COW labs called **Good Laboratory Practices** (GLPs). The GLPs emphasize quality assurance when collecting and performing blood work using waived testing kits. They are intended as an educational tool and are not mandatory. See Box 2-1 for an abbreviated form of the GLPs.

CLINICAL AND LABORATORY STANDARDS INSTITUTE

The **Clinical and Laboratory Standards Institute (CLSI)** (formerly National Committee for Clinical Laboratory Standards [NCCLS]) is a global, nonprofit, standards-developing organization with representatives from the profession, industry, and government who use a

BOX • 2-1   Good Laboratory Practices

For more information see http://www.cms.hhs.gov/clia/downloads/wgoodlab.pdf

1. Keep and make available to the testing personnel the manufacturer's current product insert for the lab test being performed.
2. Follow the manufacturer's instructions for specimen collection and handling.
3. Properly identify the patient.
4. Label the patient's specimen for testing with an identifier unique to each patient.
5. Inform the patient of any test preparation such as fasting, clean catch urines, etc.
6. Read the product insert prior to performing the test and achieving the optimal result.
7. Follow the storage requirements for the test kit.
8. Do not mix components of different kits.
9. Record the patients' test results in the proper place, such as the lab test log or the patient's chart.
10. Perform any instrument maintenance as directed by the manufacturer.

consensus process to develop voluntary guidelines and standards for all areas of the laboratory. Phlebotomy program approval, certification examination questions, and the Standard of Care are based on these important guidelines and standards.

NATIONAL ACCREDITING AGENCY FOR CLINICAL LABORATORY SCIENCES

The **National Accrediting Agency for Clinical Laboratory Sciences (NAACLS),** recognized by the United States Department of Education as an authority on educational quality, is an autonomous, nonprofit organization that provides either accreditation or approval for clinical laboratory educational programs. The accreditation process involves an external peer review of the program, including an on-site evaluation, to determine whether the program meets certain established educational standards. The NAACLS approval process for phlebotomy programs requires that the program meet educational standards called **competencies** designed to improve student outcomes and maintain quality education.

Quality Improvement

An inexpensive and flexible approach for supporting QI in Joint Commission-accredited organizations is a new program designed to standardize measurements of performance nationally. Organizations will be expected to demonstrate, for each measurement, the ability to collect dependable data, conduct reliable analyses of the data, and initiate appropriate system and process improvements.

The principal intent of Joint Commission is to identify, rather than develop, sound measurements that support the objectives of the organization's process improvement. In May 2001, the Joint Commission revealed the four initial core measurement areas for hospitals: acute myocardial infarction (heart attack), community-acquired pneumonia, pregnancy and related conditions, and heart failure. At a later date, the Surgical Care Improvement Project (SCIP) was added as another core measurement to research the area of antibiotic therapy given following heart surgery. Healthcare organizations continually collect data in the core outcome measurement areas on patients who have been discharged from their facilities. Outcome measures document the results of care for individual patients and specific patient groups in certain diagnostic categories. For example, a hospital's overall rate of postsurgical infection would be considered an outcome measure.

Some of the recommended core measures directly relate to the quality and timeliness of phlebotomy. For example, the community-acquired pneumonia measure includes blood culture collection before administration of antibiotics as one of the standardized performance measures and how the collection, processing, and reporting affects patient outcome. A core measure for acute myocardial infarction includes time elapsed between the collection of specimens at specified times for tests whose results are used for critical decision making, and the treatment or surgical procedures that may be based on the results of those tests.

Patient Safety and Sentinel Events

Part of the Joint Commission's QI program is their commitment to improving safety for patients and residents in healthcare organizations. One of the ways this is demonstrated is through its sentinel (early warning) event policy. The intent of this policy is to help healthcare organizations identify sentinel events and take steps to prevent them from happening again. A sentinel event is one that signals the need for immediate investigation and response. It includes any unfavorable event that is unexpected and results in death or serious physical or psychologic injury, or any deviation from practice that increases the chance that an undesirable outcome might recur. Loss of a limb or any of its function is specifically included as a sentinel event. According to the policy, if a sentinel event occurs, the healthcare organization is required to

- Perform a thorough and credible analysis of the root cause
- Put improvements to reduce risk into practice
- Monitor improvements to determine if they are effective

Quality Assurance in Phlebotomy

As members of the healthcare team, phlebotomists need to understand the significance of their role in providing quality patient care. Laboratory testing is an important part of patient diagnosis and consequently a major part of patient care. Doctors rely on the validity of test results. Preanalytical (before analysis) factors such as patient preparation, specimen collection procedures, and specimen handling can affect specimen quality and in turn affect the validity of test results. Many of these factors fall under the responsibility of the phlebotomist. To ensure consistent quality, specimen collection and handling policies and procedures should be based on specific guidelines such as those established by CLSI, and phlebotomists should strictly adhere to them. Established polices and procedures fall under an overall process called **quality assurance** (QA).

QA DEFINED

QA is defined as a program that guarantees quality patient care by tracking outcomes through scheduled reviews in which areas of the hospital look at the appropriateness, applicability, and timeliness of patient care. Guidelines are developed for all processes used and play a part in developing the Joint Commission's measurements of performance and quality improvement standards.

QA INDICATORS

One of the most important aspects of setting up a QA identification and evaluation process is establishing indicators or guides to monitor all aspects of patient care. **QA indicators** must be measurable, well defined, objective, specific, and clearly related to an important aspect of care. Indicators can measure quality, adequacy, accuracy, timeliness, effectiveness of patient care, customer satisfaction, and so on. They are designed to look at areas of care that tend to cause problems. For example, an indicator on the QA form shown in Figure 2-1 states: "Blood culture contamination rate will not exceed 3%." A contamination rate that increased beyond the preestablished threshold listed on the form would signify unacceptable performance, and action should be taken.

 Quality indicators should be identified and monitored for all operations in any healthcare service. CLSI's most current edition of HS1—*A Quality System Model for Health Care*—offers a prototype to assist in identifying a core set of **"quality system essentials" (QSEs)** that can be applied to steps necessary to deliver a product or service called a "path of workflow." A clinical laboratory path of workflow consists of three processes: preanalytical, analytical, and postanalytical. All clinical laboratories follow this path to deliver quality lab information. For example, in monitoring laboratory performance for arterial blood gas collection, all operations across the path of workflow should be listed, and quality indicators that monitor the workflow noted (Table 2-1).

THRESHOLDS AND DATA

Threshold values must be established for all clinical indicators. A threshold value is a level of acceptable practice beyond which quality patient care cannot be assured. Exceeding this level of acceptable practice may trigger intensive evaluation to see if there is a problem that needs to be corrected. During the evaluation process, data are collected and organized. Data sources include such information as patient records, laboratory results, incident reports, patient satisfaction reports, and direct patient observation. A corrective action plan is established if the data identify a problem or opportunity for improvement. An action plan defines what will change and when that change is expected. Even when the problem appears to be

JOHN C. LINCOLN HOSPITAL & HEALTH CENTER
QUALITY ASSESSMENT AND IMPROVEMENT TRACKING
CONFIDENTIAL A.R.S. 36-445 et. seq.

STANDARD OF CARE/SERVICE:

IMPORTANT ASPECT OF CARE/SERVICE:
LABORABORY SERVICES
COLLECTION/TRANSPORT

SIGNATURES:

_____
DIRECTOR

_____
MEDICAL DIRECTOR

_____
VICE PRESIDENT/ADMINISTRATOR

DEPARTMENTS:
DATA SOURCE(S):
METHODOLOGY: [X] RETROSPECTIVE [   ] CONCURRENT
TYPE: [   ] STRUCTURE [   ] PROCESS [X] OUTCOME
PERSON RESPONSIBLE FOR:
• DATA COLLECTION: JUDY HERRIG
• DATA ORGANIZATION: JUDY HERRIG
• ACTION PLAN: JUDY HERRIG
• FOLLOW-UP: JUDY HERRIG
DATE MONITORING BEGAN: 1990
TIME PERIOD THIS MONITOR: 2ND QUARTER 2006
MONITOR DISCONTINUED BECAUSE:
FOLLOW-UP:

INDICATORS	THLD	ACT	PREV	CRITICAL ANALYSIS/EVALUATION	ACTION PLAN
Blood Culture contamination rate will not exceed 3%				Population: All patients All monthly indicators were under threshold, 3%	Share results and analysis with Lab staff and ER staff.
APR - # of Draws: 713 # Contaminated: 13	3.00%	1.8%	1.2%	% Contamination from draws other than Line draws, by unit:	
MAY - # of Draws: 710 # Contaminated: 23	3.00%	2.8%	2.3%	APR: ER = 4.7% Lab = 0.7% MAY: ER = 11.5% Lab = 1.0%	
JUN - # of Draws: 702 # Contaminated: 17	3.00%	2.4%	1.9%	JUN: ER = 8.6% Lab = 1.1% ER was over threshold for each month of quarter.	
Total for 1st Quarter - # of Draws: 2125 # Contaminated: 50	3.00%	2.4%	1.9%		

FIGURE 2-1

Microbiology quality assessment form.   (Courtesy John C. Lincoln Hospital & Health Center.)

corrected, monitoring and evaluation continue, to ensure that care is consistent and that quality continually improves.

PROCESS AND OUTCOMES

QA has traditionally looked at outcomes. Outcomes are in numbers only. For example, an outcome measurement may give the number of times that patient specimens were redrawn because the improper tube was used for collection. It is important to know how often this occurs, but it does not explain why it happened. To improve an outcome, the process needs to be reviewed. This entails following the process from start to finish. As the Joint

TABLE 2-1 Published Laboratory Quality Indicators for ABG Collection	
Quality System Essentials (QSEs)	**Quality Indicators**
Patient assessment	• Practice guideline implementation • Duplicate test ordering
Test request	• Ordering accuracy • Accuracy of order transmission • Verbal order evaluation
Specimen collection/labeling	• Wristband evaluation
Specimen transport	• Transit time • Stat transit time
Specimen receiving/processing	• Blood gas sample acceptability • Chemistry sample acceptability
QSE: Personnel	• Competence evaluation • Employee retention
QSE: Process control	• Safety
QSE: Occurrence management	• Incidents
QSE: Internal assessment	• On-site assessments • Self-assessments

Adapted from CLSI/NCCLS document H11-A4, *Procedures for the Collection of Arterial Blood Specimens; Approved Standard – Fourth Edition* with permission.

Commission suggests, it means standardizing the way performance is measured and activities are evaluated. In the previous example, it would mean looking at what the requester did at the time he or she decided the test was needed, how it was ordered, and how the laboratory processed the request until the time the results were on the patient's chart and in the hands of the person who ordered them. To ensure that the same process is always followed, there must be checks and controls on quality along the way. The use of checks and controls is called **quality control** (QC).

QC DEFINED

QC is a component of a QI program and a form of procedure control. Consistently following national standards for phlebotomy procedures is a means of controlling the quality of results. Phlebotomy QC involves using all available quality control checks on every operational procedure to make certain it is performed correctly. In phlebotomy, it is the responsibility of the person who supervises the phlebotomist to oversee QI and ensure that checks are being done and standards are being met. It is the responsibility of the phlebotomist to meet those standards at all times.

Areas of Phlebotomy Subject to Quality Assessment

PATIENT PREPARATION PROCEDURES

Quality assurance in laboratory testing actually starts before the specimen is collected, in the preanalytical stage. To obtain a quality specimen, the patient must be prepared properly. In a hospital setting, the patient's nurse can find instructions on how to prepare a patient

TEST PROCEDURE:	**ANTI THROMBIN III ACTIVITY – PLASMA ACTIVITY**
TEST MNEMONIC:	AT3
BILLING NUMBER:	3000070
MANNER OF COLLECTION:	Drawn by Lab
SPECIMEN REQUIRED:	Citrated plasma, 1 Blue Top with Black Insert of 2 Blue Top with White Insert
SPECIAL INSTRUCTIONS:	2, 1 ml citrated plasma aliquots place in plastic tubes. Centrifuge, separate and freeze plasma immediately.
PATIENT PREPARATION:	None
AVAILABILITY:	At all times.
ROUTINE TURN-AROUND-TIME:	Dependent on Reference Laboratory's testing schedule
STAT TURN-AROUND-TIME:	N/A
LIMITATIONS:	None
NORMAL RANGE:	See Reference Laboratory Report

TEST PROCEDURE:	**APTT**
TEST MNEMONIC:	APTT (ALSO SEE PTT)
BILLING NUMBER:	3000030
MANNER OF COLLECTION:	Drawn by Lab
SPECIMEN REQUIRED:	Citrated plasma, Blue Top Tube
SPECIAL INSTRUCTIONS:	If the patient is on heparin, APTT's should be timed so that the blood is not drawn immediately after the dose is given. Draw a red tube before drawing the blue top tube. TESTING CANNOT BE PERFORMED ON OVERFILLED OR UNDERFILLED BLUE TOP TUBES. CORRECT BLOOD VOLUME IN BLUE TOP TUBE IS CRITICAL.
PATIENT PREPARATION:	None
AVAILABILITY:	At all times.
ROUTINE TURN-AROUND-TIME:	1-2 Hours
STAT TURN-AROUND-TIME:	60 Minutes
LIMITATIONS:	None
NORMAL RANGE:	Normal Range: 21.5 – 34.0 seconds

TEST PROCEDURE:	**ARSENIC, URINE**
TEST MNEMONIC:	ARSENUR
BILLING NUMBER:	
MANNER OF COLLECTION:	Urine collected by nurse
SPECIMEN REQUIRED:	Random urine
SPECIAL INSTRUCTIONS:	10 ml random urine in acid-washed container, refrigerate
PATIENT PREPARATION:	None
AVAILABILITY:	At all times.
ROUTINE TURN-AROUND-TIME:	Dependent on Reference Laboratory's testing schedule
STAT TURN-AROUND-TIME:	N/A
LIMITATIONS:	None
NORMAL RANGE:	See Reference Laboratory Report

TEST PROCEDURE:	**ASPERGILLUS SEROLOGY**
TEST MNEMONIC:	ASPTER
BILLING NUMBER:	3020090
MANNER OF COLLECTION:	Drawn by Lab
SPECIMEN REQUIRED:	1 Red Top Tube
SPECIAL INSTRUCTIONS:	Refrigerate 1 ml serum
PATIENT PREPARATION:	None
AVAILABILITY:	At all times.
ROUTINE TURN-AROUND-TIME:	Dependent on Reference Laboratory's testing schedule
STAT TURN-AROUND-TIME:	N/A
LIMITATIONS:	None
NORMAL RANGE:	See Reference Laboratory Report

TEST PROCEDURE:	**AST (SGOT)**
TEST MNEMONIC:	AST
BILLING NUMBER:	3011070
MANNER OF COLLECTION:	Drawn by Lab
SPECIMEN REQUIRED:	Plasma or Serum, 1 Green Top, Red Top or SST Tube
SPECIAL INSTRUCTIONS:	None
PATIENT PREPARATION:	None
AVAILABILITY:	At all times.
ROUTINE TURN-AROUND-TIME:	4 Hours
STAT TURN-AROUND-TIME:	60 Minutes
LIMITATIONS:	None
NORMAL RANGE:	15-37 U/L

FIGURE 2-2

Page from a nursing services manual.   (Courtesy John C. Lincoln Hospital & Health Center.)

for testing by checking the laboratory's section of the **Nursing Services Manual** (Fig. 2-2) that is electronically sent to the nursing station from the lab. This document describes patient preparation and other special instructions for specimen collection. The phlebotomist and others involved in specimen collection must stay current concerning testing, to answer inquiries correctly.

SPECIMEN COLLECTION PROCEDURES

Identification   Patient identification (as described in Chapter 8) is the most important aspect of specimen collection. Methods are being continually improved to ensure correct patient identification. An example is the use of bar code readers and accompanying labels (Fig. 2-3), which can substantially reduce human error.

Equipment
Puncture Devices

Ensuring the quality and sterility of every needle and lancet is essential for patient safety. All puncture devices come in sealed sterile containers and should be used only once. If the seal has been broken, the device should be put in a sharps container and a new one obtained. Manufacturing defects in needles, such as barbs and blunt tips, can be avoided before use by quickly inspecting the needle after unsheathing.

Evacuated Tubes

CLSI has established standards for evacuated tubes to help ensure specimen integrity. Manufacturers print expiration dates on each tube for quality assurance (see Fig. 8-12). Outdated tubes should not be used because they may not fill completely, causing dilution of the sample, distortion of the cell components, and erroneous results. In addition, anticoagulants in expired tubes may not work effectively, instead allowing small clots to form and thereby invalidating hematology and immunohematology test results. As part of QC, all new lots of evacuated tubes should be checked for adequate vacuum and additive, integrity of the stopper, ease of stopper removal, and tube strength during centrifugation. Results of these and other quality control checks should be documented.

Labeling

Labeling must be exact. Labeling requirements as outlined in Chapter 8 should be strictly followed. Inaccuracies, such as transposed letters or missing information, will result in the specimen being discarded. With computer labels (see Fig. 2-3), the phlebotomist may be assured of correctly printed patient information; however, this correct label must still be placed on the correct patient's specimen.

Technique   Proper phlebotomy technique must be carefully taught by a professional who understands the importance of following national standards and the reasons for using certain equipment or techniques. When a phlebotomist understands the rationale for maintaining the standards, quality specimens are ensured.

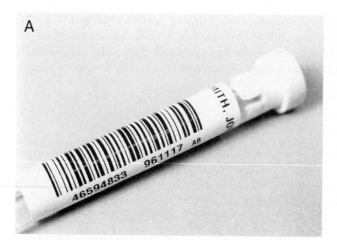

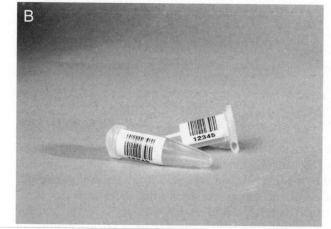

FIGURE 2-3

A. Specimen tube with bar code label. **B.** Microcollection container with bar code label. **C.** Slide with bar code label. (Courtesy Electronic Imaging Materials, Inc., Keene, NH.)

key · point No matter how experienced phlebotomists may be, a periodic review of their techniques is necessary for quality assurance and performance improvement.

Collection Priorities   Specimen collection priorities must be stressed. The importance of knowing how to recognize which specimen request is the most critical or has special collection criteria (e.g., renins or therapeutic drug monitoring [TDM]) can save the patient unnecessary medication or additional testing. It may even shorten the patient's stay in the hospital because in many instances therapy is based on test values on specimens assumed to have been collected at the right time and in the proper manner.

Delta Checks   Delta checks help ensure quality in testing. A **delta check** compares current results of a lab test with previous results for the same test on the same patient. Although some variation is to be expected, a major difference in results could indicate error and requires investigation.

Documentation

Documentation is a major part of a QA program. Different types of QA documents have been developed to standardize procedures, inform nursing and other personnel of the importance of patient preparation (Fig. 2-4), and record problems for evaluation. Documentation can be used for legal purposes as long as it is legible and includes only standard abbreviations. Most records kept in the process of providing healthcare will provide information for evaluating and monitoring outcomes used in institutional QI. Easily the most important one of these is the patient's medical record.

MEDICAL RECORD

The medical record is a chronologic documentation of a patient's care. The law requires that medical records be kept on hospital patients but does not require physicians in private practice to keep records on their patients, although most do in the form of a clinical record. Every notation in the patient's medical or clinical record should be legible, precise, and complete. The basic reasons for maintaining accurate, up-to-date medical records are as follows:

- To provide an aid to practicing medicine. Through the use of a medical record, the physician can document treatment and give a written plan for continuation of the patient's care plan
- To provide an aid to communications between the physician and others involved with the patient's care. It can also serve as a communications tool between past, present, and future physicians who care for the patient
- To serve as a legal document that may be used in a court of law. It must be a factual, legible, and objective account of the patient, past and present
- To serve as a very valuable tool for assisting the hospital in evaluating performance outcomes. The medical records include such information as a history of examinations, medical testing and laboratory reports, prescriptions written, and supplies used that are all very informative for utilization review

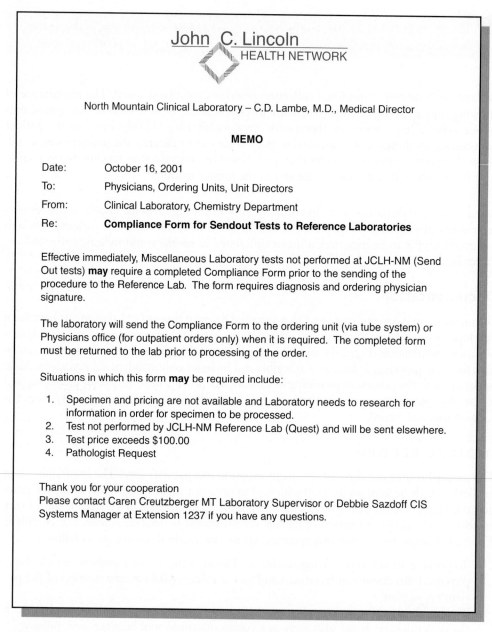

John C. Lincoln
HEALTH NETWORK

North Mountain Clinical Laboratory – C.D. Lambe, M.D., Medical Director

MEMO

Date: October 16, 2001

To: Physicians, Ordering Units, Unit Directors

From: Clinical Laboratory, Chemistry Department

Re: **Compliance Form for Sendout Tests to Reference Laboratories**

Effective immediately, Miscellaneous Laboratory tests not performed at JCLH-NM (Send Out tests) **may** require a completed Compliance Form prior to the sending of the procedure to the Reference Lab. The form requires diagnosis and ordering physician signature.

The laboratory will send the Compliance Form to the ordering unit (via tube system) or Physicians office (for outpatient orders only) when it is required. The completed form must be returned to the lab prior to processing of the order.

Situations in which this form **may** be required include:

1. Specimen and pricing are not available and Laboratory needs to research for information in order for specimen to be processed.
2. Test not performed by JCLH-NM Reference Lab (Quest) and will be sent elsewhere.
3. Test price exceeds $100.00
4. Pathologist Request

Thank you for your cooperation
Please contact Caren Creutzberger MT Laboratory Supervisor or Debbie Sazdoff CIS Systems Manager at Extension 1237 if you have any questions.

FIGURE 2-4

Procedure manual update.   (Courtesy John C. Lincoln Hospital & Health Center.)

> **c a u t i o n**   For confidentiality reasons, access to a patient's medical record is restricted to those who have a verifiable need to review the information.

COLLECTION MANUALS

The Nursing Services Manual (Fig. 2-2) and **Specimen Collection Manual**, a similar reference for outpatient settings, are examples of QA documents made available to blood collectors at all specimen collection sites. These manuals detail how to prepare the patient and collect a quality sample. They typically contain in chart form the type and minimum amount of specimen needed for testing, special handling required, reference values for the test, the days testing is available, and the normal turnaround time (TAT). The manuals also include updates and a copy of the notification of these changes to the persons who will be affected (Fig. 2-4). Both documents describe patient preparation and other special instructions for specimen collection. It is important for the phlebotomist and others involved in specimen collection to stay informed and current concerning testing protocol to be better able to answer inquiries.

THE PROCEDURE MANUAL

The **Procedure Manual** (Fig. 2-5) states the policies and procedures that apply to each test or practice performed in the laboratory. The Procedure Manual, a QA document, must be made available to all employees of the laboratory for standardization purposes. Accrediting agencies such as CAP and JCAHO demand that this manual be updated annually at a minimum. Box 2-2 lists typical information found in a procedure manual.

THE SAFETY MANUAL

The **Safety Manual** contains procedures related to chemical, electrical, fire, and radiation safety; exposure control; and disaster plans, as well as complete detailing of how to handle hazardous materials.

THE INFECTION CONTROL PROCEDURE MANUAL

The **Infection Control Procedure Manual** outlines hand washing and other decontamination procedures, precautions to take when dealing with patients or handling specimens, and how to handle accidental contamination, including postexposure incident procedures.

QA FORMS

Accreditation standards for agencies such as the Joint Commission require the facility to show documentation on all quality control checks and other quality assessment activities. These forms include equipment check forms and incident/occurrence report forms.

SECTION: LABORATORY SERVICES

TOPIC: VENIPUNCTURE

REVIEWED: 3/95, 7/06

LAST REVISION: 3/93, 8/90, 3/88, 4/87, 8/04

APPROVAL:

1.0   PURPOSE

1.1   To provide our laboratory with quality blood specimens for testing.

2.0   POLICY

2.1   Blood collection by laboratory and hospital personnel will be performed according to our laboratory procedure.

3.0   PROCEDURE

3.1   Obtain computer labels generated by orders for tests requested. For registered outpatients, use faxed order from the Outpatient Order Log or prescription.

3.2   Upon entering the patient's room, identify yourself. State that you will be drawing blood for laboratory testing and gain the patient's confidence by behaving in a professional manner.

3.3   Ensure positive patient identification.

Inpatients
3.3.1   Identify the patient to be drawn by matching each label with the patient's hospital identification armband.
3.3.2   Check for the correct match of the patient's full name and hospital medical record number and account number.
3.3.3   In the case that there is no armband present, contact the patient's nurse or charge nurse for a armband to be placed on the patient.
3.3.4   Inpatient's will **NOT** be drawn without a hospital armband.

Outpatients
3.3.5   For recurring outpatients without armbands, ask the patient for the spelling of their last name and their birth date. If the patient is a

FIGURE 2-5

Procedure manual page.   (Courtesy John C. Lincoln Hospital & Health Center.)

Equipment Check Forms   Special forms for recording equipment checks on tube additives, vacuum strength, and expiration dates are available for verification of new lot numbers. Refrigerator temperatures, which must be recorded daily, are often the responsibility of the phlebotomist. Control checks on the centrifuge require periodic documentation of the tachometer readings and maintenance performed.

BOX • 2-2   Information Found in a Procedure Manual

- Purpose of the procedure
- Policy
- Specimen type and collection method
- Equipment and supplies required
- Detailed step-by-step procedure
- Limitations and variables of the method

- Corrective actions
- Method validation
- Normal values and references
- Review and revision dates
- Approval signatures and dates

Internal Reports   Confidential incident/occurrence reports must be filled out when a problem occurs. These forms identify the problem, state the consequence, and describe the corrective action. Incident reports are not limited to situations in which an injury occurred. For example, an incident form would be filled out when a tube of blood was mislabeled. Incident reports should state facts and not feelings. The function of an incident report is not to place blame, but only to identify what took place and the corrective action taken so that such an event does not happen again. **Performance Improvement Plan** documents (Fig. 2-6) are used when counseling or suspension is necessary. The document states the deficiency, describes a specific action plan for improvement, and the next step, if necessary.

Risk Management

Risk, defined as "the chance of loss or injury," is inherent in the healthcare environment. **Risk management** is an internal process focused on identifying and minimizing situations that pose risk to patients and employees. Risk is managed in two ways: controlling risk to avoid incidents and paying for occurrences after they have happened. Generic steps in risk management involve identification of the risk, treatment of the risk using policies and procedures already in place, education of employees and patients, and evaluation of what should be done in the future.

Risk factors can sometimes be identified by looking at trends in reporting tools such as incident or occurrence reports (Fig. 2-6). Proper investigation is initiated if a situation is identified that deviates from the normal. If new procedures that reduce risk are instituted, employees are informed immediately and instructed in what to do. Evaluation of occurrences, trends, and outcomes is essential throughout the operation of a risk management program, so that risks can be identified and the appropriate changes made. Risk management procedures and other QA measures demonstrate the intent of a healthcare facility to adhere to national standards of good practice that can result in a noticeable reduction of legal issues concerning consumers of healthcare.

JOHN C. LINCOLN HOSPITAL & HEALTH CENTER
PERFORMANCE IMPROVEMENT PLAN

Employee Name:	Facility	Department	Job Title
Previous Action:	Type	Reason	Date

Current Action:
(please check one)

☐ Verbal Counseling   ☐ Written Warning   ☐ Final Written Warning
☐ Suspension – Date   ☐ Termination (check reason below)

Termination
Reason:

☐ Unexcused
Absence/Tardiness   ☐ Job Performance   ☐ Conduct   ☐ Other

I.   Describe the performance deficiency giving rise to the counseling (include specific dates, times and policies violated, etc.):

II. Describe specific job performance expectations and areas for improvement:

III. Describe the agreed upon action plan for improvement including date of follow-up to review progress, if applicable:

IV. State the next step if job performance does not improve (warning, discharge, etc.):

V.   Department director/supervisor Comments:

Department Director/Supervisor Signature:	Date

VI. Employee Comments:

I understand that all corrective action notices other than a verbal counseling will be placed in my personnel file. My signature below does not indicate agreement regarding the contents of the document; only that I have received a copy for my records.

Employee	Date	Witness	Date
Human Resources	Date	Reason	

FIGURE 2-6

Performance improvement form.   (Courtesy John C. Lincoln Hospital & Health Center.)

LEGAL ISSUES

Greater consumer awareness has led to an increase in lawsuits in all areas of society. This is especially true in the healthcare industry, where physicians and other healthcare providers were once considered above reproach. As healthcare providers go about their daily activities, there are many activities that, if performed without reasonable care and skill, could result in a lawsuit. It has been proven in past lawsuits that persons performing phlebotomy can and will be held legally accountable for their actions. Although most legal actions against healthcare workers are **civil actions** in which the alleged injured party sues for monetary damages, willful actions by healthcare workers with the intent to produce harm or death can result in criminal charges. See Table 2-2 for a description of criminal and civil actions.

fyi The same act may lead to both criminal and civil actions. For example, in assault and battery cases a guilty defendant can face imprisonment by the state and also face civil action in which the injured party tries to collect monetary damages.

Tort

The most common civil actions in healthcare are based on **tort**. A tort is a wrongful act, other than breach of contract, committed against one's person, property, reputation, or other legally protected right, for which the individual is entitled to damages awarded by the court. It is an act that is committed without just cause and may be intentional (willful) or unintentional (accidental). The following list includes definitions of tort actions and related legal terminology.

- **Assault:** An act or threat causing another to be in fear of immediate battery (harmful touching). Battery does not necessarily have to follow an assault; however the victim must believe the ability to carry out the threat is there.
- **Battery:** Intentional harmful or offensive touching of or use of force on a person without consent or legal justification. Legal justification would be, for example, when a mother gives permission to have blood drawn from her child. Intentional harm may

TABLE 2-2 Criminal and Civil Actions

Action	Definition	Punishment
Criminal	Concerned with laws designed to protect all members of society from injurious acts by others; i.e., felonies and misdemeanors	• Felony is a crime punishable by death or imprisonment; i.e., murder, assault, and rape • Misdemeanors are considered lesser offenses and usually carry a penalty of a fine or less than 1 year in jail
Civil	Concerned with actions between two private parties, such as individuals or organizations; constitute the bulk of the legal actions dealt with in the medical office or other healthcare facilities	• Damages may be awarded in a court of law and will result in monetary penalties

range from permanent disfigurement to merely grabbing something out of another person's hand without permission. Battery is usually both a tort and a crime.

> c a u t i o n A phlebotomist who attempts to collect a blood specimen without the patient's consent can be charged with assault and battery.

- **Fraud:** Deceitful practice or false portrayal of facts either by words or by conduct, often done to obtain money or property. An example includes billing for services that have not been provided.
- **Invasion of privacy:** The violation of one's right to be left alone. It can involve physical intrusion or the unauthorized publishing or release of private information, which can also be considered a breach of confidentiality.

> k e y · p o i n t Invasion of privacy by physical intrusion may be no more than opening the door and walking into a patient's room without asking permission to enter.

- **Breach of confidentiality:** Failure to keep privileged medical information private. An example is the unauthorized release of patient information such as laboratory results. This could lead to a lawsuit if it caused great embarrassment to the patient or even greater consequences, such as the loss of his or her job.
- **Malpractice:** A type of negligence (described below) committed by a professional. The training and experience of the accused individual is taken into consideration when deciding whether an act resulting in injury should be labeled negligence or malpractice. A claim of malpractice implies that a greater standard of care was owed to the injured person than the reasonable person standard associated with negligence.
- **Negligence:** Failure to exercise **due care**, the level of care that a person of ordinary intelligence and good sense would exercise under the given circumstances. In other words, negligence is doing something that a *reasonable* person would *not* do, or *not* doing something that a *reasonable* person *would* do. If a medical procedure results in injury and there is no intent to injure, it is called negligence, and the injured person has the right to sue for damages. To claim negligence the following must be present:

  1. A legal duty or obligation owed by one person to another
  2. A breaking or breach of that duty or obligation
  3. Harm done as a direct result of the action

- **Res ipsa loquitur:** A Latin phrase meaning "the thing speaks for itself," which applies to the rule of evidence in a case of negligence. When a breach of duty is so obvious that it does not need further explanation, it is said that the situation speaks for itself. For example, a homebound patient sitting on a kitchen barstool faints while having blood drawn and falls, hitting his head. A head injury develops that was obviously due to the fall. If a lawsuit results, the burden of proof is shifted to the phlebotomist who must prove that he or she was not negligent.

- **Respondeat superior:** A Latin phrase that means "let the master respond." An employer is liable (legally responsible) for the actions of an employee, even though the employee is the one at fault. This tort may be filed if a neglectful or intentional act of an employee results in some type of physical injury to a client. The key points in a claim of respondeat superior are that the employee is working within the scope of employment and has had the proper training to perform the required duties.

key • point If a neglectful act occurs while an employee is doing something that is not within his or her duties or training, the employee may be held solely responsible for that act.

- **Standard of care:** The normal level of skill and care that a healthcare practitioner would be expected to adhere to in order to provide due care for patients. This duty is established by standards of the profession and the expectations of society. It is the standard of care expected of everyone at all times; a failure to exercise due care is negligence. Employers are responsible for providing employees who possess the qualifications and training necessary to meet the standard of care and are ultimately liable if they do not.

- **Statute of limitations:** A law setting the length of time after an alleged injury in which the injured person is permitted to file a lawsuit. The time limit is specified in each state's medical malpractice law. The question for all parties involved is when does the clock start? Some of the most common occurrences given for when the statute of limitations period begins are as follows:

  1. On the day the alleged negligent act was committed
  2. When the injury resulting from the alleged negligence was actually discovered or should have been discovered by a reasonably alert patient
  3. The day the physician–patient relationship ended or the day of the last medical treatment in a series
  4. In the case of minors, the statue may not begin to run until the minor reaches the age of majority

- **Vicarious liability:** Liability imposed by law on one person for acts committed by another. One example is employer liability under respondeat superior, explained above. Another example is employer liability for negligence by an independent contractor or consultant that it hired. This is based on the fact that the contractor or consultant is acting on behalf of the employer by virtue of the contract between them.

key • point A hospital, as an employer, cannot escape liability for a patient's injury simply by subcontracting out various services to other persons and claiming it is not responsible because the party that caused the injury is not on its payroll.

Malpractice Insurance

Malpractice insurance compensates the insured in the event of malpractice liability. Individual personnel are not typically targets of lawsuits because of respondeat superior or vicarious liability, both of which involve the "deep pockets" theory (let the one with the most money pay). They can, however, be named as codefendants, in which case, the employer's malpractice insurance may not cover them. It is important for healthcare personnel to examine the possibility of a civil suit being brought against them and consider carrying malpractice insurance. The decision to purchase this insurance should be based on financial considerations as well as legal ones. From the legal point of view, it may be desirable to be covered by a separate professional liability policy because the employer may give his or her insurer the right to recover damages from an employee who is found to be negligent. Healthcare personnel may be able to purchase malpractice insurance from their professional organizations.

Avoiding Lawsuits

The best insurance against lawsuits is to take steps to avoid them. A good way to avoid lawsuits is to consistently follow the guidelines listed in Box 2-3. Above all, always remember to respect the rights of patients. This gives them control over the situation and makes them less likely to feel that they have been treated poorly.

Patient Consent

Obtaining the patient's consent before initiating a procedure is critical. There are a number of different types of patient consent including **informed consent, expressed consent,**

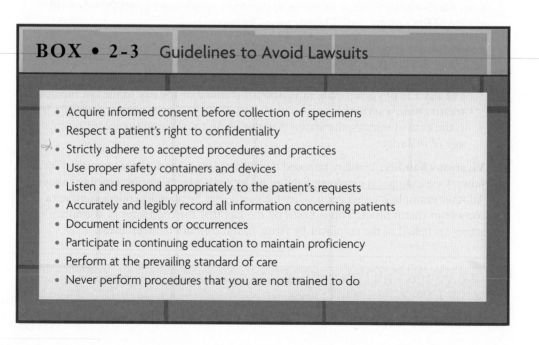

> ### BOX • 2-3 Guidelines to Avoid Lawsuits
>
> - Acquire informed consent before collection of specimens
> - Respect a patient's right to confidentiality
> - Strictly adhere to accepted procedures and practices
> - Use proper safety containers and devices
> - Listen and respond appropriately to the patient's requests
> - Accurately and legibly record all information concerning patients
> - Document incidents or occurrences
> - Participate in continuing education to maintain proficiency
> - Perform at the prevailing standard of care
> - Never perform procedures that you are not trained to do

implied consent, HIV consent, and **consent for minors.** It is important to be familiar with them all and **refusal of consent** as well.

INFORMED CONSENT

- Implies voluntary and competent permission for a medical procedure, test, or medication
- Requires that a patient be given adequate information regarding the method, risks, and consequences of a procedure before consenting to it
- Information must be given to the patient in nontechnical terms and in his or her own language, if possible, meaning an interpreter may be necessary
- The patient's permission or consent must be obtained before initiating any medical procedure
- Minors require consent of their parents or legal guardians

EXPRESSED CONSENT

- Required for treatment that involves surgery, experimental drugs, or high-risk procedures
- May be given verbally or in writing
- Written consent gives the best possible protection for both the treatment provider and the patient, must be signed by both, and witnessed by a third party
- Verbal consent for treatment should be followed by an entry in the patient's chart covering what was discussed with the patient
- Consent should cover what procedures are going to be performed and should not be in a general form that allows the physician carte blanche to do whatever he or she wants to do

fyi When a general consent issue goes to court, the court typically takes the word of the patient as to what he or she understood was to take place.

IMPLIED CONSENT

- The patient's actions imply consent without a verbal or written expression of consent
- Implied consent may be necessary in emergency procedures such as CPR to save a person's life
- Laws involving implied consent are enacted at the state level and may differ greatly from state to state

key · point If a phlebotomist tells a patient that he or she is going to collect a blood specimen and the patient holds out an arm, it is considered implied consent.

HIV CONSENT

- Legislation governing informed consent has been enacted in most states
- Laws specify exactly what type of information must be given to inform the client properly
- Generally speaking, the client must be advised on (1) the test and its purpose, (2) how the test might be used, and (3) the meaning of the test and its limitations

CONSENT FOR MINORS

- As a general rule a minor cannot give consent for the administration of medical treatment
- Parental or guardian consent is required
- Healthcare personnel who violate this rule are liable for assault and battery

fyi A minor is anyone who has not reached the age of majority determined by state law.

REFUSAL OF CONSENT

- An individual has a constitutional right to refuse a medical procedure such as venipuncture
- The refusal may be based on religious or personal beliefs and preferences
- A patient who refuses medical treatment is normally required to verify the refusal in writing on a special form

The Litigation Process

Litigation is the process used to settle legal disputes. Approximately 10% of malpractice lawsuits actually go to court. The rest are settled out of court, which can happen any time prior to the final court decision. Malpractice litigation involves the following four phases:

- **Phase one** begins when an alleged patient incident occurs or the patient becomes aware of a prior possible injury.
- **Phase two** begins when the injured party or a family member consults an attorney. The attorney requests, obtains, and reviews copies of the medical records involved and decides whether to take the case. If the attorney thinks that malpractice has occurred and takes the case, an attempt to negotiate a settlement is made. If not resolved by negotiation, a complaint is filed by the patient's attorney. Once a complaint is filed, the injured party becomes the **plaintiff** and the person/s against whom the complaint is filed becomes the **defendant**. Both sides now conduct formal **discovery**, which involves taking depositions and interrogating parties involved. Giving a **deposition** is a process in which one party questions another under oath, while a court reporter records every word. The plaintiff, the defendant, and expert witnesses for both sides may give depositions. Expert witnesses are persons who are asked to review medical records and give their opinion of whether or not the standard of care

was met. A person who lies under oath while giving a deposition can be charged with perjury.

- **Phase three** is the trial phase, the process designed to settle a dispute before a judge and jury. Both sides present their versions of the facts and the jury determines which version appears to be correct. If the jury decides in the plaintiff's favor, damages may be awarded. At this point the lawsuit may proceed to phase four.
- **Phase four** begins with an appeal of the jury decision. Although either side has the right to an appeal, the losing party is usually the one to choose this option.

The phlebotomist concerned with continuous quality improvement and safe practice reduces his or her exposure to malpractice litigation. With the rapid evolution of medicine and, more specifically, laboratory testing, safe practice includes the responsibility of the phlebotomist to stay abreast of all changes to ensure the safe collection of quality specimens. This in turn directly affects the quality of clinical laboratory services.

Legal Cases Involving Phlebotomy Procedures

The following are examples of actual legal cases involving phlebotomy procedures. They serve as a reminder that phlebotomy is not an innocuous procedure, and failure to exercise due care can result in injury to the patient and legal consequences.

CASE 1: A NEGLIGENCE CASE SETTLED THROUGH BINDING ARBITRATION

A patient had a blood specimen collected at a physician's office. Blood had been collected from him at the same office on several prior occasions with no problem. The blood drawer, who was new to the patient and seemed to be in a hurry, inserted the needle deeper into the arm and at a much steeper angle than the patient was used to. She redirected the needle several times before hitting the vein. A hematoma began to form. Meanwhile the patient told the blood drawer that he felt great pain, but she told him it would be over soon and continued the draw. The pain continued after the draw and the patient's arm later became bruised and swollen. The patient suffered permanent nerve injury from compression of the nerve by the hematoma. Plaintiff was awarded: amount unknown.

CASE 2: A NEGLIGENCE CASE SETTLED THROUGH BINDING ARBITRATION

A phlebotomist was sent to a woman's home to draw blood for insurance purposes. After missing twice, she made a third attempt that was also unsuccessful. The phlebotomist commented that she thought "she hit a muscle." The client complained of pain and suffered immediate swelling and bruising in the form of a hematoma. For up to a year after the failed venipuncture attempts, the client had restricted use of her right arm and hand due to tingling and shocking sensations. It was determined that the plaintiff suffered an injury that resulted in permanent damage because the phlebotomist was not sufficiently trained and failed to adhere to the Standard of Care. The Plaintiff was awarded one million dollars.

CASE 3: A NEGLIGENCE CASE SETTLED THROUGH BINDING ARBITRATION

A college student who had been studying for final exams and had not eaten or slept well for 2 days went to an outpatient lab to have blood drawn. The phlebotomist failed to observe the student's anxiety and complexion pallor and did not listen to her concerns. Following the blood collection, he did not ask her how she was feeling nor if she would like to lie down. As she walked alone from the blood collection area, she experienced syncope and fell face down against a stone threshold at the doorway to the outside. She suffered multiple facial fractures, permanent scarring to her face, and lost three front teeth. She was hospitalized for 2 weeks and missed her college exams. It was noted from others who were deposed that there was no bed provided for patients to use when feeling faint and there was no room set aside for emergency situations. The supervisor was not available on site at the time of the accident. The first aid administered to the student before the ambulance arrived was incorrect and resulted in additional harm to the injuries. At arbitration, the student was awarded one and a half million dollars.

CASE 4: CONGELTON VERSUS BATON ROUGE GENERAL HOSPITAL

The plaintiff went to donate blood at a hospital. She complained of pain during the procedure and the technician repositioned the needle twice. The technician offered to remove the needle but the plaintiff chose to complete the procedure. After completing the donation she complained of numbness in her arm. Later evaluation by a neurologist indicated injury to the antebrachial cutaneous nerve. Plaintiff was awarded: amount unknown.

CASE 5: JURY VERDICT AFFIRMED ON APPEAL BY KENTUCKY SUPREME COURT

The plaintiff went to the hospital to have her blood drawn. The phlebotomist placed a tourniquet on the plaintiff's arm and then left the room to answer a phone call. When she returned approximately 10 minutes later, the plaintiff's arm was swollen and had changed color. The plaintiff experienced medical complications and sought treatment. After medical consultation, three physicians concluded that the plaintiff was experiencing nerve problems with her right arm that were related to the tourniquet incident. Plaintiff was awarded $100,000.

STUDY & REVIEW QUESTIONS

1. _____ is the largest healthcare standards-setting body in the world.
   - a. CAP
   - b. CLSI
   - c. JCAHO
   - d. NAACLS

2. The CLIA federal regulations are administered by
   - a. CAP
   - b. CLSI
   - c. CMS
   - d. COW

3. _____ are set up to monitor all aspects of laboratory work.
   - a. GLPs
   - b. Quality indicators
   - c. Sentinel events
   - d. Thresholds

4. A QA program monitors
   - a. Indicators
   - b. Outcomes
   - c. Procedures
   - d. Threshold values

5. What book describes the necessary steps to follow in patient preparation?
   - a. Collection manual
   - b. Infection control manual
   - c. Procedure manual
   - d. Safety manual

6. Necessary elements of risk management are all of the following *except*
   - a. Education
   - b. Evaluation
   - c. Identification
   - d. Obligation

7. Informed consent means that a
   - a. Nurse has the right to perform a procedure on a patient even if the patient refuses
   - b. Patient agrees to a procedure after being told of the consequences associated with it
   - c. Patient has the right to look at all his or her medical records
   - d. Phlebotomist tells the patient what is ordered and the implications of the test results

8. A national organization that develops guidelines and sets standards for laboratory procedures
   - a. CAP
   - b. CLSI
   - c. JCAHO
   - d. NAACLS

9. **The physician employer of a phlebotomist who injures a patient during a blood draw is sued for negligence. This is an example of**

   a. Assault and battery
   b. Fraud
   c. Respondeat superior
   d. Vicarious liability

10. **A young adult comes to an outpatient lab to have his blood drawn. What should the phlebotomist know before drawing this patient's blood?**

    a. Age of majority in the state
    b. Date of birth of the patient
    c. Name of the patient
    d. All of the above

11. **Phlebotomists are involved in the Joint Commission's performance measurements in the area of myocardial infarction in what way?**

    a. Collecting specimens for blood cultures at specified times
    b. Collecting specimens for timed tests for cardiac enzymes
    c. Processing specimens for pneumonia testing
    d. Reporting pregnancy testing results

12. **A delta check refers to**

    a. Checking the wristband with the requisition
    b. Comparing current test results with previous one
    c. Documenting all of the QC controls
    d. Infection control precautions

13. **Which one of the following is used as a monitor or quality indicator for the process of "test requesting"?**

    a. Accuracy of ordering
    b. Safety
    c. Transit time
    d. Wristband evaluation

14. **Failure to exercise "due care" is**

    a. Assault
    b. Battery
    c. Invasion of privacy
    d. Negligence

15. **The statute of limitations timing can begin on any of the following *except***

    a. On the day the negligent act took place
    b. The day of last medical treatment
    c. The first day of counseling with a lawyer
    d. When the injury was discovered

CASE · STUDY · 2-1

Scope of Duty

A newly trained phlebotomist is sent to collect a blood specimen from a patient. The phlebotomist is an employee of a laboratory that contracts with the hospital to perform laboratory services, including specimen collection. The phlebotomist collects the specimen with no problems. Before the phlebotomist has a chance to leave the room, the patient asks for help to walk to the bathroom. The patient is a very large woman, but the phlebotomist lends an arm to help her. On the way to the bathroom, the patient slips on some liquid on the floor. The phlebotomist tries but is unable to prevent her from falling. The patient fractures her arm in the fall.

QUESTIONS

1. Was it wrong of the phlebotomist to try to help the patient? Explain why or why not.
2. Is the hospital liable for the patient' injury? Explain why or why not.
3. Can the phlebotomist be held liable for the patient's injuries? Explain why or why not.

Bibliography and Suggested Readings

American Hospital Association (AHA) http://www.aha.org/aha/resource_center/resource/resource_ethics.html

Clinical Laboratory Improvement Amendments (CLIA): http://www.cms.hhs.gov/clia/

CLSI/NCCLS document H11-A4, Procedures for the Collection of Arterial Blood Specimens; Approved Standard. Wayne, PA.

Fremgen, B. F. (2005). Medical law and ethics. Upper Saddle River, NJ: Prentice Hall.

Johns, M. L. (2006). Health information management technology- an applied approach (2nd ed.). Chicago: American Health Information Management Association.

Joint Commission on the Accreditation of Healthcare Organizations (JCAHO): http://www.joint-commission.org/

Kentucky Supreme Court, case # 2003-SC-471-DG, Baptist Healthcare Systems, Inc. D/B/A Central Baptist Hospital versus Golda H. Miller et al., opinion rendered August 25, 2005.

Mitchell, J., & Haroun, L. (2002). Introduction to health care. Albany, NY: Delmar Publishers.

Phillips, L. D. (2005). Manual of I.V. therapeutics (4th ed.). Philadelphia: F. A. Davis.

Veatch, R., & Flack, H. (1997). Case studies in allied health ethics. Upper Saddle River, NJ, Prentice Hall.

Williams, S. J. (2005). Essentials of health services. New York: Delmar Publishers.

INFECTION CONTROL, SAFETY, FIRST AID, AND PERSONAL WELLNESS

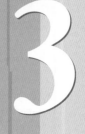

key•terms

BBP	HIV	pathogens
Biohazard	immune	percutaneous
CDC	infectious/causative agent	permucosal
chain of infection	isolation procedures	PPE
engineering controls	microbe	reservoir
EPA	MSDS	reverse isolation
fire tetrahedron	neutropenic	standard precautions
fomites	NIOSH	susceptible host
HazCom	nosocomial infection	transmission-based precautions
HBV	OSHA	vector transmission
HCV	parenteral	vehicle transmission
HICPAC	pathogenic	work practice controls

objectives

Upon successful completion of this chapter, the reader should be able to:

1. Define the key terms and abbreviations listed at the beginning of this chapter.
2. Identify the components of the chain of infection and give examples of each, describe infection control procedures used to break the chain, and identify four functions of infection control programs.
3. Describe proper procedures for hand hygiene, putting on and removing protective clothing, and entering the nursery or neonatal ICU.
4. Describe standard and transmission-based precautions and identify the organizations that developed them.
5. State safety rules to follow when working in the laboratory and in patient areas.
6. List examples of bloodborne pathogens and describe their means of transmission in a healthcare setting.

7. Discuss the major points of the bloodborne pathogens (BBP) standard, including changes required by the Needlestick Safety and Prevention Act, and identify key elements of a BBP exposure control plan.

8. Describe hazards, identify warning symbols, list actions to take if incidents occur, and specify rules to follow for proper biologic, electrical, fire, radiation, and chemical safety.

9. Identify symptoms of shock, state first aid procedures for treating external hemorrhage and shock, identify the main points of the International CPR and ECC guidelines, and identify the links in the American Heart Association chain of survival.

10. Describe the role of personal hygiene, proper nutrition, rest, exercise, back protection, and stress management in personal wellness.

INFECTION CONTROL

Although important advances have been made in understanding and treating infection, the threat of infection looms as large as it ever has. New enemies in the battle against infection emerge such as **human immunodeficiency virus** (HIV) and **hepatitis C virus** (HCV). Once conquered enemies become resistant to treatment, as in the case of *Mycobacterium tuberculosis* and methicillin-resistant *Staphylococcus aureus*. Blood collection personnel typically encounter numerous patients on a daily basis, many of whom may be harboring various infectious microorganisms. Measures to prevent the spread of infection must be taken in the course of all patient encounters. This portion of the chapter explains the infection process and describes infection control measures needed to protect blood collection personnel, patients, staff, visitors, and those doing business within healthcare facilities. Infection control involves implementing procedures and policies that prevent infection and starts with an understanding of the process of infection.

Infection

Infection is a condition that results when a microorganism (**microbe** for short) is able to invade the body, multiply, and cause injurious effects or disease. Microbes include bacteria, fungi, protozoa, and viruses. Most microbes are nonpathogenic, meaning they do not cause disease under normal conditions. Microbes that are **pathogenic** (capable of causing disease) are called **pathogens**. Infection can be local (restricted to a small area of the body) or systemic (sis-tem'ik), in which the entire body is affected.

COMMUNICABLE INFECTIONS

Some pathogenic microbes cause infections that are **communicable** (able to spread from person to person), and the diseases that result are called communicable diseases. A division of the U.S. Public Health Service called the **Centers for Disease Control and Prevention** (CDC) is charged with the investigation and control of various diseases, especially those that are communicable and have epidemic potential. The CDC develops guidelines and recommends safety precautions to protect healthcare workers and others from infection.

NOSOCOMIAL INFECTIONS

Approximately 5% of patients in the United States are exposed to and contract some sort of infection after admission to a hospital or other healthcare facility. Healthcare facility-acquired infections are called **nosocomial infections** and can result from contact with infected personnel, other patients, visitors, and contaminated equipment. The **Healthcare Infection Control Practices Advisory Committee (HICPAC)** advises the CDC on updating guidelines regarding prevention of nosocomial infections in hospitals and other healthcare facilities.

fyi Urinary tract infection (UTI) is the most common nosocomial infection in the United States.

The Chain of Infection

Infection transmission requires the presence of a number of components, which make up what is referred to as the **chain of infection** (Fig. 3-1). Six key components, or "links" in the chain are an **infectious agent, reservoir, exit pathway, means of transmission, entry pathway,** and **susceptible host.** The chain must be complete for an infection to occur. If the process of infection is stopped at any component or link in the chain, an infection is prevented. If a pathogen successfully enters a susceptible host, the chain is completed, the host becomes a new source of infectious microorganisms, and the process of infection continues.

key • point A phlebotomist, whose duties involve contact with many patients, must be fully aware of the infection process and take precautions to prevent the spread of infection.

INFECTIOUS AGENT

The infectious agent, also called the **causative agent**, is the pathogenic microbe responsible for causing an infection.

RESERVOIR

The source of an infectious agent is called a reservoir. It is a place where the microbe can survive and grow or multiply. Reservoirs include humans, animals, food, water, soil, and contaminated articles and equipment. An individual or animal infected with a pathogenic microbe is called a reservoir host. Human reservoir hosts can be patients, personnel, or visitors and include those with an active disease, those incubating a disease, and chronic carriers of a disease. Another reservoir for potentially infectious microbes is a person's own normal flora (microorganisms that normally live on the skin and other areas of the human body).

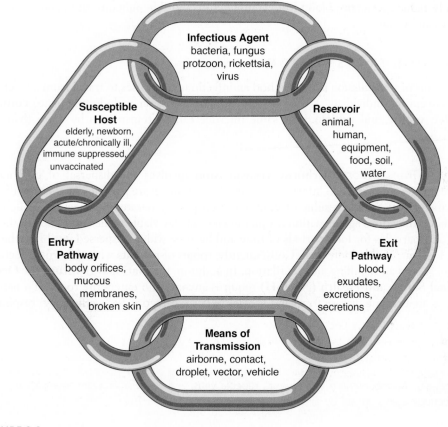

FIGURE 3-1

The chain of infection.

Contaminated articles and equipment can be a major source of infectious agents. The ability of these inanimate objects to transmit infectious agents depends upon the amount of contamination, the **viability** or ability of the microbe to survive on the object, the **virulence** or degree to which the microbe is capable of causing disease, and the amount of time that has passed since the item was contaminated. For example, HBV, the virus that causes hepatitis B, is much more virulent than human immunodeficiency virus (HIV), the virus that causes AIDS, because a smaller amount of infective material is capable of causing disease. It is also more viable because it is capable of surviving longer on surfaces than HIV. However, if enough time elapses from the time of contamination until contact by a susceptible host, it is no longer alive and therefore unable to transmit disease.

EXIT PATHWAY

An exit pathway is a way an infectious agent is able to leave a reservoir host. Infectious agents can exit a reservoir host in secretions from the eyes, nose, or mouth; exudates from wounds; tissue specimens; blood from venipuncture and skin puncture sites; and excretions of feces and urine.

MEANS OF TRANSMISSION

The means of transmission is the method an infectious agent uses to travel from a reservoir to a susceptible individual. Means of infection transmission include **airborne**, **contact**, **droplet**, **vector**, and **vehicle**. The same microbe can be transmitted by more than one route.

Airborne Transmission   **Airborne transmission** involves the dispersal of evaporated droplet nuclei containing an infectious agent. Droplet nuclei are particles smaller than 5 μm in diameter that are the residue of evaporated droplets generated by sneezing, coughing, or talking. Infectious agents within droplet nuclei can stay viable while suspended in the air or in dust particles for long periods of time and become widely dispersed until later be inhaled by a susceptible individual. Consequently, rooms of patients with airborne infections require special air handling and ventilation. In addition, the **National Institute for Occupational Safety and Health (NIOSH)** requires anyone who enters the room of a patient who has an airborne disease to wear a special N95 (N category, 95% efficiency) respirator (Fig 3-2).

fyi   *Mycobacterium tuberculosis*, rubeola virus, and varicella virus are examples of infectious agents spread by airborne transmission.

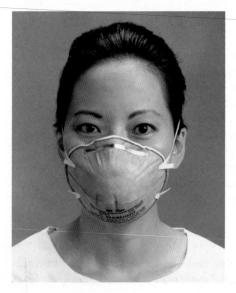

FIGURE 3-2

N95 respirator.   (Courtesy 3M Occupational Health and Environmental Safety Division. St. Paul, MN.)

Contact Transmission   **Contact transmission** is the most frequent means of infection transmission. There are two types of contact transmission, direct and indirect. **Direct contact transmission** is the physical transfer of an infectious agent to a susceptible host through close or intimate contact such as touching or kissing. **Indirect contact transmission** can occur when a susceptible host touches contaminated objects such as patient bed linens, clothing, dressings, and eating utensils. It includes contact with phlebotomy equipment such as gloves, needles, specimen tubes, testing equipment, and trays. It also includes less obvious contaminated objects such as countertops, computer keyboards, phones, pens, pencils, doorknobs, and faucet handles. The transfer of infectious agents from contaminated hands to a susceptible host is also considered indirect contact transmission.

fyi   Inanimate objects that can harbor material containing infectious agents are called **fomites** (fo'mi-tez).

Droplet Transmission   **Droplet transmission** is the transfer of an infectious agent to the mucous membranes of the mouth, nose, or conjunctiva of the eyes of a susceptible individual via infectious droplets (particles 5 μm in diameter or larger) generated by coughing, sneezing, or talking or through procedures such as suctioning or throat swab collection.

key • point   Droplet transmission differs from airborne transmission in that droplets do not travel more than 3 feet and do not remain suspended in the air.

Vector Transmission   **Vector transmission** is the transfer of an infectious agent carried by an insect, arthropod, or animal. Examples of vector transmission include the transmission of West Nile virus by mosquitoes and bubonic plague *(Yersinia pestis)* by rodent fleas.

Vehicle Transmission   **Vehicle transmission** is the transmission of an infectious agent through contaminated food, water, or drugs. Examples of vehicle transmission are salmonella infection from handling contaminated chicken and shigella infection from drinking contaminated water.

key • point   The transmission of hepatitis and HIV through blood transfusion is also considered vehicle transmission.

ENTRY PATHWAY

The entry pathway is the way an infectious agent is able to enter a susceptible host. Entry pathways include body orifices, mucous membranes of the eyes, nose. or mouth, and breaks in the skin. Entry pathways of patients can be exposed during invasive procedures such as catheterization, venipuncture, fingersticks, and heel puncture. Entry pathways of healthcare personnel can be exposed during spills and splashes of infectious specimens or created by needlesticks and injuries from other sharp objects.

SUSCEPTIBLE HOST

A **susceptible host** is someone with decreased ability to resist infection. Factors that affect susceptibility include age, health, and immune status. For example, newborns are more susceptible to infection because their immune systems are still forming, and the elderly are more susceptible because the immune system weakens with age. Disease, antibiotic treatment, immunosuppressive drugs, and procedures such as surgery, anesthesia, and insertion of catheters can all leave a patient more susceptible to infection. A healthy person who has received a vaccination against, or recovered from infection with, a particular virus has developed antibodies against that virus and is considered to be **immune**, or unlikely to develop the disease.

> **key • point** Individuals who are exposed to the hepatitis B virus (HBV) are less likely to contract the disease if they have previously completed an HBV vaccination series.

Breaking the Chain of Infection

Breaking the chain of infection involves stopping infections at the source, preventing contact with substances from exit pathways, eliminating means of transmission, blocking exposure to entry pathways, and reducing or eliminating the susceptibility of potential hosts. Examples of ways to break the chain and prevent infections are shown in Box 3-1.

BOX • 3-1 Examples of Ways to Break the Chain of Infection

- Effective hand hygiene procedures
- Good nutrition, adequate rest, and reduction of stress
- Immunization against common pathogens
- Insect and rodent control
- Isolation procedures
- Proper decontamination of surfaces and instruments
- Proper disposal of sharps and infectious waste
- Use of gloves, gowns, masks, respirators, and other personal protective equipment (PPE) when indicated
- Use of needle safety devices during blood collection

Infection Control Programs

The **Joint Commission** requires every healthcare institution to have an infection control program responsible for protecting patients, employees, visitors, and anyone doing business within healthcare institutions from infection. A typical infection control program implements procedures aimed at breaking the chain of infection, monitors and collects data on all infections occurring within the institution, and institutes special precautions in the event of outbreaks of specific infections.

EMPLOYEE SCREENING AND IMMUNIZATION

An important way infection control programs prevent infection is through employee screening and immunization programs. Screening for infectious diseases typically takes place prior to or upon employment and on a regular basis throughout employment. Screening commonly includes tuberculosis (TB) testing, also called PPD (purified protein derivative) testing. Employees with positive TB test results receive chest x-ray evaluations to determine their status. Screening may also include RPR (rapid plasma reagin) testing for syphilis and screening for diarrhea and skin diseases. Employees with certain conditions or infections may be subject to work restrictions. (Conditions requiring work restrictions are listed in Appendix F). Immunizations typically required include current hepatitis B virus (HBV), MMR (measles, mumps, rubella), diphtheria, and tetanus vaccinations or proof of immunity. Most employers provide vaccinations free of charge.

key • point OSHA regulations require employers to offer HBV vaccine free of charge to employees whose duties involve risk of exposure.

EVALUATION AND TREATMENT

An infection control program also provides for evaluation and treatment of employees who are exposed to infections on the job. This includes OSHA-mandated confidential medical evaluation, treatment, counseling, and follow-up as a result of bloodborne pathogen exposure.

SURVEILLANCE

Another major function of an infection control program is surveillance or monitoring. This involves monitoring patients and employees at risk of acquiring infections, as well as collecting and evaluating data on infections contracted by patients and employees. Infection control measures are updated, and new policies are instituted based on this information.

fyi The CDC developed the National Surveillance System for Healthcare Workers (NASH) to collaborate with healthcare facilities in the collection of information important in preventing occupational exposure and infection among healthcare workers.

Infection Control Methods

HAND HYGIENE

Hand hygiene is one of the most important means of preventing the spread of infection provided it is achieved properly and when required. Hand hygiene measures include the frequent use of antiseptic hand cleaners or hand washing, depending upon the degree of contamination. It is important that all healthcare personnel learn proper hand hygiene procedures and recognize situations when they should be performed. Box 3-2 lists situations that require hand hygiene procedures.

key • point   As part of the CDC Guidelines for Hand Hygiene in Health Care Settings it is recommended that artificial fingernails or extenders not be worn when having direct contact with high-risk patients, such as infants or those in ICU. Suggested length for natural nails should be less than $1/4$ inch long.

Use of Alcohol-Based Antiseptic Hand Cleaners   Recent CDC and HICPAC recommendations allow the use of alcohol-based antiseptic hand cleaners in place of hand washing as long as the hands are not visibly soiled with dirt or other organic material such as blood and other body substances. It is important to use enough cleaner (available in foams, gels, and rubs) to cover all surfaces and to allow the alcohol to evaporate to achieve proper antisepsis. If hands are heavily contaminated with organic material and hand- washing facilities are not available, it is recommended that hands be cleaned with detergent-containing wipes followed by the use of an alcohol-based antiseptic hand cleaner.

BOX • 3-2   Situations That Require Hand Hygiene Procedures

- Before and after each patient contact
- Between unrelated procedures such as wound care and drawing blood
- Before putting on gloves and after taking them off
- Before leaving the laboratory
- Before going to lunch or on break
- Before and after going to the restroom
- Whenever hands become visibly or knowingly contaminated

Hand Washing   There are different methods of hand washing, depending on the degree of contamination and the level of antimicrobial activity required. A routine hand-washing procedure uses plain soap and water to mechanically remove soil and transient bacteria. Hand antisepsis requires the use of an antimicrobial soap to remove, kill, or inhibit transient microorganisms. A 2-minute surgical hand scrub uses an antimicrobial soap or equivalent to remove or destroy transient microorganisms and reduce levels of normal flora prior to surgical procedures. Proper routine hand-washing procedure is described in Procedure 3-1.

PERSONAL PROTECTIVE EQUIPMENT

Protective clothing and other protective items worn by an individual are called **personal protective equipment (PPE)**. PPE provides a barrier against infection. Used properly, it protects those wearing it. Disposed of properly, it prevents spread of infection to others. PPE includes the following.

Gloves   Clean, nonsterile gloves are worn when collecting or handling blood and other body fluids, handling contaminated items, and touching nonintact skin or mucous membranes. Gloves should be pulled over the cuffs of gowns or lab coats to provide adequate protection. Three main reasons for wearing gloves are

- To prevent contamination of the hands when handling blood or body fluids or when touching mucous membranes or nonintact skin
- To reduce the chance of transmitting organisms on the hands of personnel to patients during invasive or other procedures that involve touching a patient's skin or mucous membranes
- To minimize the possibility of transmitting infectious microorganisms from one patient to another

key • point   Wearing gloves during phlebotomy procedures is mandated by the OSHA bloodborne pathogens standard.

Proper Glove Removal

After use, gloves should be removed promptly in an aseptic manner and discarded. To remove gloves properly (Fig. 3-3), grasp one glove at the wrist and pull it inside out and off the hand, ending up with it in the palm of the still-gloved hand. Slip fingers of the ungloved hand under the second glove at the wrist and pull it off the hand, ending with one glove inside the other with the contaminated surfaces inside. Hands should be sanitized immediately after glove removal and before going to another patient.

Gowns   Clean, nonsterile, fluid-resistant gowns are worn by healthcare personnel to protect their skin and prevent soiling of their clothing during patient-care activities in

Hand-Washing Technique

Purpose: Decontaminate hands to prevent the spread of infection

Equipment: Liquid soap, disposable towels, trash can

Step	Explanation/Rationale
1. Stand back so that you do not touch the sink	The sink may be contaminated
2. Turn on the faucet and wet hands under warm running water	Water should not be too hot or too cold and hands should be wet before applying soap to minimize drying, chapping, or cracking of hands from frequent hand washing

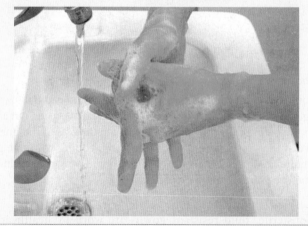

3. Apply soap and work up a lather	A good lather is needed to reach all surfaces
4. Scrub all surfaces, including between the fingers and around the knuckles	Scrubbing is necessary to dislodge micro-organisms from surfaces, especially between fingers and around knuckles

(Continued)

Step	Explanation/Rationale
5. Rub your hands together vigorously	Friction helps loosen dead skin, dirt, debris, and microorganisms. (Steps 4–5 should take at least 15 seconds, about the time it takes to sing the ABCs)
6. Rinse your hands in a downward motion from wrists to fingertips	Rinsing with the hands downward allows contaminants to be flushed from the hands and fingers into the sink rather than flowing back up the arm or wrist

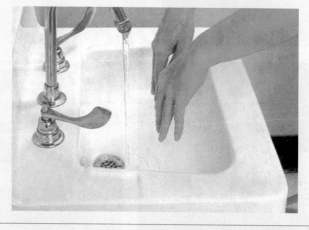

7. Dry hands with a clean paper towel	Hands must be dried thoroughly and gently to prevent chapping or cracking. Reusable towels can be a source of contamination

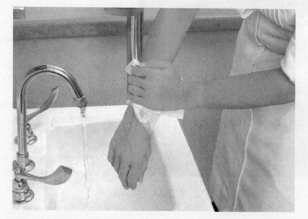

8. Use a clean paper towel to turn off the faucet unless it is foot or motion activated	Clean hands should not touch contaminated faucet handles

Images from Molle EA, Kronenberger J, West-Stack C. *Lippincott Williams & Wilkins' Clinical Medical Assisting*, 2nd edition. Baltimore: Lippincott Williams & Wilkins, 2005.

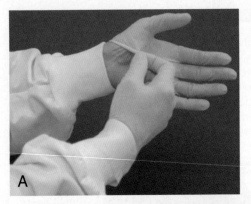
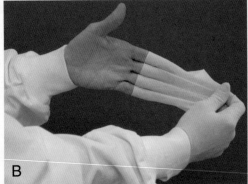
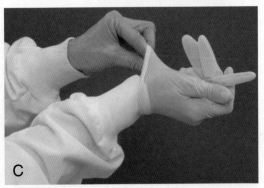
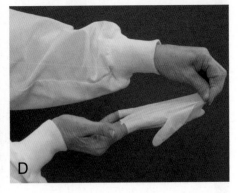
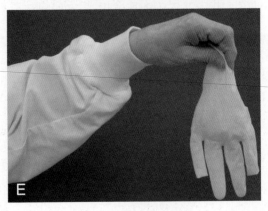

FIGURE 3-3

Glove removal. **A.** The wrist of one glove is grasped with the opposite gloved hand. **B.** The glove is pulled inside out, over, and off the hand. **C.** With the first glove held in the gloved hand, the fingers of the nongloved hand are slipped under the wrist of the remaining glove without touching the exterior surfaces. **D.** The glove is then pulled inside out over the hand so that the first glove ends up inside the second glove, with no exterior glove surfaces exposed. **E.** Contaminated gloves ready to be dropped into the proper waste receptacle.

which splashes or sprays of blood or body fluids are possible or when entering isolation rooms (See Isolation Procedures). Sterile gowns are also worn to protect certain patients (such as newborns and patients with compromised immune systems) from contaminants on the healthcare worker's clothing. Most gowns are made of disposable cloth or paper, are generous in size to adequately cover clothing, have long sleeves with knit cuffs, and fasten in the back.

Putting On and Removing Gowns

When putting on a gown, only inside surfaces of the gown should be touched. A properly worn gown has the sleeves pulled all the way to the wrist, the belt tied, and the gown overlapped, completely closed, and securely fastened. A gown is removed from the inside by sliding the arms out of the sleeves. The gown is then held away from the body and folded with the contaminated outside surface ending up inside.

Lab Coats   Lab coats, like gowns, are worn to protect skin and prevent soiling of healthcare workers' clothing during patient-care activities in which splashes or sprays of blood or body fluids are possible. They are required attire for most phlebotomy situations. Lab coats used for specimen collection and handling are generally made of fluid-resistant cotton or synthetic material, have long sleeves with knit cuffs, and come in both reusable and disposable styles.

Masks, Face Shields, and Goggles   A mask is worn to protect against droplets generated by coughing or sneezing. To put on a mask, place it over the nose and mouth. Adjust the metal band (if applicable) to fit snugly over the nose. For masks with ties, fasten the top ties around the upper portion of the head; then tie the lower ones at the back of the neck. If the mask has elastic fasteners, slip them around the ears. A face shield or a mask and goggles are worn to protect the eyes, nose, and mouth from splashes or sprays of body fluids. If an activity requires goggles, it also requires a mask. Some masks have plastic eye shields attached.

Respirators   NIOSH approved N95 respirators are required when entering rooms of patients with pulmonary tuberculosis and other diseases with airborne transmission. Respirators must fit snugly with no air leaks (see Airborne Transmission).

PUTTING ON AND REMOVING PROTECTIVE CLOTHING

When putting on complete protective clothing such as gown, mask, and gloves, the gown is put on first (Fig. 3-4A). The mask is put on next, making certain it covers the nose and mouth (Fig 3-4B). Gloves are put on last and pulled over the cuffs of the gown (Fig. 3-4C).

Protective clothing must be removed carefully in an aseptic manner to prevent contamination of the healthcare worker. When used during phlebotomy procedures it is typically removed in the opposite order from which it was put on. Gloves are removed first, being careful not to touch contaminated surfaces with ungloved hands. The mask is removed next, touching only the strings. The gown is removed last. Hands must be washed or decontaminated using an alcohol- based antiseptic promptly after removal of protective clothing.

NURSERY AND NEONATAL ICU INFECTION CONTROL TECHNIQUE

Newborns are more susceptible to infections than healthy older children and adults because their immune systems are not yet fully developed. Consequently, anyone who enters the nursery or other neonatal unit should use special infection control techniques. Most neonatal units have a separate anteroom where hand washing, gowning, and so forth are performed

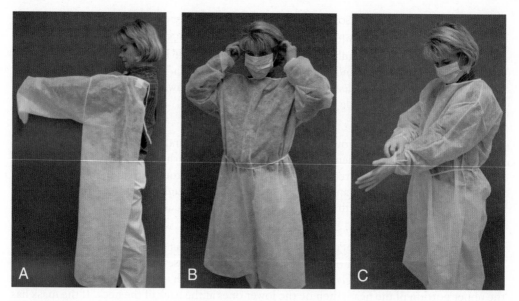

FIGURE 3-4

Protective clothing. **A.** Phlebotomist slips arms into a protective gown. **B.** A mask is applied by slipping the elastic band over the ears. **C.** Gloves are put on last and pulled over the gown cuffs.

before entering. Typical nursery and neonatal ICU infection control technique includes the following:

- Put on clean gloves, gown, and mask
- Gather only those items necessary to perform the specimen collection
- Leave the blood collection tray in the washroom outside the nursery
- Remove gloves, decontaminate hands, and put on new gloves between each patient

Isolation Procedures

One way an infection control program minimizes the spread of infection is through the establishment of **isolation procedures**. Isolation procedures separate patients with certain transmissible infections from contact with other patients and limit their contact with hospital personnel and visitors. Isolating a patient requires a doctor's order and is implemented either to prevent the spread of infection from a patient who has or is suspected of having a contagious disease or to protect a patient whose immune system is compromised. Patients are most commonly isolated in a private room. A card or sign indicating the type of isolation along with a description of required precautions is generally posted on the patient's door. A cart containing supplies needed to enter the room or care for the patient is typically placed in the hall outside the door.

PROTECTIVE/REVERSE ISOLATION

Protective or **reverse isolation** is used for patients who are highly susceptible to infections. In this type of isolation, protective measures are taken to keep healthcare workers and others from transmitting infection to the patient rather than vice versa. Patients who may require protective isolation include those with suppressed or compromised immune function such as burn patients, organ transplant patients, AIDS patients, and neutropenic (having a low neutrophil count) chemotherapy patients.

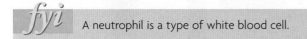

fyi   A neutrophil is a type of white blood cell.

TRADITIONAL ISOLATION SYSTEMS

At one time the CDC recommended either of two types of isolation systems: the category-specific system and the disease-specific system. The category-specific system had seven different isolation categories covering many diseases and often resulted in overisolation of patients and needless extra costs. The disease-specific system was based on the modes of transmission of common diseases. A chart listed the diseases and identified specific isolation precautions recommended for each. A diagnosis or suspicion of the presence of a transmissible disease was needed to institute either system.

UNIVERSAL PRECAUTIONS

Isolation practices were altered dramatically in 1985, when the CDC introduced a strategy called **universal precautions** (UP) after reports of healthcare workers being infected with HIV through needlesticks and other exposures to HIV-contaminated blood. UP replaced blood/body fluid precautions and were followed for all isolation categories. Under UP, the blood and certain body fluids of *all* individuals were considered potentially infectious. The introduction of UP changed the focus of infection control from prevention of patient-to-patient infection transmission, to prevention of patient-to-personnel transmission, and was a required part of an overall infection control plan.

BODY SUBSTANCE ISOLATION

Because infection transmission can occur before a diagnosis is made or even suspected, another system called **body substance isolation** (BSI) (Fig 3-5) gained acceptance. BSI incorporated elements of disease-specific and category-specific precautions and was followed for *every* patient without need for a diagnosis or suspicion of a transmissible disease. BSI went beyond universal precautions by requiring that gloves be worn when contacting *any* moist body substance.

REVISED GUIDELINE FOR ISOLATION PRECAUTIONS IN HOSPITALS

Widespread variation in the use of UP or BSI, confusion over which body fluids required precautions, lack of agreement on the importance of hand washing after glove use, and the need for additional precautions to prevent transmission of infectious agents in addition to bloodborne pathogens led to a new guideline issued jointly by the CDC and HICPAC.

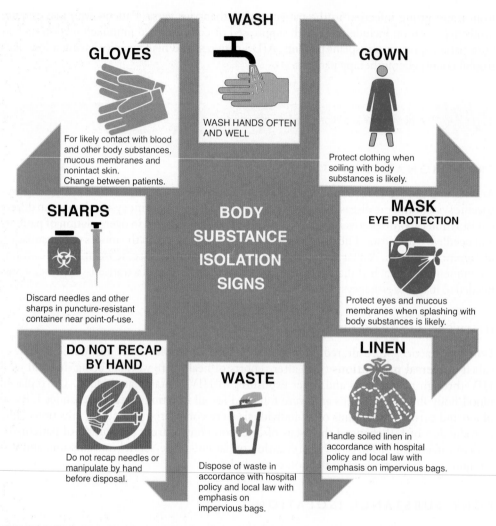

FIGURE 3-5

Body substance isolation sign. (Adapted from Briggs Corp., Des Moines, IA.)

This guideline, which is still in effect and supersedes previous CDC isolation recommendations, contains two tiers of precautions. The first tier, **standard precautions**, specifies precautions to use in caring for all patients regardless of diagnosis or presumed infection status. The second tier, **transmission-based precautions**, specifies precautions to use for patients either suspected, or known, to be infected with certain pathogens transmitted by airborne, droplet, or contact routes. The guideline also lists specific clinical conditions that are highly suspicious for infection and specifies appropriate transmission-based precautions to use for each, in addition to standard precautions, until a diagnosis can be made.

Standard Precautions   Standard precautions (Fig. 3-6) are to be used in the care of all patients and are meant to be the number-one strategy for successful nosocomial infection

STANDARD PRECAUTIONS

FOR INFECTION CONTROL

Handwashing
Wash after touching **body fluids**, after **removing gloves**, and between **patient contacts**.

Gloves
Wear **Gloves** before touching **body fluids**, **mucous membranes**, and **nonintact skin**.

Mask & Eye Protection or Face Shield
Protect eyes, nose, mouth during procedures that cause **splashes** or **sprays** of **body fluids**.

Gown
Wear **Gown** during procedures that may cause **splashes** or **sprays** of **body fluids**.

Patient-Care Equipment
Handle soiled equipment so as to prevent personal contamination and transfer to other patients.

Environmental Control
Follow hospital procedures for cleaning beds, equipment, and frequently touched surfaces.

Linen
Handle linen soiled with **body fluids** so as to prevent personal contamination and transfer to other patients.

Occupational Health & Bloodborne Pathogens
Prevent injuries from needles, scalpels, and other sharp devices.
Never recap needles using both hands.
Place sharps in puncture-proof sharps containers.
Use **Resuscitation Devices** as an alternative to mouth-to-mouth resuscitation.

Patient Placement
Use a Private Room for a patient who contaminates the environment.

"Body Fluids" include **blood**, **secretions**, and **excretions**.

Form No. **SPR-C**   BREVIS CORP., 3310 S 2700 E, SLC, UT 84109   © 1996 Brevis Corp.

Condensed Version

FIGURE 3-6

Standard precautions sign.   (Courtesy Brevis Corp., Salt Lake City, UT.)

control. They combine the major features of UP and BSI to minimize the risk of infection transmission from both recognized and unrecognized sources. Standard precautions apply to blood, *all* body fluids (including all secretions and excretions except sweat, whether or not they contain visible blood), nonintact skin, and mucous membranes.

Transmission-Based Precautions   Transmission-based precautions are to be used for patients known or suspected to be infected or colonized with highly transmissible or epidemiologically (related to the study of epidemics) significant pathogens that require special precautions in addition to standard precautions. Table 3-1 lists clinical conditions that warrant transmission-based precautions pending diagnosis. Common diseases and conditions that require transmission-based precautions are listed in Table 3-2. Precautions may be combined for diseases that have more than one means of transmission. There are three types of transmission-based precautions:

- **Airborne precautions** (Fig. 3-7) or the equivalent, which must be used in addition to standard precautions for patients known or suspected to be infected with microorganisms transmitted by airborne droplet nuclei (particles smaller than 5 μm)
- **Droplet precautions** (Fig. 3-8) or the equivalent, which must be used in addition to standard precautions for patients known or suspected to be infected with microorganisms transmitted by droplets (particles larger than 5 μm), generated when a patient talks, coughs, or sneezes and during certain procedures such as suctioning
- **Contact precautions** (Fig. 3-9) or the equivalent, which must be used in addition to standard precautions when a patient is known or suspected to be infected or colonized with epidemiologically important microorganisms that can be transmitted by direct contact with the patient or indirect contact with surfaces or patient-care items

SAFETY

Providing quality care in an environment that is safe for employees as well as patients is a concern that is foremost in the minds of healthcare providers. Safe working conditions must be ensured by employers as mandated by the Occupational Safety and Health Act (OSHA) of 1970 and enforced by the **Occupational Safety and Health Administration**, also called **OSHA.** Even so, biologic, electrical, radiation, and chemical hazards are encountered in a healthcare setting, often on a daily basis. It is important for the phlebotomist to be aware of the existence of hazards and know the safety precautions and rules necessary to eliminate or minimize them. General lab safety rules are listed in Box 3-3 Safety rules to follow when in patient rooms and other patient areas are listed in Box 3-4.

Biosafety

Biosafety is a term used to describe the safe handling of biologic substances that pose a risk to health. Biologic hazards can be encountered in a healthcare setting on a daily basis. Healthcare personnel need to be able to recognize them to take the precautions necessary to eliminate or minimize exposure to them.

TABLE 3-1   Clinical Conditions Warranting Transmission-Based Precautions Pending Confirmation of Diagnosis

Condition	Potential Pathogen	Precaution
Diarrhea		
Acute diarrhea with a likely infectious cause in an incontinent or diapered patient	Enteric pathogen	Contact
Diarrhea in an adult with a history of broad-spectrum or long-term antibiotics	*Clostridium difficile*	Contact
Meningitis	*Neisseria meningitidis*	Droplet
Rash for inflamed skin eruptions		
Petechial/ecchymotic with fever	*Neisseria meningitidis*	Droplet
Vesicular	Varicella	Airborne & contact
Maculopapular	Rubeola (measles)	Airborne
Respiratory infections		
Cough/fever/upper lobe pulmonary infiltrate in an HIV-negative patient and a patient at low risk for HIV infection	*Mycobacterium tuberculosis*	Airborne
Cough/fever/pulmonary infiltrate in any lung location in an HIV-infected patient and at high risk for HIV infection	*M. tuberculosis*	Airborne
Paroxysmal or severe persistent cough during periods of pertussis activity	*Bordetella pertussis*	Droplet
Respiratory infections, particularly bronchiolitis and croup, in infants and young children	Respiratory syncytial virus or parainfluenza virus	Contact
Risk of multidrug-resistant microorganisms		
History of infection or colonization with multidrug-resistant organisms	Resistant bacteria	Contact
Skin, wound, or urinary tract infection in a patient with a recent hospital or nursing home stay in a facility where multidrug-resistant organisms are prevalent	Resistant bacteria	Contact
Skin or wound infection		
Abscess or draining wound that cannot be covered	*Staphylococcus aureus* Group A streptococcus	Contact

TABLE 3-2 **Transmission-Based Precautions for Common Diseases and Conditions**

Airborne Precautions	Droplet Precautions	Contact Precautions
Herpes zoster (shingles)*	Adenovirus infection**	Adenovirus infection**
Measles (rubeola)	Diphtheria (pharyngeal)	Cellulitis (uncontrolled drainage)
Pulmonary tuberculosis	*Haemophilus influenzae meningitis*	*Clostridium difficile*
Varicella (chickenpox)	Influenza	Conjunctivitis (acute viral)
	Meningococcal pneumonia	Decubitus ulcer (infected, major)
	Meningococcal sepsis	Diphtheria (cutaneous)
	Mumps (infectious parotitis)	Enteroviral infections*
	Mycoplasma pneumoniae	Herpes zoster (shingles)*
	Neisseria meningitidis	Impetigo
	Parvovirus B19	Parainfluenza virus
	Pertussis (whooping cough)	Pediculosis (lice)
	Pneumonic plague	Respiratory syncytial virus
	Rubella (German measles)	Rubella (congenital)
	Scarlet fever**	Scabies
		Varicella (chickenpox)

*Widely disseminated or in immunocompromised patients
**Infants and children only

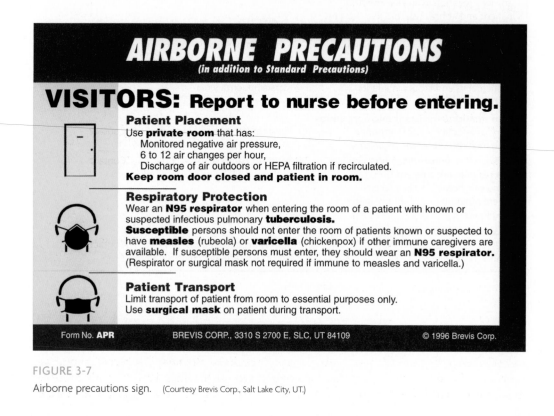

FIGURE 3-7

Airborne precautions sign.   (Courtesy Brevis Corp., Salt Lake City, UT.)

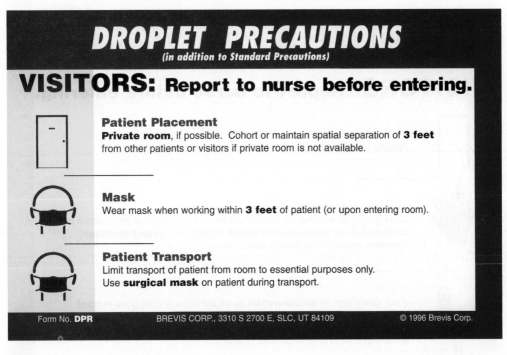

FIGURE 3-8

Droplet precautions sign.   (Courtesy Brevis Corp., Salt Lake City, UT.)

BIOHAZARD

Any material or substance harmful to health is called a **biohazard** (short for biologic hazard) and should be identified by a **biohazard symbol** (Fig. 3-10). Because most laboratory specimens have the potential to contain infectious agents they are considered biohazards.

BIOHAZARD EXPOSURE ROUTES

There are many routes by which healthcare workers can be exposed to biohazards. Ingestion is probably the most easily recognized, but routes other than the digestive tract referred to as **parenteral** (par-en'ter-al) routes can also result in biohazard exposure. The most common biohazard exposure routes are as follows.

Airborne   Biohazards can become airborne and inhaled when splashes, aerosols, or fumes are generated. Aerosols and splashes can be created when specimens are centrifuged, when tube stoppers are removed, and when preparing specimen aliquots. Dangerous fumes can be created if chemicals are improperly stored, mixed, or handled. Patients with airborne diseases can transmit infection to workers unless N95 respirators are worn when caring

CONTACT PRECAUTIONS
(in addition to Standard Precautions)

VISITORS: Report to nurse before entering.

Patient Placement
Private room, if possible. Cohort if private room is not available.

Gloves
Wear gloves when entering the room.
Change gloves after having contact with infective material that may contain high concentrations of microorganisms **(fecal** material and **wound drainage)**.
Remove gloves before leaving patient room.

Wash
Wash hands with an **antimicrobial** agent immediately after glove removal. After glove removal and handwashing, ensure that hands do not touch potentially contaminated environmental surfaces or items in the patient's room to avoid transfer of microorganisms to other patients or environments.

Gown
Wear gown when **entering** patient room if you anticipate that your clothing will have substantial contact with the patient, environmental surfaces, or items in the patient's room, or if the patient is **incontinent**, or has **diarrhea**, an **ileostomy**, a **colostomy**, or **wound drainage** not contained by a dressing. **Remove** gown before leaving the patient's environment and ensure that clothing does not contact potentially contaminated environmental surfaces to avoid transfer of microorganisms to other patients or environments.

Patient Transport
Limit transport of patient to essential purposes only. During transport, ensure that precautions are maintained to minimize the risk of transmission of microorganisms to other patients and contamination of environmental surfaces and equipment.

Patient–Care Equipment
Dedicate the use of noncritical patient–care equipment to a single patient. If common equipment is used, clean and disinfect between patients.

Form No. **CPR**　　　BREVIS CORP., 3310 S 2700 E, SLC, UT 84109　　　© 1996 Brevis Corp.

FIGURE 3-9

Contact precautions sign.　(Courtesy Brevis Corp., Salt Lake City, UT.)

BOX • 3-3 General Laboratory Safety Rules

- *Never* eat, drink, smoke, or chew gum in the laboratory. *Never* put pencils or pens in the mouth.
- *Never* place food or beverages in a refrigerator used for storing reagents or specimens.
- *Never* apply cosmetics, handle contact lenses, or rub eyes in the laboratory.
- *Never* wear long chains, large or dangling earrings, or loose bracelets.
- *Always* wear a fully buttoned lab coat when engaged in lab activities. *Never* wear a lab coat to lunch, on break, or when leaving the lab to go home. *Never* wear personal protective equipment outside the designated area for its use.
- *Always* tie back hair that is longer than shoulder length.
- *Always* keep finger nails short and well manicured. *Do not* wear nail polish or artificial nails. *Never* bite nails or cuticles.
- *Always* wear a face shield when performing specimen processing or any activity that might generate a splash or aerosol of bodily fluids.
- *Always* wear gloves for phlebotomy procedures and when processing specimens.

BOX • 3-4 Safety Rules When in Patient Rooms and Other Patient Areas

- Avoid running. It is alarming to patients and visitors and may cause an accident.
- Be careful entering and exiting patient rooms; housekeeping equipment, dietary carts, x-ray machines, and other types of equipment may be just inside the door or outside in the hall.
- Do not touch electrical equipment in patient rooms while drawing blood. Electric shock can pass through a phlebotomist and the needle and shock the patient.
- Follow standard precautions when handling specimens.
- Properly dispose of used and contaminated specimen collection supplies and return all other equipment to the collection tray before leaving the patient's room.
- Replace bedrails that were let down during patient procedures.
- Report infiltrated IVs or other IV problems to nursing personnel.
- Report unresponsive patients to nursing personnel.
- Report unusual odors to nursing personnel.
- Watch out for and report food, liquid, and other items on the floor to appropriate personnel.

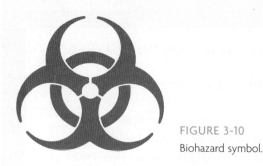

FIGURE 3-10
Biohazard symbol.

for them. Protection against airborne biohazard exposure includes following safe handling practices, wearing appropriate PPE, and working behind safety shields or splash guards.

Ingestion   Biohazards can be ingested if healthcare workers neglect to sanitize hands before handling food, gum, candy, cigarettes, or drinks. Other activities that can lead to ingestion of biohazards include covering the mouth with hands instead of tissue when coughing or sneezing, biting nails, chewing on pens or pencils, and licking fingers when turning pages in books. Frequent hand sanitization, avoiding hand to mouth activities, and refraining from holding items in the mouth or chewing on them provides the best defense against accidental ingestion of biohazardous substances.

Nonintact Skin   Biohazards can enter the body through visible and invisible preexisting breaks in the skin such as abrasions, burns, cuts, scratches, sores, dermatitis, and chapped skin. Defects in the skin should be covered with waterproof (nonpermeable) bandages to prevent contamination, even when gloves are worn.

Percutaneous   **Percutaneous** (through the skin) exposure to biohazardous microorganisms in blood or body fluid occurs through intact (unbroken) skin as a result of accidental needlesticks and injuries from other sharps including broken glass and specimen tubes. Ways to reduce the chance of percutaneous exposure include using needle safety devices properly, wearing heavy duty utility gloves when cleaning up broken glass, and never handling broken glass with the hands.

Permucosal   **Permucosal** (through mucous membranes) exposure occurs when infectious microorganisms and other biohazards enter the body through the mucous membranes of the mouth and nose and the conjunctiva of the eyes in droplets generated by sneezing or coughing, splashes, and aerosols and by rubbing or touching the eyes, nose, or mouth with contaminated hands. The chance of permucosal exposure can be reduced by following procedures to prevent exposure to splashes and aerosols and avoiding rubbing or touching the eyes, nose, or mouth.

BLOODBORNE PATHOGEN

The term **bloodborne pathogen (BBP)** is applied to any infectious microorganism present in blood and other body fluids and tissues. BBPs, which can be present in a patient's body fluids even if there are no symptoms of disease, are one of the most significant biohazards faced by healthcare workers. Although HBV, HCV, and HIV tend to receive the most attention, BBPs include other hepatitis viruses; cytomegalovirus (CMV); the microorganisms that cause syphilis, malaria, and relapsing fever; the agent that causes Creutzfeldt-Jakob disease; and more recently, West Nile virus.

HBV and Hepatitis D Virus   Hepatitis B (once called serum hepatitis) is caused by HBV, a potentially life-threatening bloodborne pathogen that targets the liver. (Hepatitis means "inflammation of the liver.") It has been the most frequently occurring laboratory-associated infection and the major occupational hazard in the healthcare industry, although the rate of infection has dropped substantially since the advent of HBV immunization programs in the 1980s. Anyone infected with HBV is at risk of also acquiring hepatitis D (delta) virus (HDV), which is a defective virus that can only multiply in the presence of HBV.

HBV Vaccination

The best defense against HBV infection is vaccination. Vaccination consists of a series of three equal intramuscular injections of vaccine: an initial dose, a second dose 1 month after the first, and a third dose 6 months following the initial dose. The vaccine also protects against HDV since it can only be contracted concurrently with HBV infection. Success of immunization and proof of immunity can be determined 1 to 2 months after the last vaccination dose by a blood test that detects the presence of the hepatitis B surface antibody (anti-HBs) in the person's serum. OSHA requires employers to offer the vaccine free to employees within 10 days of being assigned to duties with potential BBP exposure. Employees who refuse the vaccination must sign and date a declination (statement of refusal) form, which is kept in their personnel file.

fyi   The most commonly used hepatitis B vaccine does not contain live virus and poses no risk of transmitting HBV, a problem of earlier vaccines.

HBV Exposure Hazards

HBV can be present in blood and other body fluids such as urine, semen, cerebrospinal fluid (CSF), and saliva. It can survive up to a week in dried blood on work surfaces, equipment, telephones, and other objects. In a healthcare setting, it is primarily transmitted through needlesticks (a single needlestick can transmit HBV) and other sharps injuries and contact with contaminated equipment, objects, surfaces, aerosols, spills, and splashes. In nonmedical settings, it is transmitted primarily through sexual contact and sharing of dirty needles.

Symptoms of HBV Infection

HBV symptoms resemble flu symptoms, but generally last longer. They include fatigue; loss of appetite; mild fever; muscle, joint, and abdominal pain; nausea; and vomiting. Jaundice appears in about 25% of cases. About 50% of those infected show no symptoms. Some individuals become carriers who can pass the disease on to others. Carriers have an increased risk of developing cirrhosis of the liver and liver cancer. Infection is confirmed by detection of hepatitis B surface antigen (HBsAg) in an individual's serum.

Hepatitis C Virus (HCV) Hepatitis C, caused by infection with HCV has become the most widespread chronic bloodborne illness in the United States. The virus, discovered in 1988 by molecular cloning, was found to be the primary cause of non-A, non-B hepatitis. No vaccine is currently available.

HCV Exposure Hazards

HCV is found primarily in blood and serum, less frequently in saliva, and seldom in urine and semen. It can enter the body in the same manner as HBV. However, infection primarily occurs after large or multiple exposures. Like HBV, in nonmedical settings, sexual contact and needle sharing are the primary means of transmission.

Symptoms of HCV Infection

HCV symptoms are similar to those of HBV infection, although only 25% to 30% of infections even display symptoms. As with HBV, chronic and carrier states exist that can lead to cirrhosis of the liver and liver cancer. In fact, HCV infection is a leading indication for liver transplantation.

Human Immunodeficiency Virus (HIV) HIV attacks the body's immune system, causing AIDS by leaving the body susceptible to opportunistic infections. Opportunistic infections are caused by organisms that would not ordinarily be pathogens to a normal healthy individual. HIV infection has a poor prognosis and is of great concern to healthcare workers.

key • point Although the incidence of work-related HIV infection is relatively low, CDC studies have shown that phlebotomy procedures were involved in approximately 50% of the HIV exposures that have occurred so far in healthcare settings.

HIV Exposure Hazards

HIV has been isolated from blood, semen, saliva, tears, urine, cerebrospinal fluid, amniotic fluid, breast milk, cervical secretions, and tissue of infected persons. The risk to healthcare workers, however, is primarily through exposure to blood. HIV can enter the body through all the same routes as the hepatitis viruses.

Symptoms of HIV Infection

The incubation phase for HIV infection is thought to range from a few weeks up to a year or more. Initial symptoms are mild-to-severe flulike symptoms. During this phase the virus enters the T lymphocytes (T lymphs or helper T cells), triggering them to produce multiple copies of the virus. The virus then enters a seemingly inactive incubation phase while hiding in the T lymphs. Certain conditions reactivate the virus, which slowly destroys the T lymphs. Once the T lymph count is reduced to 200 or fewer per milliliter of blood, the patient is officially diagnosed as having AIDS, the third and final phase of infection. In this phase the immune system deteriorates significantly, and opportunistic infections take hold. Two symptoms of AIDS are hairy leukoplakia, a white lesion on the tongue, and Kaposi's sarcoma, a cancer of the capillaries that produces bluish-red nodules on the skin. End stages of AIDS are characterized by deterioration of the nervous system leading to neurologic symptoms and dementia.

OSHA BLOODBORNE PATHOGENS STANDARD

The OSHA **Bloodborne Pathogens Standard** was promulgated (put into force) when it was concluded that healthcare employees face a serious health risk from occupational exposure to blood and other body fluids and tissues. Enforcement of the standard, which is mandated by federal law, is meant to reduce, if not eliminate, occupational exposure to BBPs. The standard requires implementation of **engineering controls** and **work practice controls** to prevent exposure incidents, availability and use of PPE, special training, medical surveillance, and the availability of vaccination against HBV for all at risk employees.

> key • point Engineering controls are devices that isolate or remove a BBP hazard. Work practice controls are practices that change the way tasks are performed to reduce the likelihood of BBP exposure.

The BBP standard was revised in 2001 to conform to the **Needlestick Safety and Prevention Act** passed by Congress and signed into law in November 2000. The act directed OSHA to revise the BBP standard in the following four key areas:

- Revision and updating of the exposure control plan
- Solicitation of employee input in selecting engineering and work practice controls
- Modification of definitions relating to engineering controls
- New record-keeping requirements

EXPOSURE CONTROL PLAN

To comply with the OSHA standard, employers must have a written exposure control plan. The plan must be reviewed and updated at least annually to document the evaluation and implementation of safer medical devices. Nonmanagerial employees with risk of exposure must be involved in the identification, review and selection of engineering and work practice controls and their participation must be documented. Key elements of an exposure control plan are shown in Box 3-5.

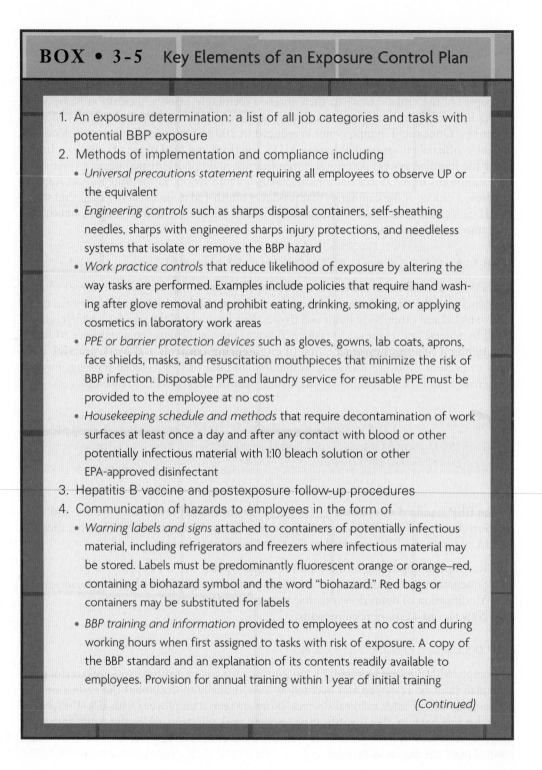

BOX • 3-5   Key Elements of an Exposure Control Plan

1. An exposure determination: a list of all job categories and tasks with potential BBP exposure
2. Methods of implementation and compliance including
   - *Universal precautions statement* requiring all employees to observe UP or the equivalent
   - *Engineering controls* such as sharps disposal containers, self-sheathing needles, sharps with engineered sharps injury protections, and needleless systems that isolate or remove the BBP hazard
   - *Work practice controls* that reduce likelihood of exposure by altering the way tasks are performed. Examples include policies that require hand washing after glove removal and prohibit eating, drinking, smoking, or applying cosmetics in laboratory work areas
   - *PPE or barrier protection devices* such as gloves, gowns, lab coats, aprons, face shields, masks, and resuscitation mouthpieces that minimize the risk of BBP infection. Disposable PPE and laundry service for reusable PPE must be provided to the employee at no cost
   - *Housekeeping schedule and methods* that require decontamination of work surfaces at least once a day and after any contact with blood or other potentially infectious material with 1:10 bleach solution or other EPA-approved disinfectant
3. Hepatitis B vaccine and postexposure follow-up procedures
4. Communication of hazards to employees in the form of
   - *Warning labels and signs* attached to containers of potentially infectious material, including refrigerators and freezers where infectious material may be stored. Labels must be predominantly fluorescent orange or orange–red, containing a biohazard symbol and the word "biohazard." Red bags or containers may be substituted for labels
   - *BBP training and information* provided to employees at no cost and during working hours when first assigned to tasks with risk of exposure. A copy of the BBP standard and an explanation of its contents readily available to employees. Provision for annual training within 1 year of initial training

(Continued)

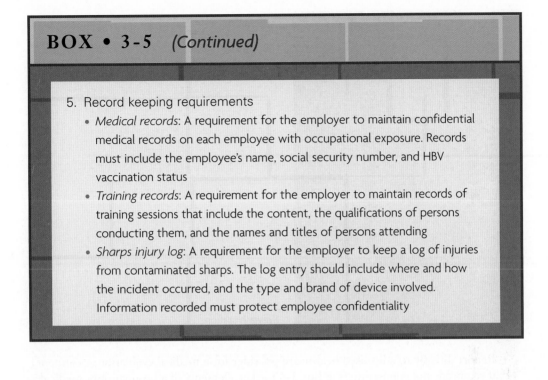

BOX • 3-5 *(Continued)*

5. Record keeping requirements
   - *Medical records*: A requirement for the employer to maintain confidential medical records on each employee with occupational exposure. Records must include the employee's name, social security number, and HBV vaccination status
   - *Training records*: A requirement for the employer to maintain records of training sessions that include the content, the qualifications of persons conducting them, and the names and titles of persons attending
   - *Sharps injury log*: A requirement for the employer to keep a log of injuries from contaminated sharps. The log entry should include where and how the incident occurred, and the type and brand of device involved. Information recorded must protect employee confidentiality

BBP EXPOSURE ROUTES

Occupational exposure to bloodborne pathogens can occur if any of the following happens while a healthcare worker is performing his or her duties.

- The skin is pierced by a contaminated needle or sharp object.
- Blood or other body fluid splashes into the eyes, nose, or mouth.
- Blood or other body fluid comes in contact with a cut, scratch, or abrasion.
- A human bite breaks the skin.

EXPOSURE INCIDENT PROCEDURE

An exposure incident requires immediate attention for the most promising outcome in the event that the exposure involves a bloodborne pathogen. The immediate response by the employee in the event of an exposure incident includes the following:

- Needlestick or other sharps injury: Carefully remove shards of glass or other objects that may be embedded in the wound and wash the site with soap and water for a minimum of 30 seconds.
- Mucous membrane exposure: Flush the site (i.e., eyes, nose, or mouth) with water or sterile saline for a minimum of 10 minutes. Use an eyewash station (Fig. 3-11) if available to adequately flush a splash to the eyes. Remove contact lenses as soon as possible and disinfect them before reuse or discard.
- Report the incident to the immediate supervisor.

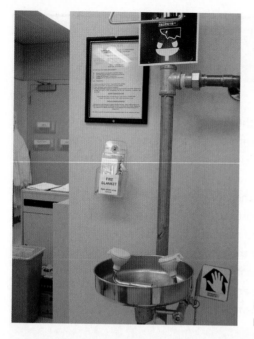

FIGURE 3-11
Eyewash station.

- Report directly to a licensed healthcare provider for a medical evaluation, treatment if required, and counseling (see Box 3-6 for key elements of a postexposure medical evaluation.)

key • point   There is currently no scientific evidence that squeezing the wound or cleaning with an antiseptic reduces the transmission of BBPs. Cleaning with bleach or other caustic agents is not recommended.

key • point   Free confidential medical evaluation following an exposure incident is required by OSHA regulations. If postexposure treatment is recommended, it should be started as soon as possible.

SURFACE DECONTAMINATION

OSHA requires surfaces in specimen collection and processing areas to be decontaminated by cleaning them with a 1:10 bleach solution or other **Environmental Protection Agency (EPA)**-approved disinfectant. Bleach solutions should be prepared daily. Cleaning must take place at the end of each shift or whenever a surface is visibly contaminated. Gloves should be worn when cleaning.

BOX • 3-6 Key Elements of a Postexposure Medical Evaluation

The employee's blood is tested for HIV in an accredited laboratory.

The source patient's blood is tested for HIV and HBV, with the patient's permission.

- If the source patient refuses testing, is HBV positive, or is in a high risk category, the employee may be given immune globulin or HBV vaccination.
- If the source patient is HIV positive, the employee is counseled and tested for HIV infection immediately and at periodic intervals, normally 6 weeks, 12 weeks, 6 months, and 1 year after exposure.

The employee may be given azidothymidine (AZT) or other HIV therapy.

The exposed employee is counseled to be alert for acute retroviral syndrome (acute viral symptoms) within 12 weeks of exposure.

BODY FLUID SPILL CLEANUP

Special EPA-approved chemical solutions and kits are available for cleanup of blood and other body fluid spills and for disinfecting surfaces. Gloves must be worn during the cleaning process. Cleanup procedures, which vary slightly depending upon the type and size of spill (see Procedure 3-2), should concentrate on absorbing the material without spreading it over a wider area than the original spill. Disposable cleanup materials must be discarded in a biohazard waste container. Reusable cleanup materials should be properly disinfected after use.

BIOHAZARD WASTE DISPOSAL

Nonreusable items contaminated with blood or body fluids are biohazardous waste and must be disposed of in special containers or bags marked with a biohazard symbol. Filled biohazard waste containers require special handling prior to decontamination and disposal. OSHA, EPA, and state and local agencies regulate biohazard waste disposal.

Electrical Safety

Fire and electric shock are potential hazards associated with the use of electrical equipment. Knowledge of the proper use, maintenance, and servicing of electrical equipment such as centrifuges can minimize hazards associated with their use. Box 3-7 contains guidelines for electrical safety.

PROCEDURE 3-2

Blood and Other Body Fluid Spill Cleanup Procedures

Type of Spill	Cleanup Procedure
Small spill (a few drops)	Carefully absorb spill with a paper towel or similar material Discard material in biohazard waste container Clean area with appropriate disinfectant
Large spill	Use a special clay or chlorine-based powder to absorb or gel (thicken) the liquid Scoop or sweep up absorbed or thickened material Discard material in a biohazard waste container Wipe spill area with appropriate disinfectant
Dried spills	Moisten spill with disinfectant (avoid scraping, which could disperse infectious organisms into the air) Absorb spill with paper towel or similar material Discard material in biohazard waste container Clean area with appropriate disinfectant
Spills involving broken glass	Wear heavy duty utility gloves (Never handle broken glass with hands) Scoop or sweep up material Discard in biohazard sharps container Clean area with appropriate disinfectant

BOX • 3-7   Electrical Safety

- *Avoid* the use of extension cords.
- *Do not* overload electrical circuits.
- Inspect cords and plugs for breaks and fraying.
- Unplug equipment when servicing, including when replacing a light bulb.
- Unplug equipment that has had liquid spilled in it. Do not plug in again until the spill has been cleaned up and you are certain the wiring is dry.
- Unplug and do not use equipment that is malfunctioning.
- *Do not* attempt to make repairs to equipment if you are not trained to do so.
- *Do not* handle electrical equipment with wet hands or when standing on a wet floor.
- Know the location of the circuit breaker box.
- *Do not* touch electrical equipment in patient rooms, especially when in the process of drawing blood. Electric shock could pass through the phlebotomist and the needle and shock the patient.

ACTIONS TO TAKE IF ELECTRIC SHOCK OCCURS

- Shut off the source of electricity.
- If the source of electricity cannot be shut off, use nonconducting material (e.g., hand inside a glass beaker) to remove the source of electricity from a victim.
- Call for medical assistance.
- Start cardiopulmonary resuscitation if indicated.
- Keep the victim warm.

Fire Safety

All employees of any institution should be aware of procedures to follow in case of fire. They should know where fire extinguishers are located and how to use them. They should know where the fire blankets (Fig. 3-12) are kept and how to use them or heavy toweling to smother clothing fires. They should know the location of emergency exits and be familiar with evacuation routes. Fire spreads rapidly and it is important for employees to know the basics of what to do and also what not to do if a fire occurs so they can react quickly and appropriately. Box 3-8 lists dos and don'ts to follow if a fire occurs.

FIRE COMPONENTS

Four components, present at the same time, are necessary for fire to occur. Three of the components, *fuel* (combustible material), *heat* to raise the temperature of the material until it ignites or catches fire, and *oxygen* to maintain combustion or burning have traditionally been referred to as the fire triangle. The fourth component, the chemical reaction that produces fire, actually creates a **fire tetrahedron** (Fig 3-13), the latest way of looking at the chemistry of fire. Basic fire safety involves keeping the components apart to prevent fire or removing one or more of the components when there is a fire to extinguish it. Fire extinguishers put out fires by removing one or more components. There are different types of fire extinguishers, depending on the class of fire involved.

FIGURE 3-12

Fire blanket storage box.

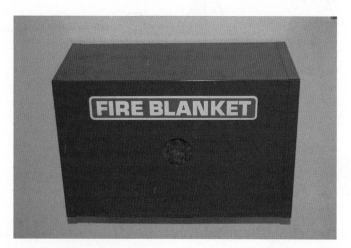

BOX • 3-8   Fire Safety Dos and Don'ts

- Do pull the nearest fire alarm.
- Do call the fire department.
- Do attempt to extinguish a small fire.
- Do close all doors and windows if leaving the area.
- Do smother a clothing fire with a fire blanket or have the person roll on the floor in an attempt to smother the fire.
- Do crawl to the nearest exit if there is heavy smoke present.
- Don't panic.
- Don't run.
- Don't use elevators.

Fire Tetrahedron

FIGURE 3-13
Fire tetrahedron.

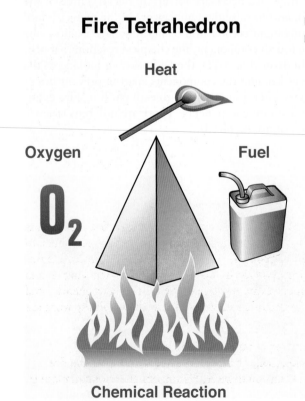

Heat

Oxygen

O$_2$

Fuel

Chemical Reaction

CLASSES OF FIRE

Five classes of fire are now recognized by the **National Fire Protection Association** (NFPA). Classification is based on the fuel source of the fire. The five classes are as follows:

- *Class A* fires occur with ordinary combustible materials such as wood, papers, or clothing, and require water or water-based solutions to cool or quench the fire to extinguish it.
- *Class B* fires occur with flammable liquids and vapors such as paint, oil, grease, or gasoline and require blocking the source of oxygen or smothering the fuel to extinguish.
- *Class C* fires occur with electrical equipment and require nonconducting agents to extinguish.
- *Class D* fires occur with combustible or reactive metals such as sodium, potassium, magnesium, and lithium and require dry powder agents or sand to extinguish (they are the most difficult fires to control and frequently lead to explosions).
- *Class K* fires occur with high-temperature cooking oils, grease, or fats and require agents that prevent splashing and cool the fire as well as smother it.

m e m o r y • j o g g e r   The following will help you remember each fire classification.
- To remember that class A fires occur with ordinary combustible materials, emphasize the "a" when saying the word "ordinary."
- To remember that class B fires occur with flammable liquids, emphasize the "b" when saying the word "flammable."
- To remember that class C fires are electrical fires, emphasize the "c" when saying the word "electrical."
- To remember class D fires, keep in mind that when you say the word "metal" quickly, it sounds like "medal," which has a "d" in it, and medals are commonly made of metal.
- To remember class K fires, keep in mind that they occur with cooking oils or fats in kitchens, which begins with a "k."

FIRE EXTINGUISHERS

There is a fire extinguisher class (Fig. 3-14) that correspond to each class of fire except class D. Class D fires present unique problems and are best left to firefighting personnel to extinguish. Using the wrong type of fire extinguisher on a fire can be dangerous. Consequently, some fire extinguishers are multipurpose to eliminate the confusion of having several different types of extinguishers. Multipurpose extinguishers are the type most frequently used in healthcare institutions. Common fire extinguisher classes and how they typically work are as follows:

- *Class A extinguishers* use soda and acid or water to cool the fire.
- *Class B extinguishers* use foam, dry chemical, or carbon dioxide to smother the fire.
- *Class C extinguishers* use dry chemical, carbon dioxide, Halon, or other nonconducting agents to smother the fire.

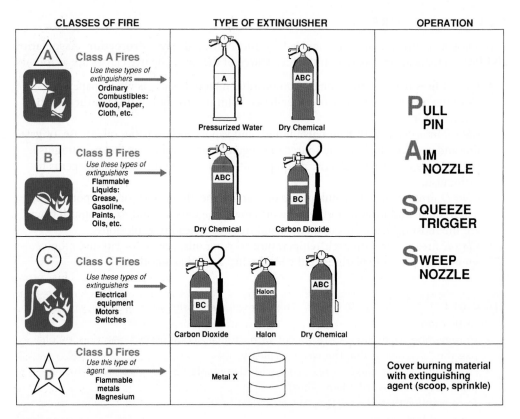

FIGURE 3-14

Classes of fire extinguishers. (Adapted with permission from the Environmental Health & Safety Department, The University of Texas, Houston, Health Science Center.)

- *Class ABC (multipurpose) extinguishers* use dry chemical reagents to smother the fire. They can be used on class A, B, and C fires.
- *Class K extinguishers* use a potassium-based alkaline liquid specifically formulated to fight high-temperature grease, oil, or fat fires by cooling and smothering them without splashing. Some class K extinguishers can also be used on class A, B, and C fires.

m e m o r y • j o g g e r   The NFPA code word for the order of action in the event of fire is RACE, where the letters stand for the following:

R = *Rescue* individuals in danger
A = *Alarm:* sound the alarm
C = *Confine* the fire by closing all doors and windows
E = *Extinguish* the fire with the nearest suitable fire extinguisher

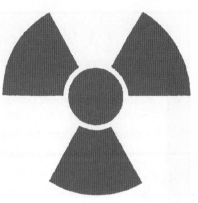

FIGURE 3-15
Radiation hazard symbol.

Radiation Safety

The principles involved in radiation exposure are *distance*, *shielding*, and *time*. This means that the amount of radiation you are exposed to depends upon how far you are from the source of radioactivity, what protection you have from it, and how long you are exposed to it. Exposure time is important because radiation effects are cumulative.

A clearly posted **radiation hazard symbol** (Fig. 3-15) is required in areas where radioactive materials are used and on cabinet or refrigerator doors where radioactive materials are stored. In addition, radioactive reagents and specimens must be labeled with a radiation hazard symbol. A radiation hazard symbol on a patient's door signifies that a patient has been treated with radioactive isotopes.

A phlebotomist may encounter radiation hazards when collecting specimens from patients who have been injected with radioactive dyes, when collecting specimens from patients in the radiology department or nuclear medicine, and when delivering specimens to radioimmunoassay sections of the laboratory. The phlebotomist should be aware of institutional radiation safety procedures. In addition, the phlebotomist should recognize the radiation hazard symbol and be cautious when entering areas displaying it. Because radiation is particularly hazardous to a fetus, pregnant employees should avoid areas displaying the radiation symbol, patients who have recently been injected with radioactive dyes, and specimens collected from patients while radioactive dye is still in their systems.

Chemical Safety

A phlebotomist may come in contact with hazardous chemicals when using cleaning reagents, adding preservatives to 24-hour urine containers, or delivering specimens to the laboratory. Inappropriate use of chemicals can have dangerous consequences. For example, mixing bleach with other cleaning compounds can release dangerous gases. In addition, many chemicals are potent acids, such as the hydrochloric acid (HCl) used as a urine preservative, or alkalis, both of which can cause severe burns. Container labels provide important information regarding the contents and should always be read carefully before use. See Box 3-9 for general chemical safety rules.

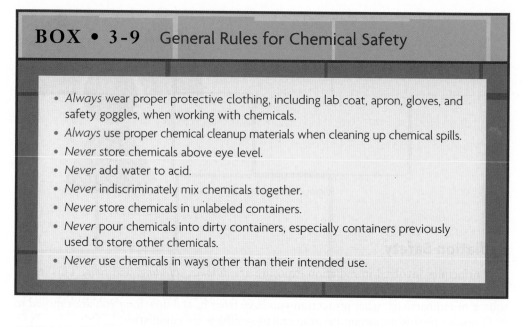

BOX • 3-9 General Rules for Chemical Safety

- *Always* wear proper protective clothing, including lab coat, apron, gloves, and safety goggles, when working with chemicals.
- *Always* use proper chemical cleanup materials when cleaning up chemical spills.
- *Never* store chemicals above eye level.
- *Never* add water to acid.
- *Never* indiscriminately mix chemicals together.
- *Never* store chemicals in unlabeled containers.
- *Never* pour chemicals into dirty containers, especially containers previously used to store other chemicals.
- *Never* use chemicals in ways other than their intended use.

OSHA HAZARD COMMUNICATION STANDARD

OSHA developed the **Hazard Communication (HazCom) Standard** to protect employees who may be exposed to hazardous chemicals. According to the law, all chemicals must be evaluated for health hazards, and all chemicals found to be hazardous must be labeled as such and the information communicated to employees.

key • point The HazCom standard is known as "The Right to Know Law" because of the labeling requirement.

HazCom Labeling Requirements Although labeling format may vary by company, all chemical manufacturers must comply with labeling requirements set by the Manufacturers Chemical Association. Labels for hazardous chemicals must contain a statement of warning such as "danger" or "poison," a statement of the hazard (e.g., toxic, flammable, combustible), precautions to eliminate risk, and first aid measures in the event of a spill or other exposure.

Material Safety Data Sheets The OSHA HazCom standard requires manufacturers to supply **material safety data sheets (MSDS)** for their products. An MSDS contains general information as well as precautionary and emergency information for the product. Every product with a hazardous warning on the label requires an MSDS to help ensure that it will be used safely and as intended.

key • point Employers are required to obtain the MSDS for every hazardous chemical present in the workplace and to make all MSDS readily accessible to employees.

DEPARTMENT OF TRANSPORTATION LABELING SYSTEM

Hazardous materials may have additional labels of precaution, including a Department of Transportation (DOT) symbol incorporating a United Nations hazard classification number and symbol (Table 3-3). The DOT labeling system uses a diamond-shaped warning sign (Fig. 3-16) containing the United Nations hazard class number, the hazard class designation or four-digit identification number, and a symbol representing the hazard.

NATIONAL FIRE PROTECTION ASSOCIATION LABELING SYSTEM

Another hazardous material rating system (Fig. 3-17) was developed by the NFPA to label areas where hazardous chemicals and other materials are stored, thus alerting firefighters in the event of a fire. This system uses a diamond-shaped symbol divided into four quadrants. Health hazards are indicated in a blue diamond on the left, the level of fire hazard is indicated in the upper quadrant in a red diamond, stability or reactivity hazards are indicated in a yellow diamond on the right, and other specific hazards are indicated in a white quadrant on the bottom.

SAFETY SHOWERS AND EYE WASH STATIONS

The phlebotomist should know the location of and be instructed in the use of safety showers and eye wash stations (Fig. 3-18) in the event of a chemical spill or splash to the eyes or other body parts. The eyes or other body parts affected should be flushed with water for a minimum of 15 minutes, followed by a visit to the emergency room for evaluation.

CHEMICAL SPILL PROCEDURES

Chemical spills require cleanup using special kits (Fig. 3-19) containing absorbent and neutralizer materials. The type of materials used depends upon the type of chemical spilled. An indicator in the cleanup materials detects when the materials have been neutralized and are safe for disposal. The EPA regulates chemical disposal.

FIRST AID

The ability to recognize and react quickly and skillfully to emergency situations may mean the difference between life and death for a victim.

TABLE 3-3 United Nations Hazard Classification Numbers and Symbols

United Nations Hazard Class	Symbol	Background Color	Examples
Class 1 Explosives	Bursting ball	Orange	Fireworks Ammunition Dynamite
Class 2 Gases (compressed, liquified, or dissolved under pressure)	Flame	*Flammable* Red	Flammable: Butane Propane
	Cylinder	*Nonflammable* Green	Nonflammable: Ammonia Chlorine
Class 3 Flammable liquids	Flame	Red	Brake fluid Camphor oil Glycol ethers Gasoline
Class 4 Flammable solids or substances	Flame	*Flammable Solid* Red and white vertical stripes	Lithium Magnesium Phosphorus Titanium
	Slashed W	*Water-Reactive Materials* Red and white vertical stripes with blue top quadrant	
Class 5 Division 5.1: oxidizing substances Division 5.2: organic peroxides	Circle with flame	Yellow	Ammonium nitrate Benzoyl peroxide Calcium chlorite
Class 6 Poisonous and infectious substances	Skull with crossbones	White	Chemical made Pesticides Cyanide AIDS specimens
Class 7 Radioactive materials	Propeller	Yellow over white	Cobalt 14 Plutonium Radioactive waste Uranium 235
Class 8 Corrosives	Test tube over hand Test tube over metal	White over black	Caustic potash Caustic soda Hydrochloric acid Sulfuric acid

(continued)

TABLE 3-3 *(continued)*

United Nations Hazard Class	Symbol	Background Color	Examples
Class 9 Miscellaneous dangerous substances	ORM-A ORM-B ORM-C ORM-D ORM-E	White	ORM-A: dry ice ORM-B: quick lime ORM-C: sawdust ORM-D: hair spray ORM-E: hazardous waste

External Hemorrhage

According to current American Red Cross guidelines, hemorrhage (abnormal bleeding) from an obvious wound can be effectively controlled by firmly applying direct pressure to the wound until bleeding stops or EMS rescuers arrive. Pressure should be applied using cloth or gauze, with additional material added if bleeding continues. It is acceptable to use an elastic bandage to hold the compress in place if pressure is applied to the bandage.

c a u t i o n   The original compress should not be removed when adding additional ones because removal can disrupt the clotting process.

FIGURE 3-16

Example of DOT hazardous materials labels (flammable, poison, corrosive, etc.). (From Jones, S. A., Weigel, A., White, R. D., et al., eds. (1992). Advanced emergency care for paramedic practice. Philadelphia: J. B. Lippincott.

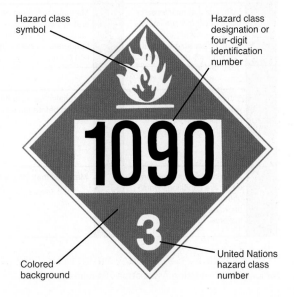

Hazard class symbol

Hazard class designation or four-digit identification number

1090

3

Colored background

United Nations hazard class number

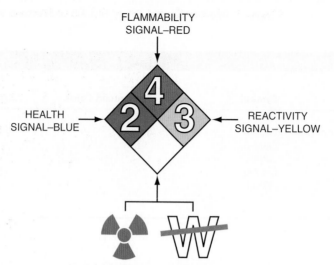

FLAMMABILITY
SIGNAL–RED

HEALTH
SIGNAL–BLUE

REACTIVITY
SIGNAL–YELLOW

RADIOACTIVE OR WATER REACTIVE

Identification of Health Hazard Color Code: **BLUE**		Identification of Flammability Color Code: **RED**		Identification of Reactivity (Stability) Color Code: **YELLOW**	
	Type of possible injury		Susceptibility of materials to burning		Susceptibility to release of energy
SIGNAL		SIGNAL		SIGNAL	
4	Materials that on very short exposure could cause death or major residual injury even though prompt medical treatment was given.	4	Materials that will rapidly or completely vaporize at atmospheric pressure and normal ambient temperature, or that are readily dispersed in air and that will burn readily.	4	Materials that in themselves are readily capable of detonation or of explosive decomposition or reaction at normal temperatures and pressures.
3	Materials that on short exposure could cause serious temporary or residual injury even though prompt medical treatment was given.	3	Liquids and solids that can be ignited under almost all ambient temperature conditions.	3	Materials that in themselves are capable of detonation or explosive reaction but require a strong initiating source or that must be heated under confinement before initiation or that react explosively with water.
2	Materials that on intense or continued exposure could cause temporary incapacitation or possible residual injury unless prompt medical treatment is given.	2	Materials that must be moderately heated or exposed to relatively high ambient temperatures before ignition can occur.	2	Materials that in themselves are normally unstable and readily undergo violent chemical change but do not detonate. Also materials that may react violently with water or that may form potentially explosive mixtures with water.
1	Materials that on exposure would cause irritation but only minor residual injury even if no treatment is given.	1	Materials that must be preheated before ignition can occur.	1	Materials that in themselves are normally stable, but that can become unstable at elevated temperatures and pressures or that may react with water with some release of energy, but not violently.
0	Materials that on exposure under fire conditions would offer no hazard beyond that of ordinary combustible material.	0	Materials that will not burn.	0	Materials that in themselves are normally stable, even under fire exposure conditions, and that are not reactive with water.

FIGURE 3-17

National Fire Protection Association 704 marking system.

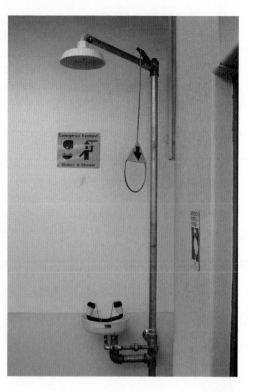

FIGURE 3-18

Combination safety shower and eye wash.

FIGURE 3-19

Spill cleanup kit.

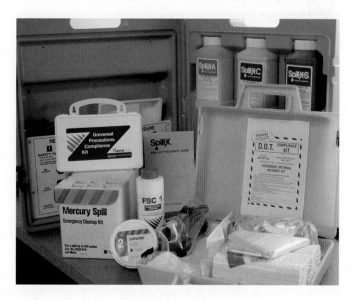

Previous guidelines added elevating the affected area and, if efforts to control bleeding were ineffective, use of arterial pressure points. Although not included now, these actions are not considered improper or harmful. Using a tourniquet to control bleeding *can* be harmful, and is not recommended. A tourniquet should only be used as a last resort to save a life after all other means to control bleeding are unsuccessful as may occur with an **avulsion** (a tearing away or amputation of a body part) or a severely mangled or crushed body part.

Shock

A state of shock results when there is insufficient return of blood flow to the heart, resulting in inadequate supply of oxygen to all organs and tissues of the body. Numerous conditions including hemorrhage, heart attack, trauma, and drug reactions can lead to some degree of shock. Because shock can be a life-threatening situation, it is important that the symptoms be recognized and dealt with immediately.

COMMON SYMPTOMS OF SHOCK

Common symptoms of shock include:

- Pale, cold, clammy skin
- Rapid, weak pulse
- Increased, shallow breathing rate
- Expressionless face and staring eyes

FIRST AID FOR SHOCK

When providing first aid to a victim of shock, be sure to do the following:

1. Maintain an open airway for the victim.
2. Call for assistance.
3. Keep the victim lying down with the head lower than the rest of the body.
4. Attempt to control bleeding or other cause of shock if known.
5. Keep the victim warm until help arrives.

> c a u t i o n   *Never* give fluids if the patient is unconscious or semiconscious or has injuries likely to require surgery and anesthesia.

Cardiopulmonary Resuscitation and Emergency Cardiovascular Care

Most healthcare institutions require their personnel to be certified in cardiopulmonary resuscitation (CPR). Consequently, most phlebotomy programs require it as a prerequisite or corequisite or include it as part of the course. The American Heart Association recommends the 6- to 8-hour Basic Lifesaving (BLS) Healthcare Provider Course for those in healthcare professions. The course includes instruction in how to perform CPR on victims of all ages, use of an automated external defibrillator (AED), and how to remove foreign body airway obstruction. Certification is good for 2 years.

American Heart Association CPR Guidelines   The American Heart Association (AHA) recently unveiled important new guidelines for CPR and Emergency Cardiovascular Care (ECC). These guidelines brought about a number of changes to lay rescuer and healthcare provider CPR training. The aim of the changes is to simplify instruction, increase chest compressions per minute, and minimize interruptions in chest compression. Highlights of the new guidelines include

- Rescue breaths simplified to normal breaths, each given over 1 second with sufficient volume to make the chest visibly rise
- Chest compression landmarks simplified to the center of the chest for adults and children, and to just below the nipple line at the center of the chest for infants
- Chest compression to ventilation ratio increased to 30:2 for adult, child, and infant
- Rate of chest compressions standardized to 100 per minute for adult, child and infant with emphasis on the importance of hard and fast chest compressions
- An automatic external defibrillator (AED) recommendation of 1 shock immediately followed by 2 minutes of CPR (5 cycles)

AMERICAN HEART ASSOCIATION CHAIN OF SURVIVAL

The AHA chain of survival is a four-step course of action used to aid victims of sudden cardiac arrest, which can optimize their chance of survival and recovery. The links in the chain are:

1. Early access to care
2. Early CPR
3. Early defibrillation
4. Advanced care

PERSONAL WELLNESS

"The doctor of the future will give no medicine but will interest his patients in the care of the human frame, in diet, and in the cause and prevention of disease."

THOMAS EDISON

Today, many people are striving for personal wellness. A century ago, such a goal was unknown, and people counted themselves lucky just to survive. For example, a person born in 1890 could expect to live only 40 years. Infectious disease took the lives of many, and environmental conditions contributed to the spread of disease. Today our most serious health threats are chronic illnesses such as heart disease or cancer—diseases that we have the power to prevent. Personal wellness requires a holistic approach, or one that meets the physical, emotional, social, spiritual, and economic needs. It is something almost everyone can have, but achieving it requires knowledge, self-awareness, motivation, and effort.

Personal Hygiene

Personal wellness starts with good personal hygiene. It is important to shower or bathe and use deodorant on a regular basis. Teeth should be brushed and mouthwash used more than once a day, if possible. Hair should be clean and neatly combed. Fingernails should be clean, short, and neatly trimmed. Personal hygiene communicates a strong impression about an individual. A fresh, clean appearance without heavily scented lotions or colognes portrays health and instills confidence in employees and their patients and employers as well.

> **key • point** Phlebotomists should pay special attention to personal hygiene not only for optimal health, but also because their job involves close patient contact.

Proper Nutrition

"Let thy food be thy medicine, and thy medicine be thy food."

HIPPOCRATES, FATHER OF MEDICINE, 500 BC

Nutrition has been defined as the "act or process of nourishing." In other words, a food is nutritious if it supplies the nutrients the body needs "to promote growth and repair and maintain vital processes." The basic purpose of nutrition is to keep us alive, but more importantly, good nutrition provides what the body needs for energy and day-to-day functioning.

Physical health requires eating well. In this fast-paced world, few of us receive the nutrition we need. Even though what we eat is described as the good American diet, in reality, what we eat is not always nutritious. Our food is often so highly processed and chemically altered that it no longer promotes healthy bodies. The American Institute for Cancer Research (AICR) recently published a recommended diet to reduce the risk of cancer. They suggested that a person choose a predominantly plant-based diet rich in a variety of vegetables, fruits, legumes, and minimally processed starchy staple foods. A healthy diet contains the widest possible variety of natural foods. It provides a good balance of carbohydrates, fat, protein, vitamins, minerals, and fiber.

> **key • point** In general, the amount of food energy (calories) supplied by diet should not exceed the amount of energy expended, so that weight remains relatively constant over time.

Rest and Exercise

Personal wellness requires a nutritional diet, exercise, and getting the right amount of rest (Fig 3-20). Healthcare workers often complain of fatigue (physical or mental exhaustion). Fatigue brought on by physical causes is typically relieved by sleep. Lack of rest and sleep can lead to medical problems. The typical frantic pace in healthcare facilities today makes

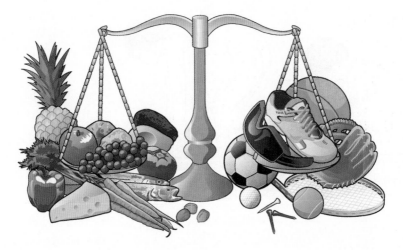

FIGURE 3-20

Wellness through proper nutrition, exercise, and rest.

it especially important to get the required hours of sleep and to take breaks during the day to rest, refresh, and stay fit.

Studies show that being physically fit increases the chance of staying healthy and living longer. The most accurate measurements of fitness consist of evaluating three components—strength (the ability to carry, lift, push, or pull a heavy load), flexibility (the ability to bend, stretch, and twist), and endurance (the ability to maintain effort for an extended period of time). No single measurement of performance classifies a person as fit or unfit. If a person becomes breathless after climbing a flight of stairs or hurrying to catch a bus but is otherwise healthy, clearly he or she could benefit from some form of conditioning or exercise.

Exercise contributes to improved quality of life on a day-to-day basis. It strengthens the immune system, increases energy, and reduces stress by releasing substances called endorphins, which create a peaceful state. People who exercise tend to relax more completely, even when under stress. Regular physical activity also appears to reduce symptoms of depression and anxiety and increase ability to perform daily tasks. Walking is a form of exercise that can be easily incorporated into almost anyone's life.

key • point If activity during work is low to moderate, AICR recommends that a person take an hour's brisk walk or similar exercise daily because there has been convincing evidence that physical activity helps prevent colon cancer.

Weight training is suggested as an excellent strength exercise. Studies have shown that using weights can build bone mass, even in the very elderly. For flexibility, yoga and Pilates are two forms of exercise that emphasize bending, stretching, and twisting. When choosing an exercise activity, it is most important is to pick one that is enjoyable so you are more apt to do it routinely.

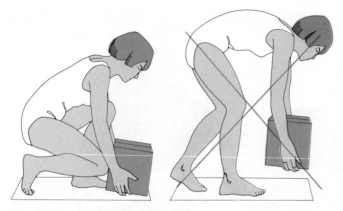

FIGURE 3-21
Lifting techniques.

Back Protection

A healthy back is necessary to lead an active and healthy life. The spine is designed to withstand everyday movement, including the demands of exercise. Improper lifting and poor posture habits, however, can reveal weaknesses. It is estimated that back injuries account for approximately 20% of all workplace injuries and illnesses. Lower back pain is a costly health problem that affects both industry and society in general. Strategies to prevent back injuries include instruction concerning back mechanics and lifting techniques (Fig. 3-21), lumbar support, and exercise. Exercise promotes strong backs; it improves back support and directly benefits the disks in the spinal column. Stress can make a person vulnerable to back problems because of muscle spasms. Keeping back muscles flexible with exercise can alleviate this stress reaction.

key • point Healthcare workers are at risk for back injury because of activities they are required to do (i.e., lift and move patients) and because of the stressful environment often associated with healthcare today.

Stress Management

Stress is a condition or state that results when physical, chemical, or emotional factors cause mental or bodily tension. It challenges our ability to cope or adapt. Stress is sometimes useful, keeping us alert and increasing our energy when we need it. Persistent or excessive stress, on the other hand, can be harmful.

Evidence suggests that "negative stress" (such as an emergency or an argument) has a damaging effect on personal wellness. Stressful situations are more likely to be damaging if they cannot be predicted or controlled. This fact is particularly apparent where job stress is concerned. Highly demanding jobs are much more stressful if an individual has no control over the workload, as is often the case in healthcare. Stress is more likely to have adverse effects on an individual if social support is lacking or there are personal or financial concerns. Although the signs of stress may not be immediately apparent, different organs and systems throughout the body are being affected. The immune system may be weakened, and other symptoms such as hypertension, ulcers, migraines, and nervous breakdowns may eventually result.

In the today's hectic healthcare environment it is necessary to manage stress to maintain personal wellness. Box 3-10 lists ways to deal with stress.

BOX • 3-10   Ways to Control Stress

- Identify your problem and talk about it with a close friend, partner, or the person at the source of the problem.
- Learn to relax throughout the day—close your eyes, relax your body, and clear your mind.
- Exercise regularly—develop a consistent exercise routine that you can enjoy.
- Avoid making too many changes at once—plan for the future to avoid simultaneous major changes.
- Spend at least 15 minutes a day thoroughly planning the time you have.
- Set realistic goals—be practical about what you can accomplish.
- Avoid procrastination by tackling the most difficult job first.

STUDY & REVIEW QUESTIONS

1. **Which of the following situations involves a nosocomial infection?**
   a. A patient admitted to the hospital with a severe urinary tract infection
   b. An employee who contracts HBV from a needlestick
   c. A patient in ICU whose surgical wound becomes infected
   d. A baby in the nursery with congenital herpes infection

2. **Reverse isolation may be used for**
   a. A pediatric patient with measles
   b. An adult patient with the flu
   c. A patient with a urinary tract infection
   d. A patient with severe burns

3. **The single most important means of preventing the spread of infection is**
   a. Proper hand antisepsis
   b. Wearing a mask
   c. Wearing gloves
   d. Infections cannot be prevented

4. **The most frequently occurring lab-acquired infection is**
   a. HBV infection
   b. HIV infection
   c. Syphilis
   d. Tuberculosis

5. **To destroy transient microorganisms when washing hands, use**
   a. Antiseptic soap
   b. Bleach solution
   c. Plain soap
   d. All of the above

6. **In the event of a body fluid splash in the eyes, the victim should immediately**
   a. Call the paramedics
   b. Flush eyes with water for 10 minutes
   c. Go to the emergency room
   d. Wipe the eyes with a tissue

7. **Which of the following items is PPE?**
   a. Biohazard bag
   b. Countertop splash shield
   c. Nonlatex gloves
   d. Sharps container

8. **All of the following examples of potential exposure to bloodborne pathogens involve a parenteral route of transmission** *except*
   a. A phlebotomist who cuts his hand on a broken tube of blood
   b. Blood leaking through the glove of a phlebotomist who has badly chapped hands
   c. Someone chewing gum while collecting blood specimens
   d. The technician in specimen processing rubbing her eye without washing her hands

9. **Specimen collection and processing area surfaces should be cleaned with**

   a. 70 % isopropyl alcohol

   b. 1:10 bleach solution

   c. Soap and water

   d. Any of the above

10. **Which of the following is a proper way to clean up a small blood spill that has dried on a counter top?**

   a. Moisten the spill with a disinfectant before carefully absorbing it with a paper towel

   b. Rub the spot with an alcohol pad; then wipe the area again with a clean alcohol pad

   c. Scrape the dried blood lose from the surface, brush it into a biohazard bag, and wash the surface with soap and water

   d. Wipe up the spot with a damp paper towel and clean the area in a circular motion using a disinfectant wipe

11. **Distance, time, and shielding are principles of**

   a. BBP safety

   b. Electrical safety

   c. Fire safety

   d. Radiation safety

12. **Safe working conditions are mandated by**

   a. CDC

   b. HazCom

   c. JCAHO

   d. OSHA

CASE · STUDY · 3-1

An Accident Waiting to Happen

A female blood drawer works alone in a clinic. It is almost time to close for lunch when a patient arrives for a blood test. The blood drawer is flustered because she has a special date for lunch. She is dressed up for the occasion, wearing a nice dress and high heels. She looks nice except for a large scratch on her left wrist that she got while playing with her cat that morning. She quickly draws the patient's blood. As she turns to put the specimen in a rack, she slips and falls. One of the tubes breaks. She does not get cut, but blood splashes everywhere, including her left wrist.

QUESTIONS

1. What is the first thing the phlebotomist should do?
2. How did the phlebotomist's actions contribute to this accident?
3. What should she have done that might have prevented the exposure, despite the tube breaking?
4. What type of exposure did she receive?

Bibliography and Suggested Readings

Linne, J., & Ringsrud, K. (1999). Clinical laboratory science, the basics and routine techniques (4th ed.). St. Louis: Mosby.

CDC: (1994). Guidelines for hand hygiene in health care settings. Department of Health and Human Services, Centers for Disease Control and Prevention.

Guidelines for preventing transmission of *Mycobacterium tuberculosis* in health-care facilities.

Hospital Infection Control Practices Advisory Committee (HICPAC) and CDC (1995) Guideline for isolation precautions in hospitals.

Larson, E. L, APIC Guidelines Committee. "APIC Guidelines for hand washing and hand antisepsis in health care setting" American Journal of Infection Control 1995;23:251–269.

Clinical and Laboratory Standards Institute, M29-A2. (2004). Protection of laboratory workers from occupationally acquired infections; approved guideline-(2nd ed.). Wayne, PA: CLSI/NCCLS.

Occupational Safety and Health Administration. (1991). Occupational exposure to bloodborne pathogens: final rule. 29CFR Part 1910.1030.

Occupational Safety and Health Administration. (2001). Occupational exposure to bloodborne pathogens: needlestick and other sharps injuries: final rule. 29 CFR Part 1910, Docket No. H370A, RIN 1218-AB85

Occupational Safety and Health Administration (OSHA): OSHA instruction. (2001). Enforcement procedures for the occupational exposure to bloodborne pathogens. Directives number CPL 2-2.69; Effective date 11/27/2001.

Overview of the Human Body

UNIT

II

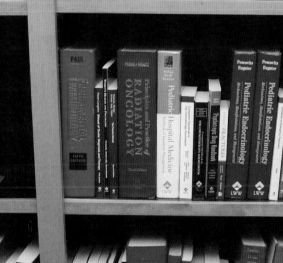
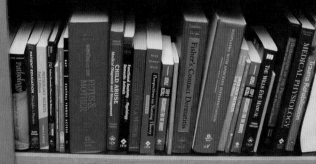
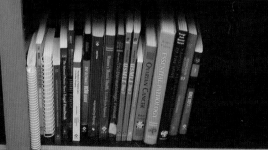

MEDICAL TERMINOLOGY

key • terms

combining form	prefix	word root
combining vowel	suffix	

objectives

Upon successful completion of this chapter, the reader should be able to:

1. Define the key terms listed at the beginning of this chapter.
2. Identify basic word elements individually and within medical terms.
3. State the meanings of common word roots, prefixes, and suffixes and identify unique plural endings.
4. State the meanings of medical terms composed of elements found in this chapter.
5. Demonstrate proper pronunciation of medical terms by using the general pronunciation guidelines found in this chapter.
6. State the meanings of common medical abbreviations listed in this chapter.
7. Identify items currently on the Joint Commission "Do Not Use" list and the list of items for possible future inclusion on the "Do Not Use" list.

Medical terminology is a special vocabulary of scientific and technical terms used in the healthcare professions to speak and write effectively and precisely. It is based on an understanding of a few basic word elements primarily derived from Greek and Latin words that are used to form most medical terms. Once the meanings of the word elements are known, the general meaning of most medical terms can be established. The basic word elements are word roots, prefixes, suffixes, and combining forms.

key • point To determine the meaning of a medical term start with the suffix, then go to the prefix, and identify the meaning of the word root or roots last.

WORD ROOTS

A **word root** (sometimes called a word stem) is the part of a medical term that establishes its basic meaning, and the foundation upon which the true meaning is built. The true meaning of a medical term is established by analyzing the other word elements such as prefixes and suffixes attached to the word root.

key • point A word root typically indicates a tissue, organ, body system, structure, substance, or condition. For example, the word root *phleb* means "vein," a body structure.

Some medical terms have more than one word root. The term *thrombophlebitis* is made up of the word root *phleb* and the word root *thromb* meaning "clot." In a few instances, a root will have several very different meanings. For example, the root *ped* appears in words derived from both Greek and Latin words for "foot" and the Greek word for "child." In addition, some words containing *ped* are derived from the Latin term *pediculus* meaning "lice." To establish the meaning of the root in these cases consider the context in which the word is used. Table 4-1 lists common medical word roots.

fyi Occasionally there will be both a Greek and Latin root with the same meaning. For example, the Greek root *nephr* and the Latin root *ren* both mean "kidney."

PREFIXES

A **prefix** is a word element that comes before a word root. A prefix modifies the meaning of the word root by adding information such as presence or absence, location, number, or size.

Example:	A/	NUCLEAR
	prefix	root
	(without)	(nucleus)

TABLE 4-1 Common Medical Word Roots

Root	Meaning	Example	Root	Meaning	Example
adip	fat	adipose	gluc	sugar, glucose	glucose
aer	air	aerobic	glyc	sugar, glucose	glycolysis
angi	vessel	angiogram	hem	blood	hemolysis
arteri	artery	arteriosclerosis	hemat	blood	hematology
arthr	joint	arthritis	hepat	liver	hepatitis
bili	bile	bilirubin	leuk	white	leukocyte
bronch	bronchus	bronchitis	lip	fat	lipemia
cardi	heart	electrocardiogram	my	muscle	myalgia
cephal	head	cephalic	necr	death	necrosis
chondr	cartilage	osteochondritis	nephr	kidney	nephritis
cry	cold	cryoglobulin	onc	tumor	oncologist
cutane	skin	percutaneous	oste	bone	osteoporosis
cyst	bladder	cystitis	path	disease	pathogen
cyt	cell	cytology	phleb	vein	phlebotomy
derm	skin	dermis	pulmon	lung	pulmonary
dermat	skin	dermatitis	ren	kidney	renal
encephal	brain	encephalitis	scler	hard	sclerotic
enter	intestines	enteritis	thromb	clot	thrombosis
erythr	red	erythrocyte	thorac	chest	thoracic
esophag	esophagus	esophagitis	tox	poison	toxicology
estr	female	estrogen	vas	vessel	vascular
fibrin	fiber	fibrinolysis	ven	vein	venipuncture
gastr	stomach	gastrointestinal			

The prefix *a-* means "without." The word root *nuclear* means nucleus. The word *anuclear* means "without a nucleus." Table 4-2 lists common medical prefixes.

SUFFIXES

A **suffix** is a word ending. It follows a word root and either changes or adds to the meaning of the word root. The best way to determine the meaning of a medical term is to first identify the meaning of the suffix.

Example: GASTR/   IC

              root   suffix

              (stomach)   (pertaining to)

The word root *gastr* means "stomach." The suffix *-ic* means "pertaining to." The word *gastric* means "pertaining to the stomach." Table 4-3 lists common medical suffixes.

> **key · point** When a suffix begins with **rh**, the **r** is doubled as in hemorrhage. When a suffix is added to a word ending in **x**, the **x** is changed to a **g** or **c** as in pharynx becoming pharyngeal and thorax becoming thoracic.

TABLE 4-2   Common Medical Prefixes

Prefix	Meaning	Example	Prefix	Meaning	Example
a-, an-, ar-	without	arrhythmia	hypo-	low, under	hypoglycemia
ana-	again, upward, back	anabolism	intra-	within	intramuscular
aniso-	unequal	anisocytosis	inter-	between	intercellular
anti-	against	antiseptic	iso-	equal, same	isothermal
bi-	two	bicuspid	macro-	large, long	macrocyte
bio-	life	biology	mal-	poor	malnutrition
brady-	slow	bradycardia	micro-	small	microcyte
cata-	down	catabolism	mono-	one	mononuclear
cyan-	blue	cyanotic	neo-	new	neonatal
dys-	difficult	dyspnea	poly-	many, much	polyuria
endo-	in, within	endothelium	post-	after	postprandial
epi-	on, over	epidermis	pre-	before	prenatal
exo-	outside	exocrine	per-	through	percutaneous
extra-	outside	extravascular	peri-	around	pericardium
hetero-	different	heterosexual	semi-	half	semilunar
homo-	same	homogeneous	sub-	below, under	subcutaneous
homeo-	same	homeostasis	tachy-	rapid	tachycardia
hyper-	too much, high	hypertension	tri-	three	tricuspid

TABLE 4-3   Common Medical Suffixes

Suffix	Meaning	Example	Suffix	Meaning	Example
-ac, -al	pertaining to	cardiac, neural	-megaly	enlargement	acromegaly
-algia	pain	neuralgia	-meter	instrument that measures or counts	thermometer
-ar, -ary	pertaining to	muscular, urinary	-ole	small	arteriole
-ase	enzyme	lipase	-oma	tumor	hepatoma
-centesis	surgical puncture to remove a fluid	thoracentesis	-osis	condition	necrosis
-cyte	cell	erythrocyte	-oxia	oxygen level	hypoxia
-emia	blood condition	anemia	-pathy	disease	cardiomyo-pathy
-gram	recording, writing	electrocardiogram	-penia	deficiency	leukopenia
-ia	state or condition	hemophilia	-pnea	breathing	dyspnea
-ic	pertaining to	thoracic	-poiesis	formation	hemopoiesis
-ism	state of or condition of	hypothyroidism	-rrhage	excess/abnormal flow	hemorrhage
-ist	one who specializes in	pharmacist	-spasm	twitch, involuntary muscle movement	arteriospasm
-itis	inflammation	tonsillitis	-stasis	stopping, controlling, standing	hemostasis
-rhage	bursting forth	hemorrhage	-tomy	cutting, incision	phlebotomy
-logist	specialist in the study of	cardiologist	-ule	small	venule
-lysis	breakdown, separation	hemolysis			

COMBINING VOWELS/FORMS

A **combining vowel** is a vowel (frequently an "o") that is added between two word roots or a word root and a suffix to make pronunciation easier. A word root combined with a vowel is called a **combining form**.

> **key • point** A combining vowel is not normally used when a suffix starts with a vowel. However, a combining vowel is kept between two word roots, even if the second root begins with a vowel.

Example 1:

GASTR /O/	ENTER /O/	LOGY
word root +	word root +	suffix
combining vowel	combining vowel	
(combining form)	(combining form)	
(stomach)	(intestines)	(study of)

The two word roots are combined by the vowel "o" to ease pronunciation, even though the second root *enter* begins with a vowel. The vowel "o" is also used between the word root *enter* and the suffix *-logy*. The term gastroenterology means "study of the stomach and intestines." The combining forms created are *gastro* and *entero*.

Example 2:

PHLEB/	ITIS
root	suffix
(vein)	(inflammation)

Because the suffix *-itis* begins with a vowel, a combining vowel is not used after the word root *phleb*. Phlebitis means "inflammation of a vein."

WORD ELEMENT CLASSIFICATION DISCREPANCIES

Medical terminology texts sometimes vary in the way they classify medical term word elements. Also, some word elements may be classified one way in one term and a different way in another term. For example, the word element *phasia*, which means "speech," is normally classified as a suffix. It functions as a word root, however, in the word *aphasia*, which means "without speech." Either way, the meaning is the same.

> **key • point** It is more important to be able to identify the meaning of a word element than to identify its classification.

UNIQUE PLURAL ENDINGS

The plural forms of some medical terms follow English rules. Others have **unique plural endings** that follow the rules of the Greek or Latin languages from which they originated. It is important to evaluate medical terms individually to determine the correct plural form. Table 4-4 lists the unique plural forms of typical singular medical term endings.

TABLE 4-4	Unique Plural Endings		
Word Ending	**Plural Ending**	**Singular Example**	**Plural Example**
-a	-ae	vena cava	vena cavae (ka've)
-en	-ina	lumen	lumina (lu'min-a)
-ex, -ix	-ices	appendix	appendices (a-pen'di-sez)
-is	-es	crisis	crises (kri'sez)
-nx	-nges	phalanx	phalanges (fa-lan'-jez)
-on	-a	protozoon	protozoa (pro''to-zo'a)
-um	-a	ovum	ova (o'va)
-us	-i	nucleus	nuclei (nu'kle-i)

PRONUNCIATION

Medical terms must be pronounced properly to convey the correct meaning, which can be changed by even one mispronounced syllable. Basic English pronunciation rules apply to most medical terms, and some may have more than one acceptable pronunciation. For example, hemophilia can be pronounced "he mo fil' e a" or "hem o fil' e a." In addition, some terms that are spelled differently are pronounced the same. For example, *ilium*, which means "hipbone," is pronounced the same as *ileum*, which means "small intestine." These terms can be confused when spoken rather than written. Verifying spelling eliminates confusion. General pronunciation guidelines are found in Table 4-5.

ABBREVIATIONS AND SYMBOLS

To save time, space, and paperwork, it is common practice in the healthcare professions to use abbreviations and symbols (such as objects and signs) to shorten words and phrases. Some of the most common abbreviations and symbols are listed in Tables 4-6 and 4-7, respectively.

TABLE 4-5	General Pronunciation Guidelines
Letter(s) Pronunciation Guideline Example(s)	

ae pronounce the second vowel only—chordae
c sounds like "s" if it precedes "e," "i," or "y" cell—circulation, cytology (in terms of Greek or Latin origin)
c has a hard sound if it precedes other vowels—capillary, colitis, culture
g sounds like "j" if it precedes "e," "i," or "y" (in terms of Greek or Latin origin)—genetic, *Giardia*, gyrate
g has a hard sound if it precedes other vowels—gallbladder, gonad, gut
ch often pronounced like a "k"—chloride, cholesterol
e may be pronounced separately if at the end of a term—syncope, diastole
es may be pronounced as a separate syllable if at the end of a term—nares
i pronounce like "eye" if at the end of a plural term—fungi, nuclei
ph pronounce with an "f" sound—pharmacy
pn pronounce the "n" sound only if at the start of a term—pneumonia
pn pronounce both letters separately if in the middle of a term—dyspnea, apnea
ps pronounce like "s"—pseudopod, psychology

TABLE 4-6　Common Abbreviations

Abbreviation	Meaning	Abbreviation	Meaning
ABGs	arterial blood gases	EBV	Epstein-Barr virus
ABO	blood group system	ECG	electrocardiogram
a.c.	before meals	EEG	electroencephalogram
ACTH	adrenocorticotropic hormone	EKG	electrocardiogram
ADH	antidiuretic hormone	ENT	ear, nose, and throat
ad lib	as desired	Eos	eosinophils
AIDS	acquired immunodeficiency syndrome	ER	emergency room
ALL	acute lymphocytic leukemia	ESR	erythrocyte sedimentation rate (sed rate)
ALT	alanine transaminase (see SGPT)	exc	excision
AML	acute myelocytic leukemia	FBS	fasting blood sugar
aq	water (aqua)	Fe	iron
AST	aspartate aminotransferase (see SGOT)	FSH	follicle stimulating hormone
		FUO	fever of unknown origin
ASO	antistreptolysin O	gluc	glucose
b.i.d.	twice a day (bis in die)	GI	gastrointestinal
bili	bilirubin	Gm, gm, g	gram
BP	blood pressure	GTT	glucose tolerance test
BUN	blood urea nitrogen	GYN	gynecology
Bx	biopsy	h	hour
C	with (cum)	Hb, Hgb	hemoglobin
Ca	calcium	HBsAg	hepatitis B surface antigen
CAD	coronary artery disease	HBV	hepatitis B virus
CBC	complete blood count	HCG	human chorionic gonadotropin
cc*	cubic centimeter	HCL	hydrochloric acid
CCU	coronary care unit	Hct	hematocrit (see crit)
chem	chemistry	HCV	hepatitis C virus
chemo	chemotherapy	HDL	high-density lipoprotein
CK	creatine kinase	Hg	mercury
cm	centimeter	HH (H & H)	hemoglobin and hematocrit
CML	chronic myelogenous leukemia	HIV	human immunodeficiency virus
CNS	central nervous system	h/o	history of
CO_2	carbon dioxide	H_2O	water
COPD	chronic obstructive pulmonary disease	h.s.	at bedtime (hora somni)
		hx	history
CPR	cardiopulmonary resuscitation	ICU	intensive care unit
crit	hematocrit (see HCT)	IM	intramuscular
C-section	cesarean section	IV	intravenous
CSF	cerebrospinal fluid	IVP	intravenous pyelogram
CT scan	computed tomography scan	K^+	potassium
CVA	cerebrovascular accident (stroke)	Kg	kilogram
CXR	chest x-ray	L	liter
DIC	disseminated intravascular coagulation	L	left
		Lat	lateral
diff	differential count of white blood cells	LD/LDH	lactic dehydrogenase
		LDL	low-density lipoprotein
dil	dilute	LE	lupus erythematosus (lupus)
DNA	deoxyribonucleic acid	lymphs	lymphocytes
DOB	date of birth	lytes	electrolytes
Dx	diagnosis		

*On the list of possible future additions to the "Do Not Use" list.

(continued)

TABLE 4-6 *(continued)*

Abbreviation	Meaning	Abbreviation	Meaning
m	meter	pt	patient
MCH	mean corpuscular hemoglobin	PVC	premature ventricular contraction
MCHC	mean corpuscular hemoglobin concentration	QNS, q.n.s.	quantity not sufficient
MCV	mean corpuscular volume	R	right
mcg	microgram	RA	rheumatoid arthritis
mets	metastases	RBC	red blood cell or red blood count (also rbc)
mg	milligram		
Mg^{++}	magnesium	req	requisition
MI	myocardial infarction	RIA	radioimmunoassay
mL	milliliter	R/O	rule out
mm	millimeter	RPR	rapid plasma reagin
mono	monocyte	RT	respiratory therapy
MRI	magnetic resonance imaging	RR	recovery room
MS	multiple sclerosis	Rx	treatment
Na^+	sodium	s̄	without
neg	negative	Sed rate	erythrocyte sedimentation rate (ESR)
NG	nasogastric		
NPO	nothing by mouth *(nulla per os)*	segs	segmented white blood cells
O_2	oxygen	SGOT	serum glutamic–oxaloacetic transaminase (see AST)
OB	obstetrics		
O&P	ova and parasite	SGPT	serum glutamic–pyruvic transaminase (see ALT)
OR	operating room		
oz	ounce	SLE	systemic lupus erythematosus
P	pulse; phosphorus	SMAC	sequential multiple analyzer computerized
Path	pathology		
p.c.	after meals	sol	solution
PCO_2	pressure of carbon dioxide in the blood	Staph	staphylococcus
		STAT, stat	immediately *(statum)*
Peds	pediatrics	STD	sexually transmitted disease
pH	hydrogen ion concentration (measure of acidity or alkalinity)	Strep	streptococcus
		Sx	symptoms
		T	temperature
PKU	phenylketonuria	T_3	triiodothyronine (a thyroid hormone)
PMNs	polymorphonuclear leukocytes		
PO_2	pressure of oxygen in the blood	T_4	thyroxine (a thyroid hormone)
p/o	postoperative	TB	tuberculosis
p.o.	orally (per os)	T cells	lymphocytes from the thymus
polys	polymorphonuclear leukocytes	T & C	type and crossmatch (type & x)
pos	positive	TIBC	total iron binding capacity
post-op	after operation	TPN	total parenteral nutrition (intravenous feeding)
PP	after a meal (postprandial)		
PPD	purified protein derivative (TB test)	TPR	temperature, pulse, and respiration
pre-op	before operation	Trig	triglycerides
prep	prepare for	TSH	thyroid-stimulating hormone
PRN, prn	as necessary *(pro re nata)*	Tx	treatment
PT	prothrombin time/protime	UA, ua	urinalysis
PTT	partial thromboplastin time	URI	upper respiratory infection

(continued)

TABLE 4-6 *(continued)*

Abbreviation	Meaning	Abbreviation	Meaning
UTI	urinary tract infection	W̶	water reactive
UV	ultraviolet	WBC, wbc	white blood cell
VCU	voiding cystourethrogram	wd	wound
VD	venereal disease	WT, wt	weight
VDRL	venereal disease research laboratory	y/o	years old

JOINT COMMISSION "DO NOT USE" LIST

To help reduce the number of medical errors related to incorrect interpretation of terminology, Joint Commission issued a minimum list of dangerous abbreviations, symbols, and acronyms that must be included on a **"Do Not Use" list** by every organization it accredits. Joint Commission also issued a list of additional abbreviations, acronyms, and symbols for possible future inclusion in the "Do Not Use" list.

fyi An Institute of Medicine (IOM) report in 1999 stated that between 44,000 and 96,000 deaths a year may be attributed to medical errors.

The list applies to all orders and all medication-related documentation that is handwritten, entered on computer, or written on preprinted forms. The list applies to handwritten laboratory reports, but does not apply to printed and electronic laboratory reports. Laboratories are also exempt from the ban on the use of trailing zeros when they are necessary to indicate the precision of test results. The Joint Commission "Do Not Use" list and possible future additions to the "Do Not Use" list are shown in Tables 4-8 and 4-9, respectively.

TABLE 4-7 Common Symbols

Symbol	Meaning	Symbol	Meaning
α	alpha	>*	greater than
β	beta	$\geq$	equal to or greater than
δ	delta	$\pm$	plus or minus, positive or negative
γ	gamma	®	registered trademark
λ	lambda	™	trademark
∞	infinity	#	number, pound
μ*	micron	%	percent
μg*	microgram (mcg)	Δ	heat
+	plus, positive	♀	female
−	minus, negative	♂	male
=	equals	↑	increase
<*	less than	↓	decrease
$\leq$	equal to or less than		

* On the list of possible future additions to the "Do Not Use" list.

TABLE 4-8   Joint Commission "Do Not Use" List

Do Not Use	Rationale	Replace with
IU	Mistaken for "IV" or "10" (ten)	Write "international unit"
U	Mistaken for "0"(zero), "4" (four), or "cc"	Write "unit"
MS	Can mean morphine sulfate or magnesium sulfate	Write "morphine sulfate" or "magnesium sulfate"
MSO_4 and $MgSO_4$	Can be confused with one another	Write "magnesium sulfate" or "morphine sulfate"
Q.D., QD, q.d., qd (daily)	Mistaken for each other	Write "daily"
Q.O.D., QOD., q.o.d, qod (every other day)	Period after the Q mistaken for "I" and the "O" mistaken for "I"	Write "every other day"
No leading zero (.X mg)	Decimal point is missed	Write 0.X mg
Trailing zero (X.0 mg) *	Decimal point is missed	Write X mg

* A trailing zero may be used when it is needed to show the level of precision of the value being reported as in laboratory test results, imaging reports on the size of lesions, and catheter/tube sizes.

TABLE 4-9   Possible Future Additions to the "Do Not Use" List

Do Not Use	Rationale	Replace with
> (greater than)	Misinterpreted as the number "7"	Write "greater than"
< (less than)	Misinterpreted as the letter "L" Confused with each other	Write "less than"
@	Mistaken for the number "2" (two)	Write "at"
Cc	Mistaken for "U" (units) if poorly written	Write "mL" or "milliliters"
μ	Mistaken for "mg" (milligrams) resulting in 1000-fold overdose	Write "mcg" or "micrograms"
Abbreviated drug names	Misinterpreted because many drugs have similar abbreviations	Write drug names in full
Apothecary units	Unfamiliar to many practitioners Confused with metric units	Use metric units

STUDY & REVIEW QUESTIONS

1. **A prefix**
   a. Comes before a word root and modifies its meaning
   b. Establishes the basic meaning of a medical term
   c. Follows a word root and adds to or changes its meaning
   d. Makes pronunciation of the term easier

2. **Which part of gastr/o/enter/o/logy is the suffix?**
   a. Enter
   b. Gastr
   c. Logy
   d. O

3. **To what part of the body does the word root *hepat* refer?**
   a. Head
   b. Heart
   c. Liver
   d. Stomach

4. **What does the suffix *-algia* mean?**
   a. Between
   b. Condition
   c. Disease
   d. Pain

5. **The plural form of atrium is**
   a. Atri
   b. Atria
   c. Atrial
   d. Atrices

6. **The medical term for red blood cell is**
   a. Erythrocyte
   b. Hepatocyte
   c. Leukocyte
   d. Thrombocyte

7. **Cystitis means**
   a. Blueness of the skin
   b. Cellular infection
   c. Inflammation of the bladder
   d. Pertaining to a cell

8. **The "e" is pronounced separately in**
   a. Diastole
   b. Syncope
   c. Systole
   d. All of the above

9. **The abbreviation NPO means**
   a. Negative patient outcome
   b. New patients only
   c. No parenteral output
   d. Nothing by mouth

10. **Which of the following abbreviations is on the current Joint Commission "Do Not Use" list?**
    a. cc
    b. IU
    c. mL
    d. UTI

CASE · STUDY · 4-1

Lab Orders

A physician orders ASAP blood cultures on an ER patient with a diagnosis of FUO.

QUESTIONS
1. When should the blood cultures be collected?
2. Where is the patient located?
3. What does the diagnosis abbreviation FUO mean?

CASE · STUDY · 4-2

Misinterpreted Instructions

A phlebotomy student was doing a clinical rotation with a laboratory in a medical clinic. A patient came in for a TB test. The phlebotomist in charge thought that it would be a good learning experience for the student to administer the test. The student was a little reluctant. The phlebotomist told her not to worry, wrote out the instructions shown below, and went about processing specimens that were ready to be centrifuged. Phlebotomist's instructions:

Choose a clean site on the inside of the arm below the elbow.

Draw .1 mL TB antigen into a tuberculin syringe.

Insert the needle just under the skin, and pull back the plunger slightly.

If you don't see blood slowly inject the antigen under the skin.

Remove the needle, but do not hold pressure or bandage the site.

The student filled the syringe with antigen. As she was injecting it into the patient, a large wheal started to form. She got scared and called the phlebotomist, who noticed that half the 1-cc syringe contained antigen. She instructed the student to pull the needle out immediately, telling her that she had used too much antigen.

QUESTIONS
1. Why would the student have used too much antigen?
2. How could the mistake have been prevented?
3. What else could have prevented the error?
4. What effect might the error have on the patient?

Bibliography and Suggested Readings

Collens, C. E. (2005). Medical terminology: the language of healthcare (2nd ed.). Philadelphia: Lippincott Williams & Wilkins.

Thomas, C. (2002). Taber's cyclopedic medical dictionary (19th ed.). Philadelphia: F. A. Davis.

Stedman's (2005) Medical dictionary for the health professions and nursing (5th ed.) Philadelphia: Lippincott Williams & Wilkins.

HUMAN ANATOMY AND PHYSIOLOGY REVIEW

key•terms

acidosis

alkalosis

alveoli

anabolism

anatomic position

anatomy

anterior

avascular

axons

body cavities

body plane

bursae

cartilage

catabolism

diaphragm

distal

dorsal

endocrine glands

exocrine glands

frontal plane

gametes

hemopoiesis

homeostasis

hormones

meninges

metabolism

mitosis

nephron

neuron

phalanges

physiology

pituitary gland

prone/pronation

proximal

sagittal plane

supine/supination

surfactant

synovial fluid

transverse plane

ventral cavities

objectives

Upon successful completion of this chapter, the reader should be able to:

1. Define the key terms and abbreviations listed at the beginning of this chapter.
2. Identify and describe body positions, planes, cavities, and directional terms.
3. Define homeostasis and the primary processes of metabolism.
4. Identify and describe the structural components of cells and the four basic types of body tissue.
5. Describe the function and identify the components or major structures of each body system.
6. List disorders and diagnostic tests commonly associated with each body system.

The human body consists of over 30 trillion cells, 206 bones, 700 muscles, approximately 5 L of blood, and about 25 miles of blood vessels. To fully appreciate the workings of this wonder, it is necessary to have a basic understanding of human **anatomy** (structural composition) and **physiology** (function). Knowledge of human anatomy and physiology (A & P) is also needed to understand the nature of the various disorders of the body and the rationale for the laboratory tests associated with them.

ANATOMIC POSITION

A person in the **anatomic position** is standing erect, arms at the side, with eyes and palms facing forward. When describing the direction or the location of a given point of the body, medical personnel normally refer to the body as if the patient is in the anatomic position, regardless of actual body position.

OTHER BODY POSITIONS

Two other body positions of particular importance to a blood drawer are **supine**, in which the patient is lying horizontal on the back with the face up, and **prone**, the opposite of supine, in which the patient is lying face down. The term prone also describes the hand with the palm facing down, a position sometimes used during blood collection.

fyi The act of turning the hand so that the palm faces down is called **pronation**. The act of turning the palm to face upward is called **supination**.

m e m o r y • j o g g e r   A way to equate supine with lying down is to think of the *ine* as in *recline*. To remember that a person who is supine is *face up,* look for the word *up* in supine.

BODY PLANES

A **body plane** (Fig. 5-1) is a flat surface resulting from a real or imaginary cut through a body in the normal anatomic position. Areas of the body are often referred to according to their location with respect to one of the following body planes:

- **Frontal (coronal) plane:** divides the body vertically into front and back portions.
- **Midsagittal (medial) plane:** divides the body vertically into equal right and left portions.
- **Sagittal plane:** divides the body vertically into right and left portions.
- **Transverse plane:** divides the body horizontally into upper and lower portions.

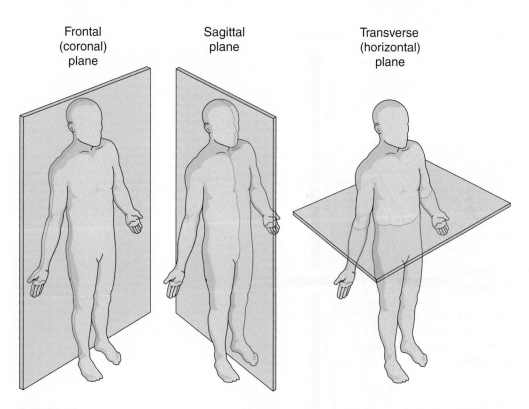

Frontal (coronal) plane   Sagittal plane   Transverse (horizontal) plane

FIGURE 5-1

Body planes. (Used with permission from Cohen, B. J. & Wood, D. L. Memmler's structure and function of the human body [7th ed.]. Philadelphia: Lippincott Williams & Wilkins, p. 7.)

fyi   A procedure called computerized axial tomography (CAT scan) produces x-rays in a transverse plane of the body. Magnetic resonance imaging (MRI) can produce images of the body in all three planes using electromagnetic waves instead of x-rays.

BODY DIRECTIONAL TERMS

Areas of the body are also identified using **directional terms** (Fig. 5-2). Directional terms describe the relationship of an area or part of the body with respect to the rest of the body or body part. Directional terms are often paired with a term that means the opposite. Table 5-1 lists common paired directional terms.

k e y • p o i n t   Directional terms are relative positions in respect to other parts of the body. For example, the ankle can be described as **distal** to the leg and **proximal** to the foot.

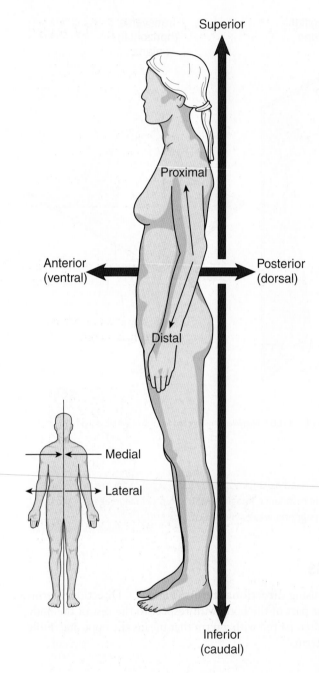

Superior

Proximal

Anterior
(ventral)

Posterior
(dorsal)

Distal

Medial

Lateral

Inferior
(caudal)

FIGURE 5-2

Directional terms. (Used with permission from Cohen, B. J. & Wood, D. L. Memmler's structure and function of the human body [7th ed.]. Philadelphia: Lippincott Williams & Wilkins, p. 6.)

TABLE 5-1   Common Paired Directional Terms

Directional Term and Meaning	Opposite Term and Meaning
Anterior (ventral): to the front of the body	Posterior (dorsal): to the back of the body
External (superficial): on or near the surface of the body	Internal (deep): within or near the center of the body
Medial: toward the midline or middle of the body	Lateral: toward the side of the body
Palmar: concerning the palm of the hand	Plantar: concerning the sole of the foot
Proximal: nearest the center of the body, origin, point of attachment	Distal: farthest from the center of the body, origin, or point of attachment
Superior (cranial): higher, or above or toward the head	Inferior (caudal): beneath, or lower or away from the head

BODY CAVITIES

Various organs of the body are housed in large, hollow spaces called **body cavities** (Fig. 5-3). Body cavities are divided into two groups, dorsal and ventral, according to their location within the body.

- **Dorsal cavities** are located in the back of the body and include the **cranial cavity**, which houses the brain, and the **spinal cavity**, which encases the spinal cord.

FIGURE 5-3

Lateral view of body cavities.   (Used with permission from Cohen, B. J. & Wood, D. L. Memmler's structure and function of the human body [7th ed.]. Philadelphia: Lippincott Williams & Wilkins, p. 8.)

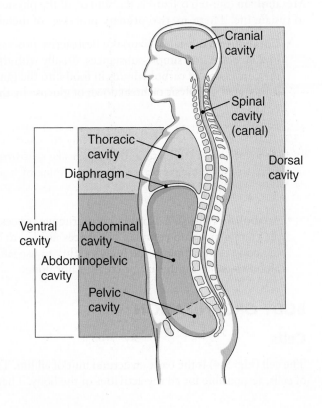

- **Ventral cavities** are located in the front of the body and include the **thoracic cavity**, which houses primarily the heart and lungs, the **abdominal cavity**, which houses numerous organs including the stomach, liver, pancreas, gallbladder, spleen, and kidneys, and the **pelvic cavity**, which houses primarily the urinary bladder and reproductive organs.

key • point   The thoracic cavity is separated from the abdominal cavity by a muscle called the **diaphragm**.

BODY FUNCTIONS

Homeostasis

The human body constantly strives to maintain its internal environment in a state of equilibrium or balance. This balanced or "steady state" condition is called **homeostasis** (ho'me-o-sta'sis), which literally translated means "standing the same." The body maintains homeostasis by compensating for changes in a process that involves feedback and regulation in response to internal and external changes.

Metabolism

Metabolism (me-tab'o-lizm) is the sum of all the physical and chemical reactions necessary to sustain life. There are two primary processes of metabolism: catabolism and anabolism.

- **Catabolism** (kah-tab'o-lizm) is a destructive process by which complex substances are broken down into simple substances, usually with the release of energy. An example is the conversion of carbohydrates in food into the glucose needed by the cells, and the subsequent glycolysis or breakdown of glucose by the cells to produce energy.

memory • jogger   A way to equate catabolism with breakdown is to remember that it begins with *cat* just like *catastrophe*. When something (your car, for example) breaks down, you often think of it as a catastrophe.

- **Anabolism** (ah-nab'o-lizm) is a constructive process by which the body converts simple compounds into complex substances needed to carry out the cellular activities of the body. An example is the body's ability to use simple substances provided by the bloodstream to synthesize or create a hormone.

BODY ORGANIZATION

Cells

The cell (Fig. 5-4) is the basic structural unit of all life. The human body consists of trillions of cells, responsible for all the activities of the body. There are many categories of cells, and

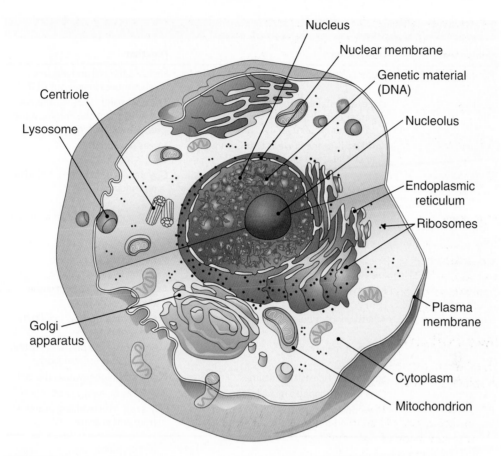

FIGURE 5-4

Cell diagram. (Used with permission from Cohen, B. J. & Wood, D. L. Memmler's structure and function of the human body [7th ed.]. Philadelphia: Lippincott Williams & Wilkins, p. 29.)

each category is specialized to perform a unique function. No matter what their function, however, all cells have the same basic structural components (Table 5-2).

key • point Most cells are able to duplicate themselves, which allows the body to grow, repair, and reproduce itself. When a typical cell duplicates itself, the DNA doubles and the cell divides by a process called **mitosis** (mi-to'sis).

Tissues

Tissues are groups of similar cells that work together to perform a special function. There are four basic tissue types: connective, **epithelial**, muscle, and nerve.

TABLE 5-2   Basic Structural Components of Cells

Component	Description	Function
Plasma membrane	Outer layer of a cell	Encloses the cell and regulates what moves in and out of it
Nucleus	Large, dark-staining organelle near the center of the cell and composed of DNA and protein	The command center of the cell that contains the chromosomes or genetic material
Nucleolus	Small body in the nucleus that is primarily RNA, DNA, and protein	Makes ribosomes
Chromosomes	Long strands of DNA organized into units called genes, occurring in humans in 26 identical pairs (46 individual)	Govern all cell activities, including reproduction
Cytoplasm	Substance within a cell composed of fluid (cytosol) and various organelles and inclusions	Site of numerous cellular activities
Organelles	Specialized structures within the cytoplasm	Varied, distinct functions depending on the type
Centrioles	Rod-shaped bodies close to the nucleus	Assist chromosome separation during cell division
Endoplasmic reticulum (ER)	A network of tubules	Synthesis and transport of lipids and proteins
Golgi apparatus	Layers of membranes	Makes, sorts, and prepares protein compounds for transport
Lysosomes	Small sacs of digestive enzymes	Digest substances within the cell
Mitochondria	Oval or rod-shaped organelles	Play a role in energy production
Ribosomes	Tiny bodies that exist singly, in clusters, or attached to ER	Play a role in assembling proteins from amino acids

- Connective tissue supports and connects all parts of the body and includes **adipose** (fat) tissue, **cartilage**, bone, and blood.
- Epithelial (ep-i-the'le-al) tissue covers and protects the body and lines organs, vessels, and cavities.
- Muscle tissue contracts to produce movement.
- Nerve tissue has the ability to transmit electrical impulses.

Organs

Organs are structures composed of tissues that function together for a common purpose.

BODY SYSTEMS

Body systems are structures and organs that are related to one another and function together. There are a number of different ways to group organs and structures together, and the number of body systems may vary in different textbooks. The following are 9 of 10 commonly recognized body systems. The tenth system, the circulatory system, is discussed in greater detail in Chapter 6.

Skeletal System

FUNCTIONS

The skeletal system is the framework that gives the body shape and support, protects internal organs, and with the muscular system provides movement and leverage. It is also responsible for calcium storage and **hemopoiesis** (he'mopoy-e'sis) or **hematopoiesis** (hem'a-to-poy-e'-sis), the production of blood cells that normally occurs in the bone marrow.

STRUCTURES

Skeletal system structures include all the bones (206), joints, and supporting connective tissue that form the skeleton (Fig. 5-5).

FIGURE 5-5

Human skeleton. (Used with permission from Cohen, B. J. & Wood, D. L. Memmler's structure and function of the human body [7th ed.]. Philadelphia: Lippincott Williams & Wilkins, p. 66.)

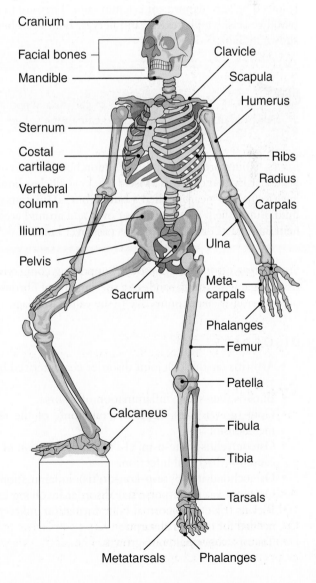

TABLE 5-3   Classification of Bones by Shape

Bone Shape	Examples
Flat	Rib bones and most skull (cranial) bones
Irregular	Back bones (vertebrae) and some facial bones
Long	Leg (femur, tibia, fibula), arm (humerus, radius, ulna), and hand bones (metacarpals, phalanges)
Short	Wrist (carpals) and ankle bones (tarsals)

Bones   Bones are a special type of dense connective tissue consisting of bone cells surrounded by hard deposits of calcium salts. They are living tissue with their own network of blood vessels, lymph vessels, and nerves. Bones can be classified by shape into four groups shown in Table 5-3.

key • point   Bones of particular importance in blood collection are the distal **phalanx** of the finger and the **calcaneus** or heel bone of the foot.

Joints   Joints are the junction or union between two or more bones. Freely movable joints have a cavity that contains a viscid (sticky) colorless liquid called **synovial fluid**. Some joints have a small sac nearby called a **bursa** (bur'sa) (pl. bursae) (bur'se) that is filled with synovial fluid. Bursae help ease movement over and around areas subject to friction, such as prominent joint parts or where tendons pass over bone.

Supporting Connective Tissue   Supporting connective tissue includes fibrous connective tissue, ligaments (thick bands of a special type of fibrous connective tissue), and a dense type of hard, nonvascular connective tissue called cartilage.

DISORDERS

- Arthritis (ar-thri'tis): joint disorder characterized by joint inflammation, pain, and swelling.
- Bursitis (bur-si'tis): inflammation of a bursa.
- Gout (gowt): joint disorder (commonly of the feet) caused by faulty uric acid metabolism.
- Osteomyelitis (os'te-o-mi'el-i'tis): inflammation of the bone (especially the marrow), caused by bacterial infection.
- Osteochondritis (os'te-o-kon-dri'tis): inflammation of the bone and cartilage.
- Osteoporosis (os'te-por-o'sis): disorder involving loss of bone density.
- Rickets (rik'ets): abnormal bone formation indirectly resulting from lack of vitamin D needed for calcium absorption.
- Tumors: abnormal bone growth.

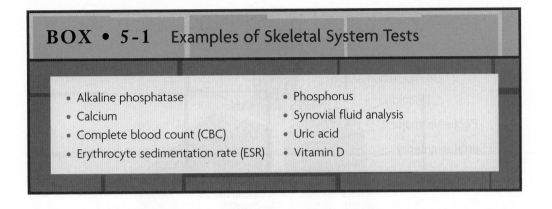

BOX • 5-1 Examples of Skeletal System Tests

- Alkaline phosphatase
- Calcium
- Complete blood count (CBC)
- Erythrocyte sedimentation rate (ESR)
- Phosphorus
- Synovial fluid analysis
- Uric acid
- Vitamin D

DIAGNOSTIC TESTS

Examples of diagnostic tests associated with the skeletal system are listed in Box 5-1.

Muscular System

FUNCTIONS

The muscular system (Fig. 5-6) gives the body the ability to move, maintain posture, and produce heat. It also plays a role in organ function and blood circulation.

> **key • point**   Skeletal muscle movement helps keep blood moving through your veins. For example, moving your arms helps move blood from your fingertips back to your heart.

STRUCTURES

The muscular system includes all the muscles of the body, of which there are three types: cardiac, skeletal, and smooth (visceral). Muscle type is determined by location, **histologic** (microscopic) cellular characteristics, and how muscle action is controlled (see Table 5-4).

DISORDERS

- Atrophy (at'ro-fe): decrease in size (wasting) of a muscle, usually due to inactivity.
- Muscular dystrophy (dis'tro-fe): genetic disease in which the muscles waste away or atrophy.
- Myalgia (mi-al'je-ah): painful muscle.
- Tendonitis (ten'dun-'tis): inflammation of muscle tendons, usually due to overexertion.

DIAGNOSTIC TESTS

Examples of diagnostic tests associated with the muscular system are listed in Box 5-2.

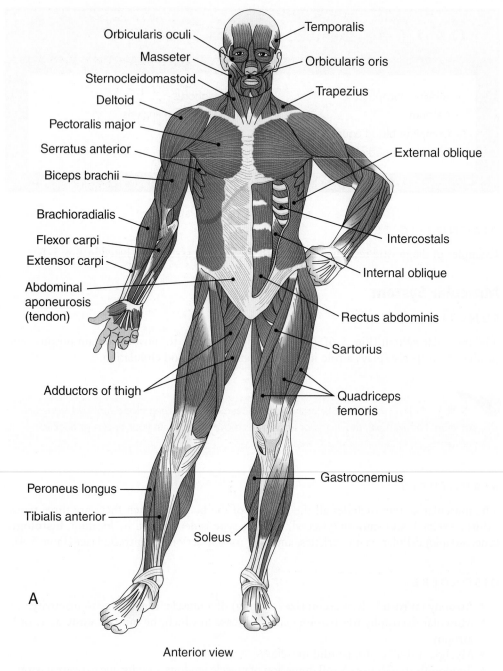

Orbicularis oculi
Masseter
Sternocleidomastoid
Deltoid
Pectoralis major
Serratus anterior
Biceps brachii

Brachioradialis
Flexor carpi
Extensor carpi
Abdominal aponeurosis (tendon)

Adductors of thigh

Peroneus longus
Tibialis anterior

Temporalis
Orbicularis oris
Trapezius

External oblique

Intercostals

Internal oblique

Rectus abdominis
Sartorius

Quadriceps femoris

Gastrocnemius

Soleus

A

Anterior view

FIGURE 5-6

Muscular system. **A.** Superficial muscles, anterior view. Associated structures are labeled in parentheses.

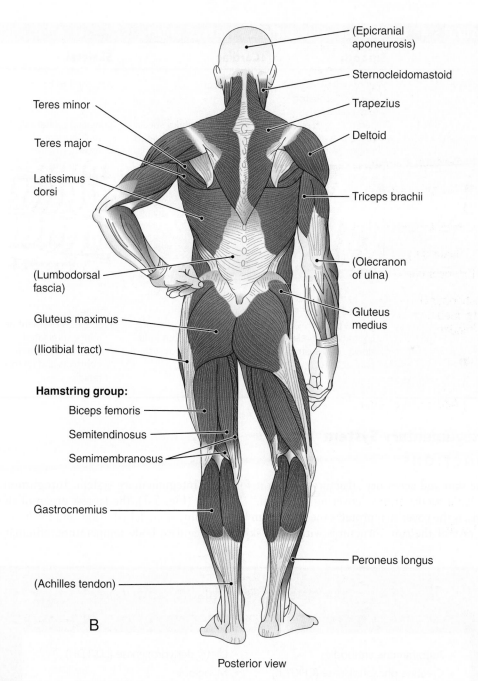

(Epicranial aponeurosis)

Sternocleidomastoid

Teres minor

Trapezius

Teres major

Deltoid

Latissimus dorsi

Triceps brachii

(Lumbodorsal fascia)

(Olecranon of ulna)

Gluteus maximus

Gluteus medius

(Iliotibial tract)

Hamstring group:

Biceps femoris

Semitendinosus

Semimembranosus

Gastrocnemius

Peroneus longus

(Achilles tendon)

B

Posterior view

FIGURE 5-6 *(Continued)*

B. Superficial muscles, posterior view. Associated structures are labeled in parentheses.

TABLE 5-4 Comparison of the Different Types of Muscle

	Smooth	Cardiac	Skeletal
Location	Wall of hollow organs, vessels, respiratory passageways	Wall of heart	Attached to bones
Cell characteristics	Tapered at each end, branching networks, nonstriated	Branching networks; special membranes (intercalated disks) between cells; single nucleus; lightly striated	Long and cylindrical; multinucleated heavily striated
	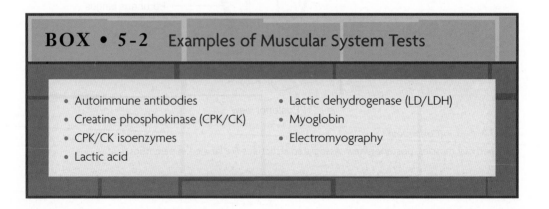		
Control	Involuntary	Involuntary	Voluntary
Action	Produces peristalsis; contracts and relaxes slowly; may sustain contraction	Pumps blood out of heart; self-excitatory but influenced by nervous system and hormones	Produces movement at joints; stimulated by nervous system; contracts and relaxes rapidly

Integumentary System

FUNCTIONS

The skin and accessory structures within it form the integumentary system. **Integument** (in-teg'u-ment) means "covering" or "skin." The skin (Fig. 5-7), the largest organ of the body, is the cover that protects the body from bacterial invasion, dehydration, and the harmful rays of the sun. Structures within the skin help regulate body temperature, eliminate

BOX • 5-2 Examples of Muscular System Tests

- Autoimmune antibodies
- Creatine phosphokinase (CPK/CK)
- CPK/CK isoenzymes
- Lactic acid
- Lactic dehydrogenase (LD/LDH)
- Myoglobin
- Electromyography

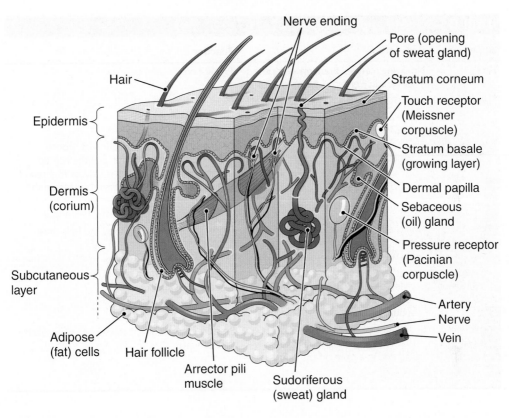

FIGURE 5-7

Cross section of the skin.   (Used with permission from Cohen, B. J. & Wood, D. L. Memmler's structure and function of the human body [10th ed.]. Philadelphia: Lippincott Williams & Wilkins, p. 102.)

small amounts of waste through sweat, receive environmental stimuli (sensation of heat, cold, touch, and pain), and manufacture vitamin D from sunlight.

STRUCTURES

The integumentary system consists of the skin and associated structures referred to as appendages (Table 5-5), which include **exocrine glands** (oil and sweat glands), hair, and nails. It also includes blood vessels, nerves, and sensory organs within the skin.

SKIN LAYERS

There are two main layers of the skin, the **epidermis** (ep'i-der'mis) and the **dermis**. The dermis lies on top of a layer of **subcutaneous** tissue.

Epidermis   The epidermis is the outermost and thinnest layer of the skin. It is primarily made up of **stratified** (layered), **squamous** (scalelike**)** epithelial cells. The epidermis is

	TABLE 5-5	Skin Appendages	
Appendage	**Description**		**Function**
Hair	Nonliving material primarily composed of **keratin** (ker'a-tin), a tough protein		Protection
Hair follicles	Sheaths that enclose hair and contain a bulb of cells at the base from which hair develops		Produce hair
Arrector pili	Tiny, smooth muscles attached to hair follicles		Responsible for the formation of "goose bumps" as they react to pull the hair up straight when a person is cold or frightened. When the muscle contracts it presses on the nearby sebaceous gland, causing it to release sebum to help lubricate the hair and skin
Nails	Nonliving keratin material that grows continuously as new cells form from the nail root		Protect the fingers and toes and help grasp objects
Sebaceous (oil) glands	Glands connected to hair follicles; called oil glands because they secrete an oily substance called **sebum** (se'bum)		Sebum helps lubricate the skin and hair to keep it from drying out
Sudoriferous (sweat) glands	Coiled dermal structures with ducts that extend through the epidermis and end in a pore on the skin surface		Produce perspiration, a mixture of water, salts, and waste

avascular, meaning it contains no blood or lymph vessels. The only living cells of the epidermis are in its deepest layer, the **stratum germinativum** (ger-mi-na-ti'vum), also called stratum **basale** (ba'sal'e), which is the only layer where mitosis (cell division) occurs. It is also where the skin pigment **melanin** is produced. Cells in the stratum germinativum are nourished by diffusion of nutrients from the dermis. As the cells divide they are pushed toward the surface, where they gradually die from lack of nourishment and become **keratinized** (hardened), which helps thicken and protect the skin.

Dermis   The dermis, also called corium or true skin, is the inner layer of the skin. It is much thicker than the epidermis and is composed of elastic and fibrous connective tissue. Elevations called **papillae** (pa-pil'e) and resulting depressions in the dermis where it joins the epidermis give rise to the ridges and grooves that form fingerprints. This area is often referred to as the **papillary dermis**. The dermis contains blood and lymph vessels, nerves, **sebaceous** (se-ba'shus) and **sudoriferous** (su-dor-if'er-us) **glands**, and **hair follicles**. These structures can also extend into the subcutaneous layer.

Subcutaneous   The **subcutaneous** (beneath the skin) **layer** is composed of connective and adipose (fat) tissue that connects the skin to the surface muscles.

fyi   Aging causes thinning of the epidermis, dermis, and subcutaneous layer. This makes the skin more translucent and fragile and leaves the blood vessels less well protected. As a result the elderly bruise more easily.

DISORDERS

- Acne (ak'ne): inflammatory disease of the sebaceous gland and hair follicles.
- Cancer (kan'ser): basal cell, squamous, melanoma.
- Dermatitis (der'ma-ti'tis): skin inflammation.
- Fungal infections: including tinea and ringworm.
- Herpes (her'pez): including cold sore or viral infection.
- Impetigo (im-pe-ti'go): staph or strep infection.
- Keloid (ke'loyd): fibrous tissue growth at a scar area.
- Pediculosis (pe-dik'u-lo'sis): lice infestation.
- Pruritus (proo-ri'tus): itching.
- Psoriasis (so-ri'a-sis): chronic skin condition of unknown origin characterized by clearly defined red patches of scaly skin.

DIAGNOSTIC TESTS

Examples of diagnostic tests associated with the integumentary system are listed in Box 5-3.

BOX • 5-3   Examples of Integumentary System Tests

- Biopsy
- Microbiology cultures
- Skin scrapings for fungal culture
- Skin scrapings for KOH (potassium hydroxide) preparation
- Tissue cultures

Nervous System

FUNCTIONS

The nervous system (Fig. 5-8) controls and coordinates activities of the various body systems by means of electrical impulses and chemical substances sent to and received from all parts of the body. The nervous system has two functional divisions, the somatic nervous system and the autonomic nervous system, identified by the type of control (voluntary or involuntary), and according to the type of tissue stimulated (Table 5-6).

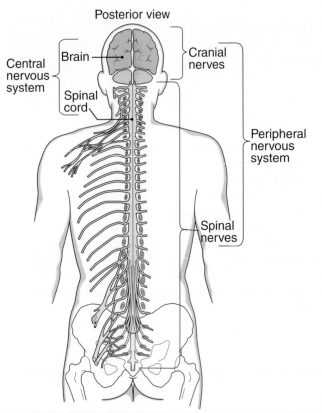

Posterior view

Central nervous system

Brain

Spinal cord

Cranial nerves

Peripheral nervous system

Spinal nerves

FIGURE 5-8

Structural divisions of the nervous system. (Used with permission from Cohen, B. J. & Wood, D. L. Memmler's structure and function of the human body [10th ed.]. Philadelphia: Lippincott Williams & Wilkins, p.187.)

STRUCTURES

The fundamental unit of the nervous system is the **neuron** (Fig. 5-9). The two main structural divisions of the nervous system are the **central nervous system (CNS)** and the **peripheral nervous system (PNS)**.

Neurons   Neurons are highly complex cells that are capable of conducting messages in the form of impulses that enable the body to interact with its internal and external environment.

TABLE 5-6   Functional Nervous System Divisions

Division	Function	Type of Control	Tissue Stimulated
Autonomic	Conducts impulses that affect activities of the organs, vessels, and glands	Involuntary	Cardiac muscle, smooth muscle, and glands
Somatic	Conducts impulses that allow an individual to consciously control skeletal muscles	Voluntary	Skeletal muscle

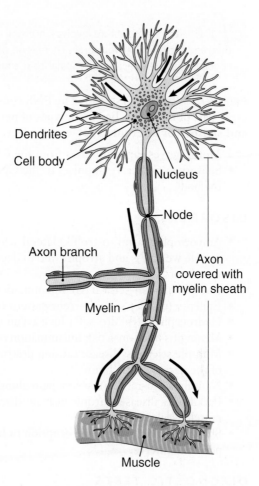

FIGURE 5-9

Diagram of a motor neuron. The break in the axon denotes length. The *arrows* show the direction of the nerve impulse.   (Used with permission from Cohen, B. J. & Wood, D. L. Memmler's structure and function of the human body [10th ed.]. Philadelphia: Lippincott Williams & Wilkins, p. 181.)

Labels in figure: Dendrites, Cell body, Nucleus, Node, Axon branch, Axon covered with myelin sheath, Myelin, Muscle

Neurons have a cell body containing a nucleus and organelles typical of other cells, but are distinguished by unique threadlike fibers called **dendrites** and **axons** that extend out from the cell body. The dendrites carry messages to the nerve cell body, while axons carry messages away from it.

Central Nervous System   The CNS consists of the brain, the nervous system command center that interprets information and dictates responses, and the spinal cord. Every part of the body is in direct communication with the CNS by means of its own set of nerves, which come together in one large trunk that forms the spinal cord.

The brain and spinal cord are surrounded and cushioned by a cavity filled with a clear, plasmalike fluid called **cerebrospinal** (ser'e-bro-spi'nal) **fluid (CSF).** The cavity is completely enclosed and protected by three layers of connective tissue called the **meninges** (me-nin'jez). When CSF is needed for testing, a physician performs a **lumbar puncture** (spinal tap) to enter the cavity and obtain a CSF sample.

fyi Lumbar puncture involves inserting a hollow needle into the space between the third and forth lumbar vertebrae. There is no danger of injuring the spinal cord with the needle in this area because the spinal cord ends at the first lumbar vertebra.

Peripheral Nervous System　The PNS consists of all the nerves that connect the CNS to every part of the body. Two main types of nerves are **motor** or **efferent** (ef'fer-ent) **nerves and sensory or afferent (a'fer-ent) nerves.**

- Motor nerves carry impulses from the CNS to organs, glands, and muscles.
- Sensory nerves carry impulses to the CNS from sensory receptors in various parts of the body.

DISORDERS

- Amyotrophic (a-mi'-o-tro'fik) lateral sclerosis (skle-ro'sis)(ALS): a disease involving muscle weakness and atrophy due to degeneration of portions of the brain and spinal cord.
- Encephalitis (en-sef-a-li'tis): inflammation of the brain.
- Epilepsy (ep'i-lep'se): recurrent pattern of seizures.
- Hydrocephalus (hi'dro-sef'a-lus): accumulation of cerebrospinal fluid in the brain.
- Meningitis (men-in-ji'tis): inflammation of the membranes of the spinal cord or brain.
- Multiple sclerosis: disease causing destruction of the myelin sheath (fatlike covering) of the nerves of the brain.
- Neuralgia (nu-ral'je-a): severe pain along a nerve.
- Parkinson's disease: chronic nervous disease characterized by fine muscle tremors and muscle weakness.
- Shingles (shing'gelz): acute eruption of herpes blisters along the course of a peripheral nerve.

DIAGNOSTIC TESTS

Examples of nervous system diagnostic tests are listed in Box 5-4.

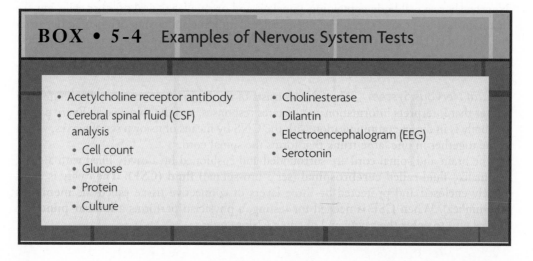

BOX • 5-4　Examples of Nervous System Tests

- Acetylcholine receptor antibody
- Cerebral spinal fluid (CSF) analysis
  - Cell count
  - Glucose
  - Protein
  - Culture
- Cholinesterase
- Dilantin
- Electroencephalogram (EEG)
- Serotonin

Endocrine System

FUNCTIONS

The word **endocrine** comes from the Greek words *endon*, meaning "within" and *"krinein,"* meaning "to secrete." The endocrine system (Fig. 5-10) consists of a group of ductless glands that secrete substances called **hormones** directly into the bloodstream. Hormones are powerful chemical substances that have a profound effect on many body processes such as metabolism, growth and development, reproduction, personality, and the ability of the body to react to stress and resist disease.

STRUCTURES

Endocrine system structures include various hormone secreting glands and other organs and structures that have endocrine function. The **pituitary** (pi-tu'i-tar-ee) **gland** is often called the master gland of this system because it secretes hormones that stimulate the

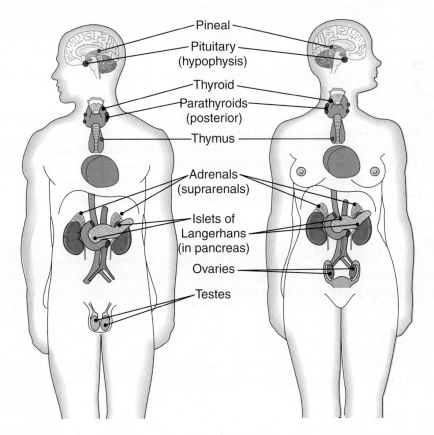

Pineal
Pituitary
(hypophysis)
Thyroid
Parathyroids
(posterior)
Thymus
Adrenals
(suprarenals)
Islets of
Langerhans
(in pancreas)
Ovaries
Testes

FIGURE 5-10

Endocrine system.   (Used with permission from Cohen, B. J. & Wood, D. L. Memmler's structure and function of the human body [7th ed.]. Philadelphia: Lippincott Williams & Wilkins, p. 166.)

other glands. However, release of hormones by the pituitary is actually controlled by chemicals called releasing hormones sent from the hypothalamus of the brain. Table 5-7 lists the various hormone secreting glands and organs, their location in the body, the major hormones they secrete, and the principal function of each hormone.

fyi   Interesting facts about hormones:

- Adrenal hormones adrenaline and noradrenaline are known as the "fight-or-flight" hormones because of their effects when the body is under stress. They act by increasing blood pressure, heart activity, metabolism, and glucose release, permitting the body to do an extraordinary amount of work.
- Because the pineal hormone melatonin plays a role in promoting sleep, travelers sometimes take melatonin pills to help overcome the effects of jet lag brought on by crossing different time zones.
- Production of thyroid hormones requires the presence of adequate amounts of iodine in the blood. Iodine was first added to salt to prevent goiter, an enlargement of the thyroid gland sometimes caused by a lack of iodine in the diet.

Other Structures with Endocrine Function   There are a number of other body structures with endocrine function. For example:

- The heart ventricles secrete a hormone called B-type natriuretic peptide (BNP) in response to volume expansion and pressure overload.
- The kidneys secrete erythropoietin (e-rith'ro-poy'e-tin), which stimulates red blood cell production when oxygen levels are low.
- The lining of the stomach secretes a hormone that stimulates digestion.
- The placenta secretes several hormones that function during pregnancy.

key • point   Pregnancy tests are based on a reaction with a hormone called **human chorionic** (ko-re-on'ik) **gonadotropin** (gon-ah-do-tro'pin) (hCG) secreted by embryonic cells that eventually give rise to the placenta.

DISORDERS

Endocrine disorders are most commonly caused by tumors, which can cause either **hypersecretion** (secreting too much) or **hyposecretion** (secreting too little) of the gland.

Pituitary Disorders

- Acromegaly (ak'ro-meg'a-le): overgrowth of the bones in the hands, feet, and face caused by excessive GH in adulthood.

TABLE 5-7 Endocrine Glands

Gland	Location	Hormone	Principle Function
Pituitary (pi-tu'i-tar-ee)	In the brain	Adrenocorticotropic (ad-re'no-kor'ti-ko-trop'ik) hormone (ACTH)	Stimulates the adrenal glands
		Antidiuretic (an'ti-di-u-ret'ik) hormone (ADH)	Decreases urine production
		Follicle-stimulating hormone (FSH)	Stimulates development of ova and sperm and the secretion of reproductive hormones
		Growth hormone (GH)	Regulates growth
		Thyroid-stimulating hormone (TSH)	Controls thyroid activity
Pineal (pin'eal)	In the brain, posterior to the pituitary	Melatonin	Helps set diurnal (daily) rhythm with levels lowest around noon and peaking at night; thought to play a role in seasonal affective disorder (SAD)
Thyroid (thi'royd)	In the throat near the larynx	Calcitonin (kal'si-to'nin)	Lowers blood calcium levels
		Triiodothyronine (tri-i-o-do-thi'ro-nin) or T_3	Increases metabolic rate
		Thyroxine (thi-roks'in) or T_4	Increases metabolic rate
Parathyroids (par-a-thi'royds)	In the throat behind the thyroid gland, two on each side	Parathyroid hormone (PTH)	Regulates calcium exchange between blood and bones; increases blood calcium levels
Thymus (thi'mus)	In the chest behind the sternum (breastbone	Thymosin (thi'mo-sin)	Promotes maturation of specialized WBCs called T lymphocytes (T cells) and the development of immunity
Adrenals	One on top of each kidney	Epinephrine (ep-i-nef'rin), also called adrenalin (a-dren'a-lin)	Increases blood pressure, heart rate, metabolism, and release of glucose
		Norepinephrine, also called noradrenaline	Increases blood pressure, heart rate, metabolism, and release of glucose
		Cortisol (kor'ti-sol)	Active during stress, aids carbohydrate, protein, and fat metabolism
		Aldosterone (al-dos'ter-on)	Helps the kidneys regulate sodium and potassium in the bloodstream
Islets (i'lets) of Langer-hans (lahng'er-hanz)	Pancreas	Insulin	Needed for movement of glucose into the cells and decreases blood glucose levels
		Glucagon (gloo'ka-gon)	Increases blood glucose levels by stimulating the liver to release glucose (stored as glycogen) into the bloodstream

(continued)

TABLE 5-7	(continued)		
Gland	**Location**	**Hormone**	**Principle Function**
Testes	Scrotum	Testosterone (tes-tos'ter-on)	Stimulates growth and functioning of the male reproductive system and development of male sexual characteristics
Ovaries	Pelvic cavity	Estrogens (es'tro-jens)	Stimulates growth and functioning of the female reproductive system and development of female sexual characteristics
		Progesterone (pro'jes-ter-on)	Prepares the body for pregnancy

- Diabetes insipidus (di'a-be'tez in-sip'id-us): condition characterized by increased thirst and increased urine production caused by inadequate secretion of ADH, also called **vasopressin** (vas'o-pres'in).
- Dwarfism: condition of being abnormally small, one cause of which is growth hormone (GH) deficiency in infancy.
- Gigantism: excessive development of the body or of a body part due to excessive GH.

Thyroid Disorders

- Congenital hypothyroidism: insufficient thyroid activity in a newborn, from either a genetic deficiency or maternal factors such as lack of dietary iron during pregnancy.
- Cretinism (kre'tin-izm): severe untreated congenital hypothyroidism in which the development of the child is impaired, resulting in a short, disproportionate body, thick tongue and neck, and mental handicap.
- Goiter (goy'ter): enlargement of the thyroid gland.
- Hyperthyroidism (Graves' disease): condition characterized by weight loss, nervousness, and protruding eyeballs, due to an increased metabolic rate caused by excessive secretion of the thyroid gland.
- Hypothyroidism: condition characterized by weight gain and lethargy due to a decreased metabolic rate caused by decreased thyroid secretion.
- Myxedema (hypothyroid syndrome): condition characterized by anemia, slow speech, mental apathy, drowsiness, and sensitivity to cold, resulting from decreased functioning of the thyroid gland.

Parathyroid Disorders
Hypersecretion of the parathyroids can lead to kidney stones and bone destruction. Hyposecretion can cause muscle spasms and convulsions.

Adrenal Disorders

- Addison's disease: condition characterized by weight loss, dehydration, and hypotension (abnormally low blood pressure) caused by decreased glucose and sodium levels due to hyposecretion of the adrenal glands.

- Aldosteronism: condition characterized by hypertension (high blood pressure) and edema caused by excessive sodium and water retention due to hypersecretion of aldosterone.
- Cushing's syndrome: condition characterized by a swollen, "moon-shaped" face and redistribution of fat to the abdomen and back of the neck caused by an excess of cortisone.

Pancreatic Disorders

- Diabetes mellitus (di'a-be'tez mel-i-tus): condition in which there is impaired carbohydrate, fat, and protein metabolism due to a deficiency of insulin.
- Diabetes mellitus type I or insulin-dependent diabetes mellitus (IDDM): type of diabetes in which the body is totally unable to produce insulin. This type is often called juvenile-onset diabetes because it usually appears before 25 years of age.
- Diabetes mellitus type II or non-insulin-dependent diabetes mellitus (NIDDM): type of diabetes in which the body is able to produce insulin, but either the amount produced is insufficient or there is impaired use of the insulin produced. This type of diabetes occurs predominantly in adults.
- Hyperglycemia (hi'per-gli-se'me-a): Increased blood sugar that often precedes diabetic coma if not treated.
- Hyperinsulinism: Too much insulin in the blood due to excessive secretion of insulin or an overdose of insulin (insulin shock).
- Hypoglycemia (hi'po-gli-se'me-a): Abnormally low glucose (blood sugar) often due to hyperinsulinism.

DIAGNOSTIC TESTS

Examples of diagnostic tests associated with the endocrine system are listed in Box 5-5.

BOX • 5-5　Examples of Endocrine System Tests

- Adrenocorticotropic hormone (ACTH)
- Aldosterone
- Antidiuretic hormone (ADH)
- Cortisol
- Erythropoietin
- Glucagon
- Glucose tolerance test (GTT)
- Glycosylated hemoglobin
- Growth hormone (GH)
- Insulin level
- Thyroid function studies:
  - T_3 (triiodothyronine)
  - T_4 (thyroxine)
  - TSH (thyroid-stimulating hormone)

Digestive System

FUNCTIONS

The digestive system (Fig. 5-11) provides the means by which the body takes in food, breaks it down into usable components for absorption, and eliminates waste products from this process.

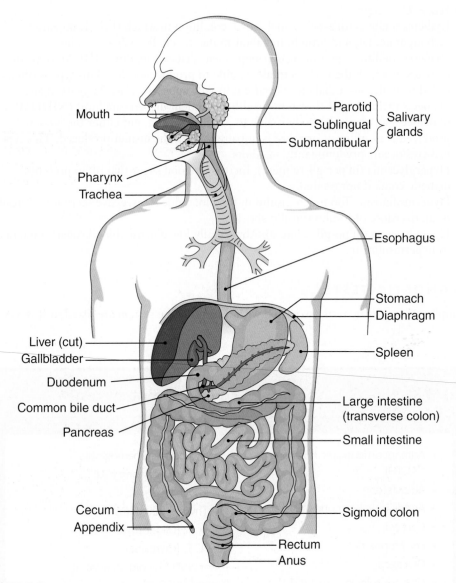

FIGURE 5-11

Digestive system. (Used with permission from Cohen, B. J. & Wood, D. L. Memmler's structure and function of the human body [10th ed.]. Philadelphia: Lippincott Williams & Wilkins, p. 389.)

STRUCTURES

The digestive system components form a continuous passageway called the digestive or **gastrointestinal (GI) tract**, which extends from the mouth to the anus through the **pharynx**, **esophagus**, stomach, and small and large intestines.

ACCESSORY ORGANS AND STRUCTURES

The digestive system also includes and is assisted by a number of accessory organs and structures: lips, teeth, tongue, **salivary glands**, **liver**, **pancreas**, and **gallbladder**.

ACCESSORY ORGAN FUNCTIONS

The lips, teeth, and tongue aid in chewing and swallowing food. The salivary glands secrete saliva, a substance that moistens food and also contains an enzyme that begins the process of starch digestion. Important digestive functions of the liver include glycogen storage, protein catabolism, detoxification of harmful substances, and the secretion of bile necessary for the digestion of fat. Bile is concentrated and stored in the gallbladder. Digestive functions of the pancreas include the secretion of insulin and glucagon and the production of digestive enzymes, including **amylase**, **lipase**, and **trypsin**.

DISORDERS

- Appendicitis (a-pen'di-si'tis): inflammation of the appendix.
- Cholecystitis (ko'le-sis-ti'tis): inflammation of the gallbladder.
- Colitis (ko-li'tis): inflammation of the colon.
- Diverticulosis (di'ver-tik'u-lo'sis): pouches in the walls of the colon.
- Gastritis (gas-tri'tis): inflammation of the stomach lining.
- Gastroenteritis (gas'tro-en-ter-i'tis): inflammation of the stomach and intestinal tract.
- Hepatitis (hep'a-ti'tis): inflammation of the liver.
- Pancreatitis (pan'kre-a-ti'tis): inflammation of the pancreas.
- Peritonitis (per'i-to-ni'tis): inflammation of the abdominal cavity lining.
- Ulcer: open sore or lesion.

fyi   Some stomach ulcers are caused by the *Helicobacter pylori* microorganism and are treated with antibiotics in addition to antacids.

DIAGNOSTIC TESTS

Examples of diagnostic tests associated with the gastrointestinal tract of the digestive system are listed in Box 5-6. Examples of tests associated with the accessory organs of the digestive system are listed in Box 5-7.

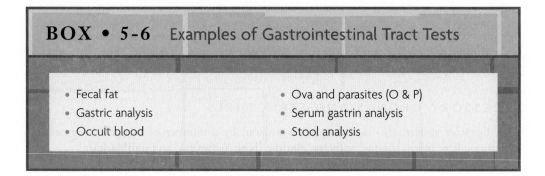

BOX • 5-6 Examples of Gastrointestinal Tract Tests

- Fecal fat
- Gastric analysis
- Occult blood
- Ova and parasites (O & P)
- Serum gastrin analysis
- Stool analysis

Reproductive System

FUNCTIONS

The reproductive system (Fig. 5-12) produces the **gametes** (gam'eets), **sex** or **germ cells**, that are needed to form a new human being. In males, the gametes are called **spermatozoa** (sper'mat-o-zo'a), or sperm. In females, the gametes are called **ova** (o'va), or eggs. Reproduction occurs when an **ovum** (singular of ova) is fertilized by a sperm.

STRUCTURES

The reproductive system consists of glands called **gonads** (go'nads) and their associated structures and ducts. The gonads manufacture and store the gametes and produce hormones (see Endocrine System) that regulate the reproductive process.

Structures of the female reproductive system include the ovaries (female gonads), fallopian (fa-lo'pe-an) tubes, uterus, cervix, vagina, and vulva.

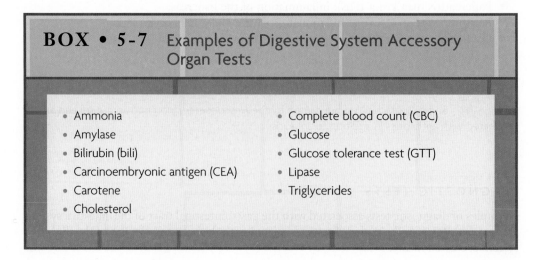

BOX • 5-7 Examples of Digestive System Accessory Organ Tests

- Ammonia
- Amylase
- Bilirubin (bili)
- Carcinoembryonic antigen (CEA)
- Carotene
- Cholesterol
- Complete blood count (CBC)
- Glucose
- Glucose tolerance test (GTT)
- Lipase
- Triglycerides

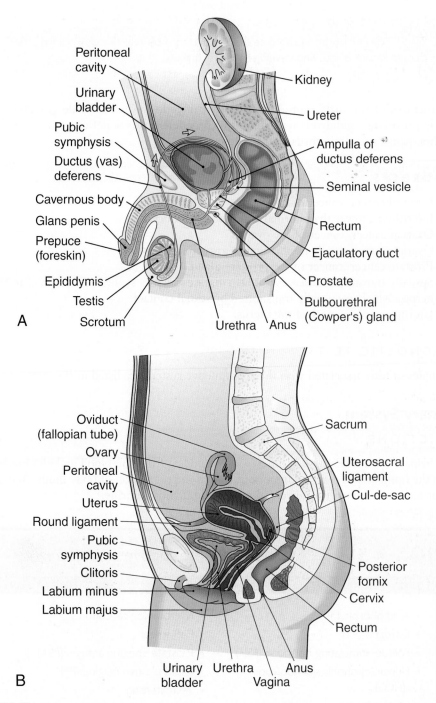

FIGURE 5-12

Reproductive system. **A.** Male. **B.** Female. (Used with permission from Cohen, B. J. & Wood, D. L. Memmler's structure and function of the human body [7th ed.]. Philadelphia: Lippincott Williams & Wilkins, pp. 314, 321.)

Structures of the male reproductive system include the testes (male gonads), seminal vesicles, prostate, epididymis (ep'i-did'i-mis), vas deferens (vas def'er-enz), seminal ducts, urethra, penis, spermatic cords, and scrotum.

DISORDERS

- Cervical cancer: cancer of the cervix.
- Infertility: a lower than normal ability to reproduce.
- Ovarian cancer: cancer of the ovaries.
- Ovarian cyst: a usually nonmalignant growth in an ovary.
- Prostate cancer: cancer of the prostate gland.
- Sexually transmitted diseases (STDs): diseases such as syphilis, gonorrhea, and genital herpes, which are usually transmitted by sexual contact.
- Uterine cancer: cancer of the uterus.

DIAGNOSTIC TESTS

Examples of tests associated with the reproductive system are listed in Box 5-8.

Urinary System

FUNCTIONS

The urinary system (Fig. 5-13) filters waste products from the blood and eliminates them from the body. It also plays an important role in the regulation of body fluids. Activities of the urinary system result in the creation and elimination of urine.

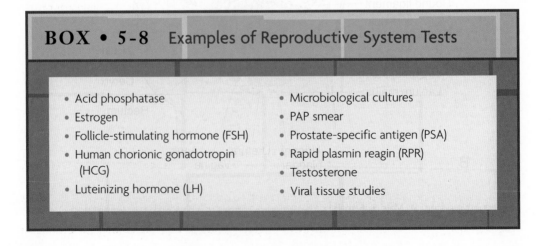

BOX • 5-8 Examples of Reproductive System Tests

- Acid phosphatase
- Estrogen
- Follicle-stimulating hormone (FSH)
- Human chorionic gonadotropin (HCG)
- Luteinizing hormone (LH)
- Microbiological cultures
- PAP smear
- Prostate-specific antigen (PSA)
- Rapid plasmin reagin (RPR)
- Testosterone
- Viral tissue studies

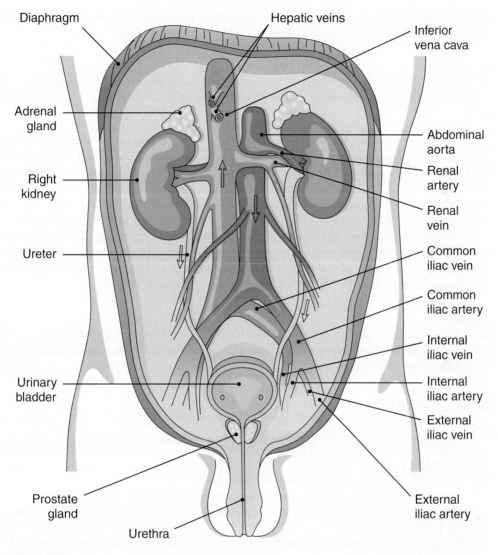

FIGURE 5-13

Urinary system (male). (Used with permission from Cohen, B. J. & Wood, D. L. Memmler's structure and function of the human body [7th ed.]. Philadelphia: Lippincott Williams & Wilkins, p. 294.)

STRUCTURES

The main structures of the urinary system are two **kidneys**, two **ureters**, a **urinary bladder**, and a **urethra**.

The kidneys are bean-shaped organs located at the back of the abdominal cavity, just above the waistline, one on each side of the body. The kidneys help maintain water and electrolyte balance and eliminate urea (a waste product of protein metabolism). They also produce erythropoietin, a hormone that stimulates red blood cell production, and the enzyme renin, which plays a role in regulating blood pressure.

fyi Electrolytes include sodium, potassium, chloride, bicarbonate, and calcium ions and are essential to normal nerve, muscle, and heart activity.

The functional or basic working unit of the kidney is the **nephron**, of which each kidney contains nearly a million. As blood travels through a nephron, water and dissolved substances including wastes are filtered from it through a tuft of capillaries called the **glomerulus** (pl. glomeruli). The resulting glomerular filtrate travels through other structures within the nephron, where water and essential amounts of substances such as sodium, potassium, and calcium are reabsorbed into the bloodstream. The remaining filtrate is called urine.

The ureter is a narrow, muscular tube that transports urine from the kidney to the urinary bladder, located in the anterior portion of the pelvic cavity. The urinary bladder is a muscular sac that serves as a reservoir for the urine. Urine is voided (emptied) from the bladder to the outside of the body through a single tube called the urethra.

key • point Blood creatinine is a measure of kidney function because creatinine is a waste product normally removed from the blood by the kidneys. If kidney function declines, creatinine accumulates in the blood.

DISORDERS

- Cystitis (sis–ti'tis): Bladder inflammation.
- Kidney stones: uric acid, calcium phosphate, or oxalate stones in the kidneys, ureter, or bladder.
- Nephritis (nef–ri'tis): inflammation of the kidneys.
- Renal (re'nal) failure: sudden, severe impairment of renal function.
- Uremia (u–re'me-a): impaired kidney function with a buildup of waste products in the blood.
- Urinary (u'ri-nar'e)tract infection (UTI): infection involving the organs or ducts of the urinary system.

DIAGNOSTIC TESTS

Examples of urinary system tests are listed in Box 5-9.

Respiratory System

FUNCTIONS

The respiratory system (Fig. 5-14) delivers a constant supply of oxygen (O_2) to all the cells of the body and removes carbon dioxide (CO_2), a waste product of cell metabolism. This is accomplished with the help of the circulatory system through respiration.

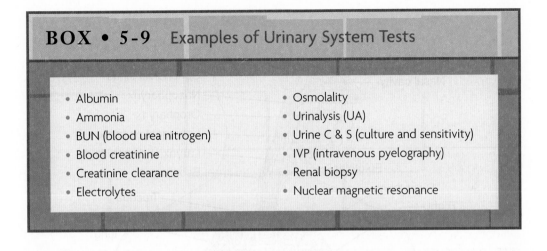

BOX • 5-9 Examples of Urinary System Tests

- Albumin
- Ammonia
- BUN (blood urea nitrogen)
- Blood creatinine
- Creatinine clearance
- Electrolytes
- Osmolality
- Urinalysis (UA)
- Urine C & S (culture and sensitivity)
- IVP (intravenous pyelography)
- Renal biopsy
- Nuclear magnetic resonance

Respiration   Respiration permits the exchange of O_2 and CO_2 between the blood and the air and involves two processes, **external respiration** and **internal respiration**. During external respiration, O_2 from the air enters the bloodstream in the lungs and CO_2 leaves the bloodstream and is breathed into the air from the lungs. During internal respiration, O_2 leaves the bloodstream and enters the cells in the tissues, and CO_2 from the cells enters the bloodstream.

fyi   Although the nose provides the main airway for external respiration, some air enters and leaves through the mouth.

Gas Exchange and Transport   During normal external respiration (Fig. 5-15), oxygen and carbon dioxide are able to diffuse (go from an area of higher concentration to an area of lower concentration) through the walls of the air sacs and the tiny, one-cell-thick capillaries of the lungs. Blood in lung capillaries is low in O_2 and high in CO_2. Therefore, O_2 from the alveoli diffuses into the capillaries while CO_2 diffuses from the capillaries into the alveoli to be expired (breathed out).

The amount of O_2 that can be carried in the blood plasma is not enough to meet the needs of the body. Fortunately, hemoglobin (a protein in red blood cells) has the ability to bind O_2, increasing the amount the blood can carry by more than 70%. Most of the O_2 that diffuses into the capillaries in the lungs binds to the iron-containing heme portion of hemoglobin molecules. Very little is dissolved in the blood plasma. O_2 combined with hemoglobin is called **oxyhemoglobin**.

Hemoglobin also has the ability to bind with CO_2. Hemoglobin combined with CO_2 is called **carbaminohemoglobin**. However, only about 20% of the CO_2 from the tissues is carried to the lungs in this manner. Approximately 10% is carried as gas dissolved in the blood plasma. The remaining 70% is carried as **bicarbonate ion**, which is formed in the red blood cells and released into the blood plasma. In the lungs, the bicarbonate ion reenters

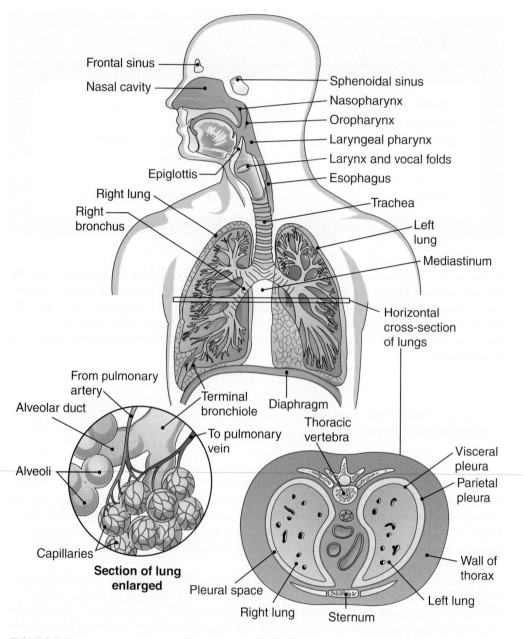

FIGURE 5-14

Respiratory system.   (Used with permission from Cohen, B. J. & Wood, D. L. Memmler's structure and function of the human body
[7th ed.]. Philadelphia: Lippincott Williams & Wilkins, p. 248.)

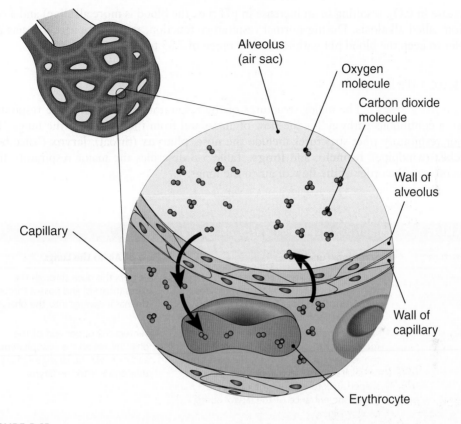

FIGURE 5-15

External respiration. (Used with permission from Cohen, B. J. & Wood, D. L. Memmler's structure and function of the human body [7th ed.]. Philadelphia: Lippincott Williams & Wilkins, p. 255.)

the red blood cells and is released as CO_2 again so it can diffuse into the alveoli and be exhaled by the body.

Whether oxygen or hemoglobin associates (combines) with or disassociates (releases) from hemoglobin depends upon the partial pressure (P) of each gas. Partial pressure is defined as the pressure exerted by one gas in a mixture of gases. Oxygen associates with hemoglobin in the lungs, where the **partial pressure of oxygen (PO_2)** is increased, and disassociates from hemoglobin in the tissues, where the PO_2 is decreased. Carbon dioxide associates with hemoglobin in the tissues, where the **partial pressure of carbon dioxide (PCO_2)** is increased, and disassociates with hemoglobin in the lungs, where the PCO_2 is decreased.

Acid–Base Balance CO_2 levels play a major role in the acid–base (pH) balance of the blood. If CO_2 levels increase, blood pH decreases (i.e., becomes more acidic), which can lead to a dangerous condition called **acidosis**. The body responds by increasing the rate of respiration (hyperventilation) to increase O_2 levels. Prolonged hyperventilation causes a decrease in CO_2, resulting in an increase in pH (i.e., the blood is more alkaline) and a condition called **alkalosis**. During normal respiratory function, the bicarbonate ion acts as a buffer to keep the blood pH within a steady range of 7.35 to 7.45.

STRUCTURES

Respiratory Tract   The major structures of the respiratory system form the respiratory tract, a continuous pathway for the flow of air to and from the air sacs in the lungs. The major respiratory tract structures include the nose, **pharynx** (throat), **larynx** (voice box), **trachea** (windpipe), **bronchi**, and **lungs**. Table 5-8 describes the major respiratory tract structures in the order of the flow of air to the lungs.

TABLE 5-8	Major Structures of Respiratory Tract	
Structure	**Description/Function**	**Flow of Air to the Lungs**
Nose	Provides the main airway for respiration; warms, moistens and filters air; provides a resonance chamber for the voice; and contains receptors for the sense of smell	Air enters the nose through the nares (nostrils) and passes through the nasal cavities into the pharynx
Pharynx	A funnel-shaped passageway that receives food from the mouth and delivers it to the esophagus, and air from the nose and carries it into the larynx. (A thin, leaf-shaped structure called the **epiglottis** covers the entrance of the larynx during swallowing)	Air enters the upper end of the pharynx, called the nasopharynx, and exits via the laryngeal pharynx that opens into the larynx
Larynx	The enlarged upper end of the trachea that houses the vocal cords, the ends of which mark the division between the upper and lower respiratory tracts	Air passes through the larynx into the lower trachea
Trachea	A tube that extends from the larynx into the upper part of the chest and carries air to the lungs	Air moves through the trachea into the bronchi in the lungs
Lungs	Organs that house the bronchial branches and the alveoli where gas exchange takes place	Air moves throughout the lungs within the bronchi
Bronchi (sing. bronchus)	Two airways that branch off the lower end of the trachea and lead into the lungs; one branch each into the left and right lungs, where they subdivide into secondary bronchi that divide into smaller and smaller branches	Air moves through the branches of the bronchi, referred to as the *bronchial tree*, until it reaches the terminal bronchioles
Terminal bronchioles	The smallest divisions of the bronchi, the ends of which contain the alveoli	Air flows out of the terminal bronchioles into the alveoli
Alveoli (singular alveolus)	Tiny air sacs covered with blood capillaries where the exchange of gases in the lungs takes place	Oxygen leaves the alveoli and enters the capillaries. Carbon dioxide leaves the capillaries and enters the alveoli to be expired

Lungs   The human body has two lungs, a right with three lobes and a left with only two lobes because of the space needed for the heart. The lungs are encased in a thin membrane consisting of several layers called **pleura**. An infinitely small space between the layer that covers the lungs and one that lines the inner thoracic cavity is called the **pleural space** or cavity.

> *fyi*   Fluid within the pleural cavity (pleural fluid) helps keep the lungs expanded by reducing surface tension. It also helps prevent friction as the lungs expand and contract.

Alveoli   The **alveoli** (al-ve'o-li) (sing. alveolus) are the tiny air sacs in the lungs where the exchange of oxygen and carbon dioxide takes place. The walls of the alveoli are a single layer of squamous (flat) epithelial cells surrounded by a thin membrane. The thinness of the walls allows gases to easily pass between the alveoli and the blood in the tiny capillaries that cover them. The thinness of the walls would ordinarily leave them prone to collapse. However, a coating of fluid called **surfactant** lowers the surface tension (or pull) on the walls and helps to stabilize them.

> k e y • p o i n t   A deficiency of surfactant in premature infants causes the alveoli to collapse leading to a condition called **infant respiratory distress syndrome**, or IRDS. Premature infants can be given animal or synthetic surfactant through inhalation, for example, in an effort to treat this life-threatening condition.

DISORDERS

- Apnea (ap'ne-ah): a temporary cessation of breathing.
- Asthma (az'ma): difficulty in breathing accompanied by wheezing caused by spasm or swelling of the bronchial tubes.
- Bronchitis (brong-ki'tis): inflammation of the mucous membrane of the bronchial tubes.
- Cystic fibrosis (sis'tik fi-bro'sis): genetic endocrine disease causing excess production of mucus.
- Dyspnea (disp'ne-ah): difficult or labored breathing.
- Emphysema (em'fi-se'ma): chronic obstructive pulmonary disease (COPD).
- Hypoxia (hi-pok'se-ah): deficiency of oxygen.
- Infant respiratory distress syndrome (IRDS): severe impairment of respiratory function in the newborn due to a lack of a substance called surfactant in the baby's lungs.
- Pleurisy (ploo'ris-e): inflammation of the pleural membrane.
- Pneumonia (nu-mo'ne-a): inflammation of the lungs.
- Pulmonary edema (pul'mo-ne-re e-de'ma): accumulation of fluid in the lungs.
- Respiratory syncytial (sin-si'shal) virus (RSV): virus that is a major cause of respiratory distress in infants and children.
- Rhinitis (ri-ni'tis): inflammation of the nasal mucous membranes.
- Tonsillitis (ton-sil-i'tis): infection of the tonsils.

- Tuberculosis (tu-ber'ku-lo'sis)(TB): infectious disease affecting the respiratory system. caused by the bacterium *Mycobacterium tuberculosis.*
- Upper respiratory infection (URI): infection of the nose, throat, larynx, or upper trachea such as that caused by a cold virus.

DIAGNOSTIC TESTS

Examples of tests associated with the respiratory system are listed in Box 5-10.

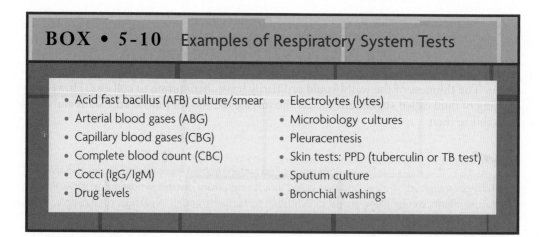

BOX • 5-10 Examples of Respiratory System Tests

- Acid fast bacillus (AFB) culture/smear
- Arterial blood gases (ABG)
- Capillary blood gases (CBG)
- Complete blood count (CBC)
- Cocci (IgG/IgM)
- Drug levels
- Electrolytes (lytes)
- Microbiology cultures
- Pleuracentesis
- Skin tests: PPD (tuberculin or TB test)
- Sputum culture
- Bronchial washings

STUDY & REVIEW QUESTIONS

1. **The transverse plane divides the body**

   a. Diagonally into upper and lower portions
   b. Horizontally into upper and lower portions
   c. Vertically into front and back portions
   d. Vertically into right and left portions

2. **Proximal is defined as**

   a. Away from the middle
   b. Closest to the middle
   c. Farthest from the center
   d. Nearest to the point of attachment

3. **The process by which the body maintains a state of equilibrium is**

   a. Anabolism
   b. Catabolism
   c. Homeostasis
   d. Venostasis

4. **Which part of a cell contains the chromosomes or genetic material?**

   a. Cytoplasm
   b. Golgi apparatus
   c. Nucleus
   d. Organelles

5. **What type of muscle lines the walls of blood vessels?**

   a. Cardiac
   b. Skeletal
   c. Striated
   d. Visceral

6. **Which of the following is an accessory organ of the digestive system?**

   a. Heart
   b. Liver
   c. Lung
   d. Ovary

7. **Evaluation of the endocrine system involves**

   a. Blood gas studies
   b. Drug monitoring
   c. Hormone determinations
   d. Spinal fluid analysis

8. **The spinal cord and brain are covered by protective membranes called**

   a. Meninges
   b. Neurons
   c. Papillae
   d. Viscera

9. **Which statement is not true? Sebaceous glands**

   a. Are also called oil glands
   b. Help lubricate the skin
   c. Secrete sebum
   d. Are part of the endocrine system

10. **Most gas exchange between blood and tissue takes place in the**

    a. Arterioles
    b. Capillaries
    c. Pulmonary vein
    d. Venules

CASE · STUDY · 5-1

Body System Structures and Disorders

A college student found that she was studying many hours a day after she arrived home and did most of it on the floor leaning on her elbows. She found no time to exercise except weekends when she hit the pavement for 10+ miles both days because she loved running and had been a marathon runner in the past. On Monday mornings she would experience pain in her leg muscles and tendons. After a few months, she noticed a very large, fluid-filled sac on her elbow.

QUESTIONS

1. What are the names of the conditions she is experiencing in her leg muscles and tendons?
2. What is that fluid-filled sac on her elbow called and why is it there?
3. What most likely caused her problems?

CASE · STUDY · 5-2

Body Systems, Disorders, Diagnostic Tests, and Directional Terms

A phlebotomist responded to a call from the ER to collect STAT glucose and insulin levels on a patient. The patient was unconscious, but the patient's husband granted permission for the blood draw. The patient had an IV in the left arm and a pulmonary function technician had just collected ABGs in the right wrist, so the phlebotomist elected to draw the sample distal to the IV.

QUESTIONS

1. What body systems of the patient are being evaluated?
2. What is most likely wrong with the patient?
3. Where did the phlebotomist collect the specimen?

Bibliography and Suggested Readings

Cohen, B. J., & Wood, D. L. (2000). Memmler's structure and function of the human body (7th ed.). Philadelphia: Lippincott Williams & Wilkins.

Cohen, B. J., & Wood, D. L. (2005). Memmler's the human body in health and disease (10th ed.). Philadelphia: Lippincott Williams & Wilkins.

Fischbach, F. (2003). Laboratory diagnostic tests (7th ed.). Philadelphia: Lippincott Williams & Wilkins.

Herlihy, B., & Maebius, N. K. (2000). The human body in health and illness. Philadelphia: W. B. Saunders.

Mahon, C., Smith, L., & Burns, C. (1998). An introduction to clinical laboratory science. Philadelphia: W. B. Saunders.

THE CIRCULATORY SYSTEM

key • terms

arrhythmia

atria

basilic vein

blood pressure

cardiac cycle

cephalic vein

coagulation

crossmatch

diastole

ECG/EKG

erythrocyte

extrinsic pathway

fibrinolysis

hemostasis

intrinsic pathway

leukocyte

median cubital vein

pulmonary circulation

sphygmomanometer

systemic circulation

systole

thrombocyte

vasoconstriction

ventricles

objectives

Upon successful completion of this chapter, the reader should be able to:

1. Define the key terms and abbreviations listed at the beginning of the chapter.
2. Identify the layers and other structures of the heart and describe their function.
3. Describe the cardiac cycle and how an ECG tracing relates to it and explain the origins of heart sounds and pulse rates.
4. Describe how to take blood pressure readings and explain what they represent.
5. Identify the two main divisions of the vascular system, describe the function of each, and trace the flow of blood throughout the system.
6. Identify the different types of blood vessels and describe the structure and function of each.
7. Name and locate major arm and leg veins and describe the suitability of each for venipuncture.
8. List the major constituents of blood, describe the function of each of the formed elements, and differentiate between serum, plasma, and whole blood.
9. Describe how ABO and Rh blood types are determined, and the importance of compatibility testing prior to transfusion.
10. Define hemostasis and describe basic coagulation and fibrinolysis processes.
11. Identify the structures and vessels and describe the function of the lymphatic system.
12. List the disorders and diagnostic tests of the circulatory system.

The **circulatory system** consists of the cardiovascular system (heart, blood, and blood vessels) and the lymphatic system (lymph, lymph vessels, and nodes). The circulatory system is the means by which oxygen and food are carried to the cells of the body. It is also the means by which carbon dioxide and other wastes are carried away from the cells to the excretory organs: the kidneys, lungs, and skin. The circulatory system also aids in the coagulation process, assists in defending the body against disease, and plays an important role in the regulation of body temperature.

THE HEART

The heart (Fig. 6-1) is the major structure of the circulatory system. It is the "pump" that circulates blood throughout the body. It is located in the center of the thoracic cavity between the lungs with the apex (tip) pointing down and to the left of the body.

Heart Structure

The heart is a four-chambered, hollow, muscular organ, slightly larger than a man's closed fist. It is surrounded by a thin, fluid-filled sac called the **pericardium** (per'i-kar'de-um), and its walls have three distinct layers. The heart has two sides, a right and a left. Each side has two chambers, an upper and a lower. One-way valves between the chambers help prevent the back-flow of blood and keep it flowing through the heart in the right direction. The right and left chambers are separated from each other by partitions called **septa** (sing. **septum**).

LAYERS

The three layers of the heart (Table 6-1) are the **epicardium** (ep'-i-kar'de-um), the thin outer layer; **myocardium** (mi-o-kar'de-um), the middle muscle layer; and **endocardium** (en' do-kar'de-um), the thin inner layer.

CHAMBERS

The upper chambers on each side of the heart are called **atria** (a'tre-a), and the lower chambers are called **ventricles** (ven'trik-ls). The atria (sing. atrium) are receiving chambers, and the ventricles are pumping or delivering chambers. The location and function of the chambers of the heart are described in Table 6-2.

VALVES

The valves at the entrance to the ventricles are called **atrioventricular** (a'tre-o-ven-trik'u-lar) **(AV) valves**.

> *fyi* The atrioventricular valves are attached to the walls of the ventricles by thin threads of tissue called **chordae** (kor'de) **tendineae** (ten-din'e-e), which keep the valves from flipping back into the atria.

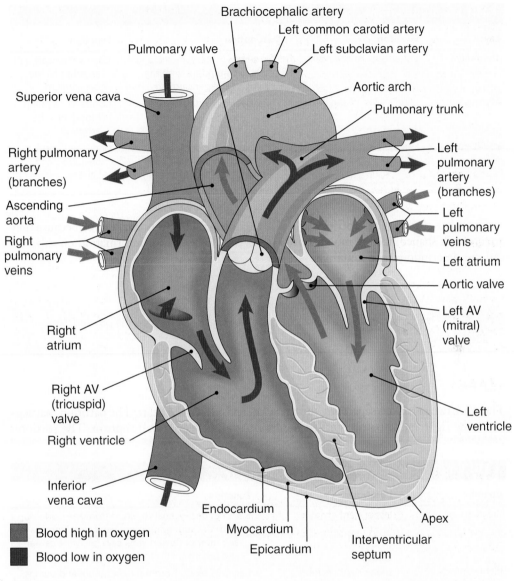

Brachiocephalic artery
Left common carotid artery
Left subclavian artery
Pulmonary valve
Aortic arch
Pulmonary trunk
Superior vena cava
Right pulmonary artery (branches)
Left pulmonary artery (branches)
Ascending aorta
Left pulmonary veins
Right pulmonary veins
Left atrium
Aortic valve
Right atrium
Left AV (mitral) valve
Right AV (tricuspid) valve
Left ventricle
Right ventricle
Inferior vena cava
Blood high in oxygen
Blood low in oxygen
Endocardium
Myocardium
Epicardium
Apex
Interventricular septum

FIGURE 6-1
Heart and great vessels.

TABLE 6-1	Layers of the Heart		
Layer	Location	Description	Function
Epicardium	Outer layer of the heart	Thin serous (watery) membrane that is continuous with the lining of the pericardium	Covers the heart and attaches to the pericardium
Myocardium	Middle layer of the heart	Thick layer of cardiac muscle	Contracts to pump blood into the arteries
Endocardium	Inner layer of the heart	Thin layer of epithelial cells that is continuous with the lining of the blood vessels	Lines the interior chambers and valves

The valves that exit the ventricles are called **semilunar** (sem'e-lu'nar) **valves** because they are crescent shaped like the moon (Latin, *luna*). See Table 6-3 for information on valve locations, descriptions, and functions.

fyi The term mitral valve comes from its resemblance to a miter, the pointed, two-sided hat worn by bishops.

SEPTA

There are two partitions separating the right and left sides of the heart. The partition that separates the right and left atria is called the **interatrial** (in-ter-a'tre-al) **septum**. The partition

TABLE 6-2	Chambers of the Heart	
Chamber	Location	Function
Right atrium	Upper right chamber	Receives deoxygenated blood from the body via both the **superior (upper) vena cava** (ve'na ka'va) and **inferior (lower) vena cava** (pl., vena cavae) and pumps it into the right ventricle
Right ventricle	Lower right chamber	Receives blood from the right atrium and pumps it into the **pulmonary artery** which carries it to the lungs to be oxygenated
Left atrium	Upper left chamber	Receives oxygenated blood from the lungs via the **pulmonary veins** and pumps it into the left ventricle
Left ventricle	Lower left chamber	Receives blood from the left atrium and pumps it into the **aorta** (a-or'ta). The walls of the left ventricle are nearly three times as thick as the right ventricle owing to the force required to pump the blood into the arterial system

TABLE 6-3	Heart Valves		
Valve	**Location**	**Description**	**Function**
Right AV valve (also called the **tricuspid** (tri-kus'pid) **valve**)	Between the right atrium and right ventricle	Has three cusps (flaps), hence the name tricuspid	Closes when the right ventricle contracts and prevents blood from flowing back into the right atrium
Left AV valve (also called the **bicuspid** or **mitral valve**)	Between the left atrium and left ventricle	Has two cusps, hence the name bicuspid	Closes when the left ventricle contracts and prevents blood from flowing back into the left atrium
Right semilunar valve (also called pulmonary or pulmonic valve)	At the entrance to the pulmonary artery	Has three half-moon–shaped cusps	Closes when the right ventricle relaxes and prevents blood from flowing back into the right ventricle
Left semilunar valve (also called aortic valve)	At the entrance to the aorta	Has three half-moon–shaped cusps	Closes when the left ventricle relaxes and prevents blood from flowing back into the left ventricle

that separates the right and left ventricles is called the **interventricular** (in-ter-ven-trik'u-lar) **septum**. Each septum consists mostly of myocardium.

CORONARY CIRCULATION

The heart muscle does not receive nourishment or oxygen from blood passing through the heart. It receives its blood supply via the right and left **coronary arteries** that branch off of the aorta, just beyond the aortic semilunar valve. Partial obstruction of a coronary artery or one of its branches can reduce blood flow to a point where it is not adequate to meet the oxygen needs of the heart muscle, a condition called myocardial **ischemia** (is-kee'me-ah).

Complete obstruction or prolonged ischemia leads to **myocardial** (mi'o-kar'de-al) **infarction** (MI) or "heart attack" because of necrosis (ne-kro'sis) or death of the surrounding tissue from lack of oxygen.

fyi   Fatty plaque buildup from a condition called atherosclerosis can lead to severe narrowing of coronary arteries. This condition is sometimes treated using a coronary bypass procedure. In this surgical procedure, a vein (commonly the saphenous vein from the leg) is grafted onto the artery to divert the blood around the affected area.

Heart Function

CARDIAC CYCLE

One complete contraction and subsequent relaxation of the heart lasts about 0.8 seconds and is called a **cardiac cycle**. The contracting phase of the cardiac cycle is called **systole** (sis'to-le), and the relaxing phase is called **diastole** (di-as'to-le).

ELECTRICAL CONDUCTION SYSTEM

To be effective at pumping blood the heart contractions must be synchronized (coordinated) so that both atria contract simultaneously, followed by contraction of both ventricles. Synchronization is achieved by means of specialized muscle cells that form the electrical conduction system (Fig. 6-2). Instead of contracting, these cells act like nerve tissue in that

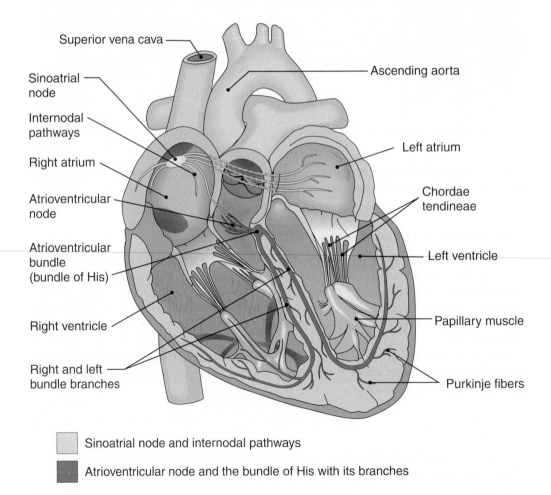

FIGURE 6-2

Electrical conduction system of the heart.

TABLE 6-4	The Electrical Conduction System Pathway	
Structure	**Location**	**Function**
Sinoatrial (SA) node	Upper wall of the right atrium	Begins the heart beat by generating the electrical pulse that travels through the muscles of both atria, causing them to contract simultaneously and push blood through the atrioventricular valves into the ventricles
Internodal pathway fibers	Wall of the right atrium	Relay the impulse to the **atrioventricular (AV) node**
Atrioventricular (AV) node	Bottom of the right atrium in the interatrial septum	Picks up the impulse, slows it down while the atria finish contracting, and then relays it through the **AV bundle (bundle of His)**
AV bundle (bundle of His)	Top of the interventricular septum	Relays impulse throughout the ventricular walls by means of bundle branches and **Purkinje fibers.** This causes the ventricles to contract, forcing blood through the semilunar valves. Both atria and ventricles relax briefly before the entire cycle starts again

they initiate and distribute electrical impulses throughout the myocardium to coordinate the cardiac cycle. The specialized tissues create an electrical conduction system pathway and include two tissue masses called nodes and a network of specialized fibers that branch throughout the myocardium. Heart contraction is initiated by an electrical impulse generated from the **sinoatrial** (sin'o-a'tre-al) **node** or SA node, also called the **pacemaker**, at the start of the pathway. The electrical conduction system pathway is described in Table 6-4.

fyi   The SA node is called the pacemaker because it sets the basic pace or rhythm of the heart beat.

ELECTROCARDIOGRAM

The cardiac cycle can be recorded by means of an **electrocardiogram** (ECG or EKG), an actual record of the electrical currents that correspond to each event in heart muscle contraction. The recording is called an ECG tracing (Fig. 6-3). Heart contractions are recorded as waves when electrodes (leads or wires) are placed on the skin. The P wave of the tracing represents the activity of the atria and is usually the first wave seen. The QRS complex (a collection of three waves), along with the T wave, represents the activity of the ventricles. An ECG is useful in diagnosing heart muscle damage and abnormalities in heart rate.

ORIGIN OF THE HEART SOUNDS (HEART BEAT)

As the ventricles contract (systole), the atrioventricular valves close, resulting in the first heart sound: a long, low-pitched sound commonly described as a "lubb." The second heart

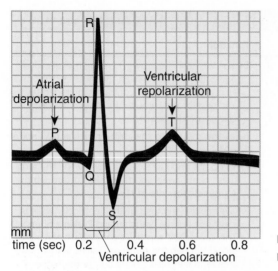

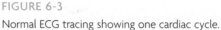

FIGURE 6-3

Normal ECG tracing showing one cardiac cycle.

sound comes at the beginning of ventricular relaxation (diastole) and is due to the closing of the semilunar valves. It is shorter and sharper and described as a "dupp." Abnormal heart sounds are called **murmurs**, and are often due to faulty valve action.

HEART RATE AND CARDIAC OUTPUT

The **heart rate** is the number of heart beats per minute. Normal adult heart rate averages 72 beats per minute. The volume of blood pumped by the heart in 1 minute is called the **cardiac output** and averages 5 liters per minute.

An irregularity in the heart rate, rhythm, or beat is called an **arrhythmia** (ah-rith'me-ah). A slow rate, less than 60 beats per minute, is called **bradycardia** (brad'e-kar'de-ah). A fast rate, over 100 beats per minute, is called **tachycardia** (tak'e-kar'de-ah). Extra beats before the normal beat are called **extrasystoles**. Rapid, uncoordinated contractions are called **fibrillations** and can result in lack of pumping action.

PULSE

The **pulse** is the palpable rhythmic throbbing caused by the alternating expansion and contraction of an artery as a wave of blood passes through it. It is created as the ventricles contract and blood is forced out of the heart and through the arteries. In normal individuals, the pulse rate is the same as the heart rate. The pulse is most easily felt by compressing the radial artery on the thumb side of the wrist.

BLOOD PRESSURE

Blood pressure is a measure of the force (pressure) exerted by the blood on the walls of blood vessels. It is commonly measured in a large artery (such as the brachial artery in the upper arm), using a **sphygmomanometer** (sfig'mo-mah-nom'e-ter), more commonly known as a "blood pressure cuff." Blood pressure results are expressed in millimeters of mercury (mm Hg) and are read from a manometer that is either a gauge or a mercury column, depending upon the type of blood pressure cuff used. The two components of blood pressure measured are

- **Systolic** (sis-tol'ik) **pressure**: the pressure in the arteries during contraction of the ventricles.
- **Diastolic** (di-as-tol'ik) **pressure**: the arterial pressure during relaxation of the ventricles.

fyi A blood pressure reading is expressed as the systolic pressure over the diastolic pressure. Average normal blood pressure is verbally expressed as 120 over 80, and is written 120/80.

A brachial blood pressure reading is taken by placing a blood pressure cuff around the upper arm and a stethoscope over the brachial artery. The cuff is inflated until the brachial artery is compressed and the blood flow is cut off. Then the cuff is slowly deflated until the first heart sounds are heard with the stethoscope. The pressure reading at this time is the systolic pressure. The cuff is then slowly deflated until a muffled sound is heard. The pressure at this time is the diastolic pressure.

Heart Disorders

- Angina pectoris (an'-ji'na pek'to-ris): also called ischemic heart disease (IHD); pain on exertion, caused by inadequate blood flow to the myocardium from the coronary arteries.
- Aortic stenosis (a-or'tik ste-no'sis): narrowing of the aorta or its opening.
- Bacterial endocarditis (en'do-kar-di'tis): an infection of the lining of the heart, most commonly caused by streptococci.
- Congestive heart failure (CHF): impaired circulation caused by inadequate pumping of a diseased heart, resulting in fluid buildup (edema) in the lungs or other tissues.
- Myocardial infarction (MI): heart attack or death of heart muscle due to obstruction (occlusion) of a coronary artery.
- Myocardial ischemia (is-kee'me-ah): insufficient blood flow to meet the needs of the heart muscle.
- Pericarditis (per-i-kar-di'tis): inflammation of the pericardium.

Diagnostic Tests

Examples of heart tests are shown in Box 6-1.

fyi When a person has a heart attack the heart muscle is damaged, releasing the enzymes CK and AST into the bloodstream. A sample of blood can be tested for these enzymes. If the results are elevated, a heart attack is suspected.

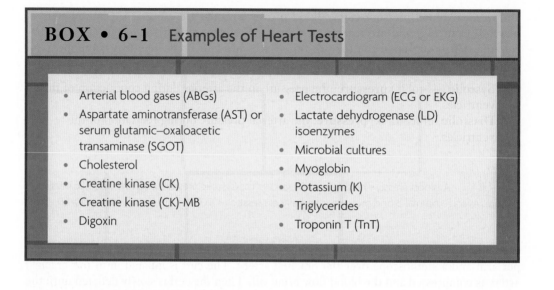

BOX • 6-1 Examples of Heart Tests

- Arterial blood gases (ABGs)
- Aspartate aminotransferase (AST) or serum glutamic–oxaloacetic transaminase (SGOT)
- Cholesterol
- Creatine kinase (CK)
- Creatine kinase (CK)-MB
- Digoxin
- Electrocardiogram (ECG or EKG)
- Lactate dehydrogenase (LD) isoenzymes
- Microbial cultures
- Myoglobin
- Potassium (K)
- Triglycerides
- Troponin T (TnT)

THE VASCULAR SYSTEM

Functions

The vascular system is the system of blood vessels that, along with the heart, form the closed system by which blood is circulated to all parts of the body. There are two divisions to this system, the pulmonary circulation and the systemic circulation.

THE PULMONARY CIRCULATION

The **pulmonary circulation** carries blood from the right ventricle of the heart to the lungs to remove carbon dioxide and pick up oxygen, and returns oxygenated blood to the left atrium of the heart.

THE SYSTEMIC CIRCULATION

The **systemic circulation** serves the rest of the body, carrying oxygenated blood and nutrients from the left ventricle of the heart to the body cells and returning to the right atrium of the heart with blood that is carrying carbon dioxide and other waste products of metabolism from the cells.

Structures

The structures of the vascular system are the various blood vessels that, along with the heart, form the closed system for the flow of blood. Blood vessels are tubelike structures capable of expanding and contracting. There are three types of blood vessels: arteries, veins, and capillaries.

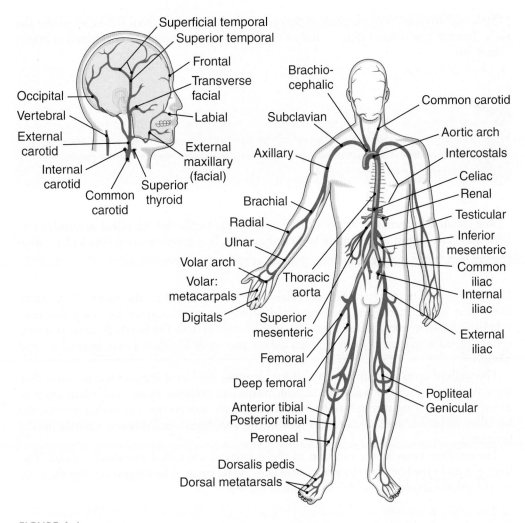

FIGURE 6-4
Principal arteries of the body.

ARTERIES

Arteries (Fig. 6-4) are blood vessels that carry blood away from the heart. They have thick walls because the blood that moves through them is under pressure from the contraction of the ventricles. This pressure creates a pulse that can be felt, distinguishing them from veins.

key • point   When arterial blood is collected by syringe, the pressure normally causes the blood to "pump" or pulse into the syringe under its own power.

Systemic arteries carry oxygenated (oxygen-rich) blood away from the heart to the tissues. Because it is oxygen rich, or full of oxygen, normal systemic arterial blood is bright cherry red.

> **key·point** The pulmonary artery is the only artery that carries deoxygenated, or oxygen-poor, blood. It is part of the pulmonary circulation and carries deoxygenated blood from the heart to the lungs. It is classified as an artery because it carries blood away from the heart.

The smallest branches of arteries that join with the capillaries are called **arterioles** (ar-te're-olz). The largest artery in the body is the **aorta**. It is approximately 1 inch (2.5 cm) in diameter.

Veins **Veins** (Fig. 6-5) are blood vessels that return blood to the heart. Veins carry blood that is low in oxygen (deoxygenated or oxygen poor), except for the pulmonary vein, which carries oxygenated blood from the lungs back to the heart. Because systemic venous blood is oxygen poor, it is much darker and more bluish red than normal arterial blood.

The walls of veins are thinner than arteries because the blood is under less pressure than arterial blood. Since the walls are thinner, veins can collapse more easily than arteries. Blood is kept moving through veins by skeletal muscle movement, valves that prevent the backflow of blood, and pressure changes in the abdominal and thoracic cavities during breathing.

The smallest veins at the junction of the capillaries are called **venules** (ven'ulz). The largest veins in the body are the **vena cavae** (sing. **vena cava**). The longest veins in the body are the **great saphenous** (sa-fe'nus) **veins** in the leg.

Capillaries **Capillaries** are microscopic, one-cell-thick vessels that connect the arterioles and venules, forming a bridge between the arterial and venous circulation. Blood in the capillaries is a mixture of both venous and arterial blood. In the systemic circulation, arterial blood delivers oxygen and nutrients to the capillaries. The thin capillary walls allow the exchange of oxygen for carbon dioxide and nutrients for wastes between the cells and the blood (Fig. 6-6). Carbon dioxide and wastes are carried away in the venous blood. In the pulmonary circulation, carbon dioxide is delivered to the capillaries in the lungs and exchanged for oxygen.

The Flow of Blood

The network of arteries, veins and capillaries form the pathway for the flow of blood (Fig. 6-7) throughout the body that allows for the delivery of oxygen and nutrients to the body cells and the removal of carbon dioxide and other waste products of metabolism.

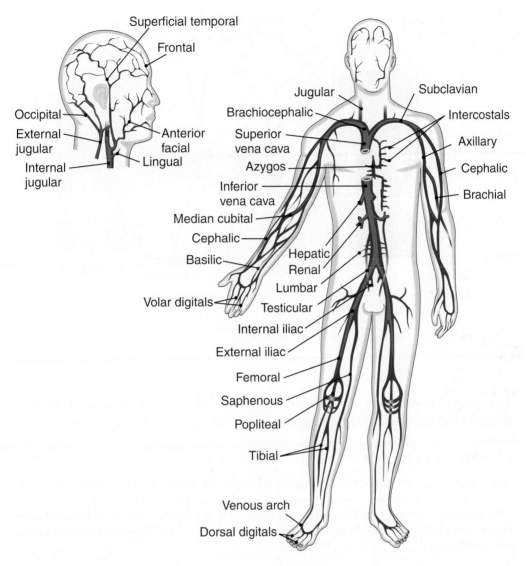

FIGURE 6-5

Principal veins of the body.

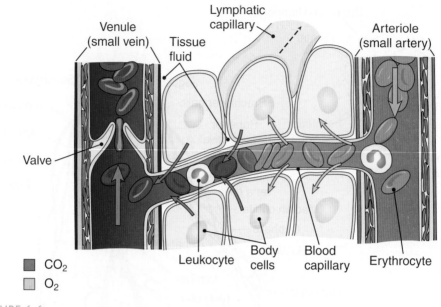

FIGURE 6-6

Oxygen and carbon dioxide exchange in the tissue capillaries.

The order of vascular flow starting with the return of oxygen poor blood to the heart is shown in Box 6-2.

BLOOD VESSEL STRUCTURE

Arteries and veins are composed of three main layers. The thickness of the layers varies with the size and type of blood vessel. Figure 6-8 shows a cross-section of an artery and a vein as seen through a microscope. Capillaries are composed of a single layer of endothelial cells enclosed in a basement membrane. (See Fig. 6-9 for a comparison diagram of arteries, veins, and capillaries.)

Layers

- **Tunica** (tu'ni-ka) **adventitia** (ad'ven-tish'e-a): the outer layer of a blood vessel, sometimes called the tunica externa. It is made up of connective tissue and is thicker in arteries than in veins.
- **Tunica media**: the middle layer of a blood vessel. It is made up of smooth muscle tissue and some elastic fibers. It is much thicker in arteries than in veins.
- **Tunica intima** (in'ti-ma): the inner layer or lining of a blood vessel, sometimes called the tunica interna. It is made up of a single layer of endothelial cells with an underlining basement membrane, a connective tissue layer, and an elastic internal membrane.

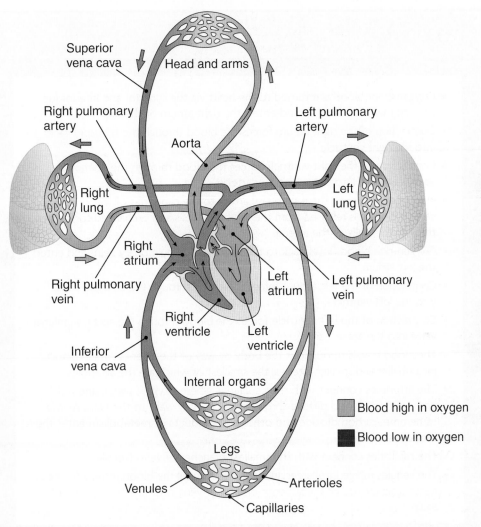

FIGURE 6-7
Representation of the vascular flow.

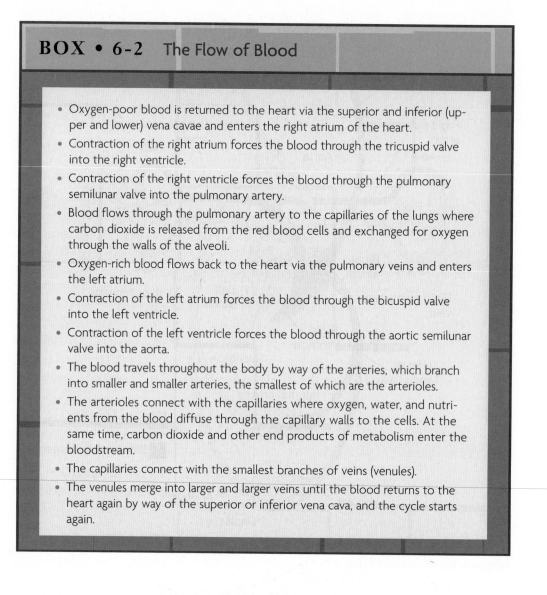

BOX • 6-2   The Flow of Blood

- Oxygen-poor blood is returned to the heart via the superior and inferior (upper and lower) vena cavae and enters the right atrium of the heart.
- Contraction of the right atrium forces the blood through the tricuspid valve into the right ventricle.
- Contraction of the right ventricle forces the blood through the pulmonary semilunar valve into the pulmonary artery.
- Blood flows through the pulmonary artery to the capillaries of the lungs where carbon dioxide is released from the red blood cells and exchanged for oxygen through the walls of the alveoli.
- Oxygen-rich blood flows back to the heart via the pulmonary veins and enters the left atrium.
- Contraction of the left atrium forces the blood through the bicuspid valve into the left ventricle.
- Contraction of the left ventricle forces the blood through the aortic semilunar valve into the aorta.
- The blood travels throughout the body by way of the arteries, which branch into smaller and smaller arteries, the smallest of which are the arterioles.
- The arterioles connect with the capillaries where oxygen, water, and nutrients from the blood diffuse through the capillary walls to the cells. At the same time, carbon dioxide and other end products of metabolism enter the bloodstream.
- The capillaries connect with the smallest branches of veins (venules).
- The venules merge into larger and larger veins until the blood returns to the heart again by way of the superior or inferior vena cava, and the cycle starts again.

LUMEN

The internal space of a blood vessel through which the blood flows is called the **lumen** (lu'men).

VALVES

Venous valves are thin membranous leaflets composed primarily of epithelium similar to the semilunar valves of the heart. Most of the venous system is flowing against the pull of gravity. As blood is moved forward by skeletal muscle movement, for example, the valves help keep it flowing toward the heart by allowing blood flow in only one direction (Fig. 6-10).

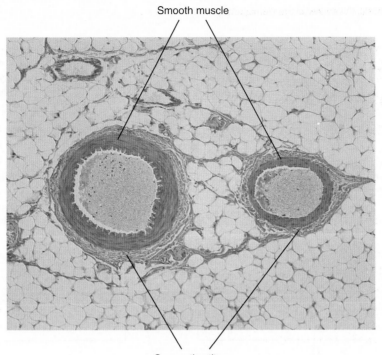

Smooth muscle

Connective tissue

FIGURE 6-8

Cross section of an artery and a vein as seen through a microscope.

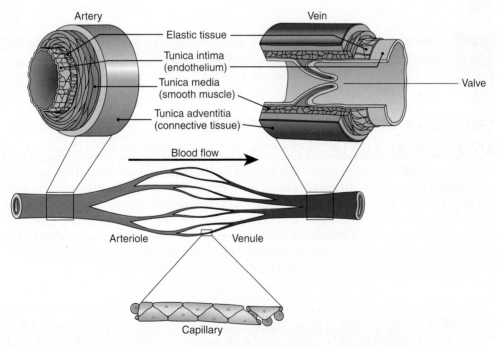

Artery

Vein

Elastic tissue

Tunica intima (endothelium)

Tunica media (smooth muscle)

Tunica adventitia (connective tissue)

Valve

Blood flow

Arteriole

Venule

Capillary

FIGURE 6-9

Artery, vein, and capillary structure.

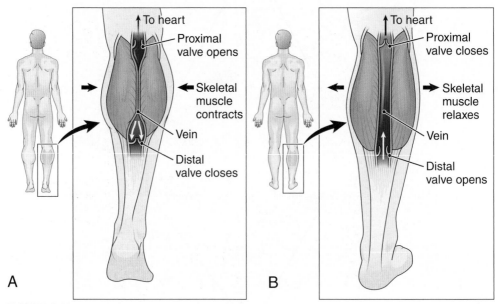

FIGURE 6-10

Role of skeletal muscles and valves in blood return. **A.** Contracting skeletal muscle compresses the vein and drives blood forward, opening the proximal valve, while the distal valve closes to prevent backflow of blood. **B.** When the muscles relaxes again, the distal valve opens, and the proximal valve closes until blood moving in the vein forces it open again.

key·point The presence of valves within veins is a major structural difference between arteries and veins.

Phlebotomy-Related Vascular Anatomy

ANTECUBITAL FOSSA

The major veins for venipuncture are located in the arm in what is referred to as the **antecubital** (an'te-ku'bi-tal) **fossa**. This is the area of the arm that is anterior to (in front of) and below the bend of the elbow. Several major arm veins lie close to the surface in this area, making them easier to locate and penetrate with a needle. These major superficial veins are referred to as **antecubital veins**. Anatomic arrangement of antecubital veins varies slightly from person to person; however, two basic vein arrangements referred to as the H- and M-shaped patterns (Fig. 6-11) are seen most often.

fyi The vein distribution patterns are so named because the major antecubital veins on the arm resemble the shape of either an "H" or an "M."

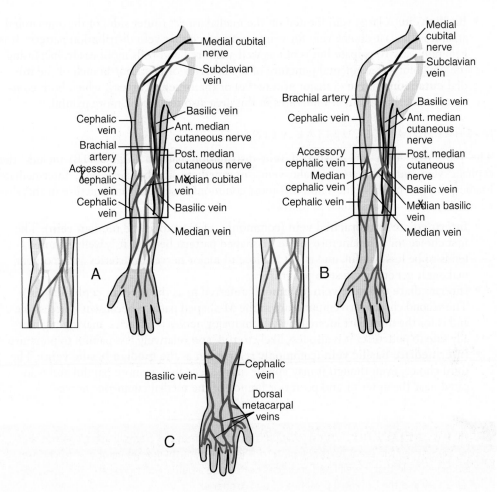

FIGURE 6-11

Principal veins of the arm including major antecubital veins. **A.** H-shaped pattern of antecubital veins of the right arm in anatomic position. **B.** M-shaped pattern of antecubital veins of the right arm in anatomic position. **C.** Right forearm, wrist, and hand veins in prone position.

H-SHAPED ANTECUBITAL VEINS

The H-shaped vein distribution pattern (Fig. 6-11A) is displayed by approximately 70% of the population and includes the median cubital vein, cephalic vein, and basilic vein.

- **Median cubital vein**: Located near the center of the antecubital area, it is the preferred vein for venipuncture in the H-shaped pattern. It is typically larger, closer to the surface, and more stationary than the others, making it the easiest and least painful to puncture and the least likely to bruise.
- **Cephalic vein**: Located in the lateral aspect of the antecubital area, it is the second-choice vein for venipuncture in the H-shaped pattern. It is often harder to palpate than the median cubital but is fairly well anchored and often the only vein that can be palpated (felt) in obese patients.

- **Basilic vein**: A large vein located on the medial aspect (inner side) of the antecubital area, it is the last-choice vein for venipuncture in either vein distribution pattern. It is generally easy to palpate but is not as well anchored and rolls more easily, increasing the possibility of accidental puncture of the anterior or posterior branch of the **medial cutaneous nerve** (a major arm nerve) or the **brachial artery**, which both commonly underlie this area. Punctures in this area also tend to be more painful.

M-SHAPED ANTECUBITAL VEINS

The veins that form the M-shaped vein distribution pattern (Fig. 6-11B) include the cephalic vein, intermediate cephalic vein, intermediate antebrachial vein, intermediate basilic vein, and basilic vein. The veins most commonly used for venipuncture in this distribution pattern are described as follows:

- **Intermediate antebrachial vein** (commonly referred to as the **median vein**): The first choice for venipuncture in the M-shaped pattern because it is well anchored, tends to be less painful, and is not as close to major nerves or arteries as the others, making it generally safest to puncture.
- **Intermediate cephalic vein** (commonly referred to as the **median cephalic vein**): The second choice for venipuncture in the M-shaped pattern because it is accessible and is for the most part located away from major nerves or arteries, making it generally safe to puncture. It is also less likely to roll, and relatively less painful to puncture.
- **Intermediate basilic vein** (commonly referred to as the **median basilic vein**): The third choice, even though it may appear more accessible, is more painful and is located near the anterior and posterior branch of the medial cutaneous nerve.

key • point Vein location may differ somewhat from person to person, and you may not see the exact textbook pattern. The important thing to remember is to choose a prominent vein that is well fixed and does not overlie a pulse, which indicates the presence of an artery and the potential presence of a major nerve.

OTHER ARM AND HAND VEINS

According to CLSI, although the larger and fuller median cubital and cephalic veins are used most frequently, veins on the back of the hand and wrist are also acceptable for venipuncture (Fig. 6-11C).

caution Veins on the underside of the wrist are never acceptable for venipuncture.

LEG, ANKLE, AND FOOT VEINS

Because of the potential for significant medical complications such as phlebitis or thrombosis, leg, ankle, and foot veins (Fig. 6-12) must not be used for venipuncture without

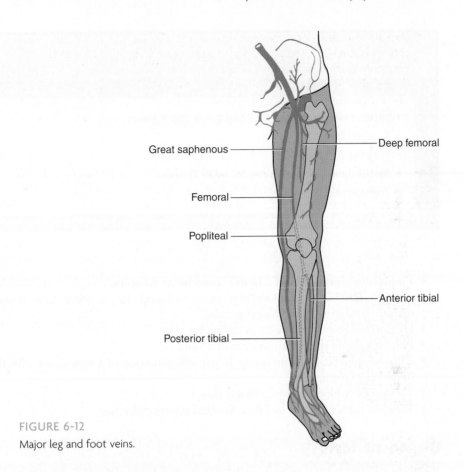

FIGURE 6-12

Major leg and foot veins.

permission of the patient's physician. Puncture of the femoral vein is performed only by physicians or specially trained personnel.

ARTERIES

Arterial puncture requires special training to perform, is more painful and hazardous to the patient, and is generally limited to the collection of arterial blood gas (ABG) specimens for evaluating respiratory function. Arterial puncture for ABG collection is explained in Chapter 12.

Vascular System Disorders

- Aneurysm (an'u-rizm): a localized dilation or bulging in the wall of a blood vessel, usually an artery.
- Arteriosclerosis (ar-te're-o-skle-ro'sis): thickening, hardening, and loss of elasticity of artery walls.
- Atherosclerosis (ath'er-o'skle-ro'sis): a form of arteriosclerosis involving changes in the intima of the artery due to accumulation of lipids and so on.

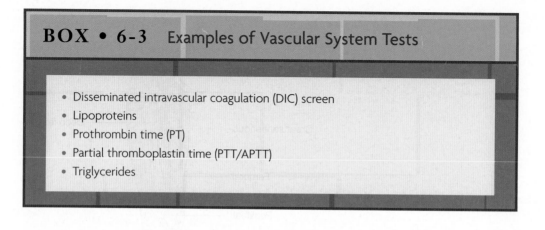

BOX • 6-3   Examples of Vascular System Tests

- Disseminated intravascular coagulation (DIC) screen
- Lipoproteins
- Prothrombin time (PT)
- Partial thromboplastin time (PTT/APTT)
- Triglycerides

- Embolism: obstruction of a blood vessel by an embolus.
- Embolus (em'bo-lus): a blood clot, part of a blood clot, or other mass of undissolved matter circulating in the bloodstream.
- Hemorrhoids: varicose veins in the rectal area.
- Phlebitis (fle-bi'tis): inflammation of a vein.
- Thrombophlebitis (throm'bo-fle-bi'tis): inflammation of a vein along with thrombus (blood clot) formation.
- Thrombus: a blood clot in a blood vessel.
- Varicose veins (varices): swollen, knotted superficial veins.

Diagnostic Tests

Examples of vascular system tests are shown in Box 6-3.

THE BLOOD

Blood has been referred to as "the river of life," flowing throughout the circulatory system delivering nutrients, oxygen, and other substances to the cells and transporting waste products away from the cells for elimination.

Blood Composition

Blood is a mixture of fluid and cells that is about five times thicker than water, salty to the taste, and slightly alkaline with a pH of about 7.4 (pH is the degree of acidity or alkalinity on a scale of 1 to 14, with 7 being neutral). In vivo (in the living body), the fluid portion of the blood is called **plasma**, and the cellular portion is referred to as the **formed elements**. The average adult weighing 70 kg (approximately 154 pounds) has a blood volume of about 5 liters (5.3 quarts), of which approximately 55% is plasma and 45% is formed elements. Accordingly, approximately one half of a blood specimen will be serum or plasma and the other half will be blood cells.

🔑 **k e y • p o i n t** Testing personnel typically prefer specimens that contain roughly 2½ times the amount of sample required to perform the test; so the test can be repeated if needed, with some to spare. Consequently, a test that requires 1 mL of serum or plasma would require a 5-mL blood specimen because only half the specimen will be fluid, while a test that requires 1 mL of whole blood would require a 2½-mL specimen.

PLASMA

Normal plasma is a clear, pale-yellow fluid that is nearly 90% water (H_2O) and 10% solutes (dissolved substances). Composition of the solute includes the following:

- Gases, such as oxygen (O_2), carbon dioxide (CO_2), and nitrogen (N).
- Minerals such as sodium (Na), potassium (K), calcium (Ca), and magnesium (Mg). Sodium helps maintain fluid balance, pH, and calcium and potassium balance necessary for normal heart action. Potassium is essential for normal muscle activity and the conduction of nerve impulses. Calcium is needed for proper bone and tooth formation, nerve conduction, and muscle contraction. In addition, calcium is essential to the clotting process.
- Nutrients, which supply energy. Plasma nutrients include carbohydrates such as glucose, and lipids (fats) such as triglycerides and cholesterol.
- Proteins, such as albumin, which is manufactured by the liver and functions to help regulate osmotic pressure, or the tendency of blood to attract water; antibodies, which combat infection; and fibrinogen, which is also manufactured by the liver and functions in the clotting process.
- Waste products of metabolism such as urea (BUN), creatinine, and uric acid.
- Other substances such as vitamins, hormones, and drugs.

FORMED ELEMENTS

Erythrocytes **Erythrocytes** (e-rith'ro-sites), or red blood cells (RBCs) (Fig. 6-13), are the most numerous cells in the blood, averaging 4.5 to 5 million per cubic millimeter of blood. Their main function is to carry oxygen from the lungs to the cells. They also carry carbon dioxide from the cells back to the lungs to be exhaled.

FIGURE 6-13

Red blood cells as seen under a scanning electron microscope.

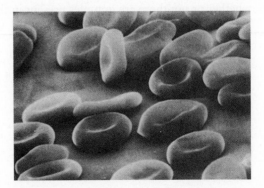

key · point   The main component of RBCs is **hemoglobin** (Hgb or Hb), an iron-containing pigment that enables them to transport oxygen and carbon dioxide and also gives them their red color.

RBCs are produced in the bone marrow. They are formed with a nucleus, which they lose as they mature and enter the bloodstream. Normally a few **reticulocytes** (re-tik'u-lo-sits) or **retics** (immature RBCs that still contain remnants of material from their nuclear stage), also enter the bloodstream. Mature RBCs have a life span of approximately 120 days, after which they begin to disintegrate and are removed from the bloodstream by the spleen and liver. They are described as anuclear (no nucleus) biconcave (indented from both sides) disks approximately 7 to 8 microns in diameter. RBCs have **intravascular** (within blood vessels) function, which means that they do their job within the bloodstream.

Leukocytes   **Leukocytes**, or white blood cells (WBCs), contain a nucleus. The average adult has from 5,000 to 10,000 WBCs per cubic millimeter of blood. WBCs are formed in the bone marrow and lymphatic tissue. They are said to have **extravascular** (outside the blood vessels) function because they are able to leave the bloodstream and do their job in the tissues. WBCs may appear in the bloodstream for only 6 to 8 hours but reside in the tissues for days, months, or even years. The life span of WBCs varies with the type.

fyi   The process by which WBCs are able to slip through the walls of the capillaries to enter the tissues is called **diapedesis** (di'a-ped-e'sis). Dia (Greek for through), ped from "pedan" (leap), esis (condition or state).

The main function of WBCs is to neutralize or destroy pathogens. Some accomplish this by **phagocytosis** (fag'o-si-to'sis), a process in which a pathogen or foreign matter is surrounded, engulfed, and destroyed by the WBC. (WBCs also use phagocytosis to remove disintegrated tissue.) Some WBCs produce antibodies that destroy pathogens indirectly or release substances that attack foreign matter.

There are different types of WBCs, each identified by size, shape of the nucleus, and whether or not there are granules present in the cytoplasm when the cells in a blood smear are stained with a special blood stain called Wright's stain (Fig. 6-14). WBCs containing

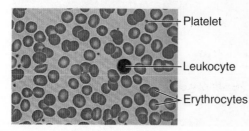
— Platelet

— Leukocyte

— Erythrocytes

FIGURE 6-14

Blood cells in a stained blood smear as seen under a microscope.

Granulocytes

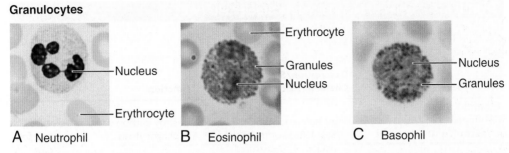

FIGURE 6-15

Granulocytes. **A.** Neutrophil. **B.** Eosinophil. **C.** Basophil.

easily visible granules are called **granulocytes** (gran'u-lo-sites'). WBCs that lack granules or have extremely fine granules that are not easily seen are called **agranulocytes**.

Granulocytes

Granulocytes can be differentiated by the color of their granules when stained with Wright's stain. There are three types of granulocytes (Fig. 6-15): **neutrophils, eosinophils** (eos), and **basophils** (basos). Neutrophils are normally the most numerous WBC in adults. A typical neutrophil is a **polymorphonuclear**, meaning it has several lobes or segments, and is also called a poly, PMN, or seg for short.

k e y • p o i n t The presence of increased numbers of neutrophils is associated with bacterial infection.

Agranulocytes

There are two types of agranulocytes (Fig. 6-16): **monocytes** (monos) and **lymphocytes** (lymphs). Lymphocytes are normally the second most numerous WBC and the most numerous agranulocyte. Two main types of lymphocytes are **T lymphocytes** and **B lymphocytes**. Monocytes are the largest WBC. (The various types of granulocytes and agranulocytes are listed and described in Table 6-5.)

FIGURE 6-16

Agranulocytes. **A.** Lymphocyte. **B.** Monocyte.

Agranulocytes

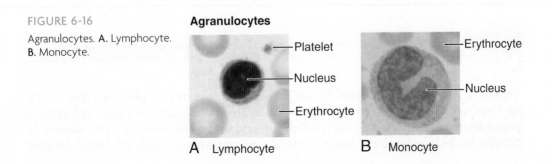

	TABLE 6-5	**Types of Normal White Blood Cells (WBCs)**		

WBC Types	Average Percentage of WBC Total (Adults)	Description/Staining Characteristics	Function	Life Span
Granulocytes				
Neutrophils (nu'tro-fils)	65%	Most numerous WBC. Segmented or multilobed nucleus. Fine-textured lavender-staining granules	Destroy pathogens by phagocytosis	6 hours to a few days
Eosinophils (e'o-sin'o-fils)	Up to 3%	Bead-like granules that stain bright orange–red. Two-lobed nucleus	Ingest and detoxify foreign protein; help help turn off immune reactions; increase with allergies and pinworm infestations	8–12 days
Basophils (ba'so-fils)	Less than 1%	Least numerous WBC: Large dark blue-staining granules that often obscure a typically S-shaped nucleus	Release histamine and heparin, which enhance the inflammatory response	Thought to live several days
Agranulocytes				
Monocytes	1–7%	Largest WBC; fine, gray–blue cytoplasm and a large, dark-staining nucleus	Destroy pathogens by phagocytosis; first line of defense in the inflammatory process	Several months
Lymphocytes	15–30%	Second most numerous WBC; typically have a large, round, dark-purple nucleus that occupies most of the cell and is surrounded by a thin rim of pale-blue cytoplasm	T lymphocytes, directly attack infected cells; B lymphocytes, rise to plasma cells that produce immunoglobulins (antibodies) that are released into the bloodstream to circulate and attack foreign cells	Varies from a few hours to a number of years

fyi   Monocytes are sometimes called macrophages after they leave the bloodstream.

Thrombocytes   **Thrombocytes** (throm'bo-sits), better known as **platelets** (Fig. 6-17), are the smallest of the formed elements. Platelets are actually parts of a large cell called a **megakaryocyte** (meg'a-kar'e-o-sit'), which is found in the bone marrow. The number of platelets in the blood (platelet count) of the average adult ranges from 150,000 to 400,000

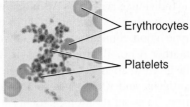

Erythrocytes

Platelets

FIGURE 6-17
Platelets (thrombocytes) in a stained blood smear.

Platelets

per cubic millimeter. Platelets are essential to **coagulation** (the blood clotting process) and are the first cell on the scene when an injury occurs (see Hemostasis). The life span of a platelet is about 10 days.

Blood Type

An individual's blood type (also called blood group) is inherited and is determined by the type of antigen present on his or her red blood cells. Some blood type antigens cause formation of antibodies to the opposite blood type. If a person receives a blood transfusion of the wrong type, the person's antibodies may react with the donor RBCs and cause them to **agglutinate** (a-gloo'tin-ate) (clump together) and **lyse** (līs) (disintegrate). An adverse reaction between donor cells and a recipient, which can be fatal, is called a **transfusion reaction**. A person will not normally produce antibodies against his or her own RBC antigens. The most commonly used method of blood typing recognizes two blood group systems: the ABO system and the Rh factor system.

ABO BLOOD GROUP SYSTEM

The **ABO blood group system** recognizes four blood types, A, B, AB, and O, based on the presence or absence of two antigens identified as A and B. An individual who is type A has the A antigen; type B has the B antigen; type AB has both antigens; and type O has neither A nor B. Type O is the most common type, and type AB is the least common.

Unique to the ABO system are preformed antibodies (also called agglutinins) in a person's blood that are directed against the opposite blood type. Type A blood has an antibody (agglutinin) directed against type B, called anti-B. A person with type B has anti-A; type O has both anti-A and anti-B; and type AB has neither. Table 6-6 shows the antigens and antibodies present in the four ABO blood types.

TABLE 6-6	**ABO Blood Group System**	
Blood Type	**RBC Antigen**	**Plasma Antibodies (Agglutinins)**
A	A	Anti-B
B	B	Anti-A
AB	A and B	Neither anti-A nor anti-B
O	Neither	Anti-A and anti-B

Individuals with type AB blood were once referred to as universal recipients because they have neither A nor B antibody to the RBC antigens and can theoretically receive any ABO type blood. Similarly, type O individuals were once called universal donors because they have neither A nor B antigen on their RBCs, and in an emergency their blood can theoretically be given to anyone. However, type O blood does contain plasma antibodies to both A and B antigens, and when given to an A or B type recipient, it can cause a mild transfusion reaction. To avoid reactions, patients are now given type-specific blood, even in emergencies.

RH BLOOD GROUP SYSTEM

The **Rh blood group system** is based upon the presence or absence of an RBC antigen called the D antigen, also known as **Rh factor**. An individual with the D antigen present on red blood cells is said to be positive for the Rh factor, or **Rh positive** (Rh+). An individual whose RBCs lack the D antigen is said to be **Rh negative** (Rh−). A patient must receive blood with the correct Rh type as well as the correct ABO type. Approximately 85% of the population is Rh+.

Unlike the ABO system, antibodies to the Rh factor (anti-Rh antibodies) are not pre-formed in the blood of Rh− individuals. However, an Rh− individual who receives Rh+ blood can become sensitized. This means that the individual may produce antibodies against the Rh factor. In addition, an Rh− woman who is carrying an Rh+ fetus may become sensitized by the RBCs of the fetus, most commonly by leakage of the fetal cells into the mother's circulation during childbirth. This may lead to the destruction of the RBCs of a subsequent Rh+ fetus because Rh antibodies produced by the mother can cross the placenta into the fetal circulation. When this occurs, it is called **hemolytic disease of the newborn** (HDN).

fyi An unsensitized Rh− woman can be given Rh immune globulin (RhIg), such as RhoGam, at certain times during her pregnancy and soon after an Rh+ baby's birth. RhIg will destroy Rh+ fetal cells that may have entered her bloodstream and prevent sensitization.

COMPATIBILITY TESTING/CROSSMATCH

Other factors in an individual's blood can cause adverse reactions during a blood transfusion, even with the correct ABO and Rh type blood. For this reason, a **compatibility** test or **crossmatch** (a test to determine suitability of the donor and recipient blood to be mixed together) is performed using the patient's serum and cells as well as the donor's serum and cells before a unit of blood is determined compatible for transfusion. Recently invented artificial blood, made by chemically altering donor blood, is being tested on humans. This blood is designed to be given to individuals of any blood type and poses no risk of transmitting disease.

Types of Blood Specimens

SERUM

Blood that has been removed from the body will coagulate or clot within 30 to 60 minutes. The clot consists of the blood cells enmeshed in a fibrin network (see Hemostasis). The remaining fluid portion is called **serum** and can be separated from the clot by centrifugation (spinning the clotted blood at high rpms in a machine called a centrifuge). Normal fasting serum is a clear, pale-yellow fluid. Serum has the same composition as plasma except it does not contain fibrinogen, because the fibrinogen was used in the formation of the clot. Many laboratory tests, especially chemistry and immunology tests, are performed on serum.

PLASMA

Not all tests can be performed on serum. For example, most coagulation tests cannot be performed on serum because the coagulation factors, particularly fibrinogen, are used up in the process of clot formation. Some chemistry tests such as ammonia and potassium cannot be performed on serum because clotting releases these substances from the cells. In addition, some chemistry test results are needed STAT (immediately) to respond to emergency situations; having to wait 30 minutes or more for a specimen to clot before centrifuging it to get serum would be unacceptable. If clotting is prevented, however, coagulation factors and other substances affected by clotting are preserved, and the specimen can be centrifuged immediately. Blood can be prevented from clotting by adding a substance called an anticoagulant (See Anticoagulants, Chapter 7). Adding an anticoagulant initially creates a whole blood specimen. When a whole blood specimen is centrifuged, it will separate into three distinct layers (Fig. 6-18): a bottom layer of red blood cells; a thin, fluffy-looking, whitish colored middle layer of WBCs and platelets referred to as the **buffy coat**; and a top layer of clear liquid called plasma that can be separated from the cells and used for testing. Normal fasting plasma is a clear to slightly hazy, pale-yellow fluid visually indistinguishable from serum. The major difference between plasma and serum is that plasma contains fibrinogen. Many laboratory tests can be performed on either serum or plasma.

FIGURE 6-18

Separated whole blood specimen.

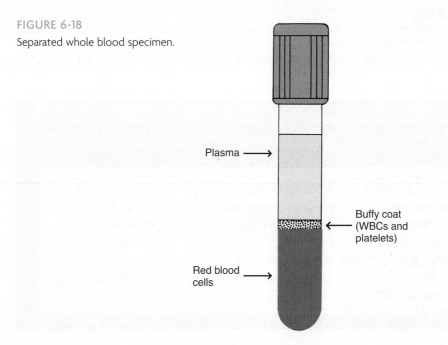

Plasma ⟶

Buffy coat
(WBCs and
platelets) ⟵

Red blood ⟶
cells

WHOLE BLOOD

Some tests, including most hematology tests and some chemistry tests such as glycohemo-globin, cannot be performed on serum or plasma. These tests need to be performed on **whole blood** (blood in the same form as it is in the bloodstream). This means that the blood specimen must not be allowed to clot or separate. To obtain a whole blood specimen, it is necessary to add an anticoagulant. In addition, because the components will separate if the specimen is allowed to stand undisturbed, the specimen must be mixed for a minimum of 2 minutes immediately prior to performing the test.

Blood Disorders

- Anemia: an abnormal reduction in the number of RBCs in the circulating blood.
- Leukemia: an increase in WBCs characterized by the presence of a large number of abnormal forms.
- Leukocytosis: an abnormal increase in WBCs in the circulating blood.
- Leukopenia: an abnormal decrease in WBCs.
- Polycythemia: an abnormal increase in RBCs.
- Thrombocytosis: increased number of platelets.
- Thrombocytopenia: decreased number of platelets.

Diagnostic Tests

Examples of diagnostic tests for blood disorders are listed in Box 6-4.

HEMOSTASIS

Hemostasis (he'mo-sta'sis) (Fig. 6-19) is the process by which the body stops the leakage of blood from the vascular system after injury. If an injury occurs to a blood vessel, the

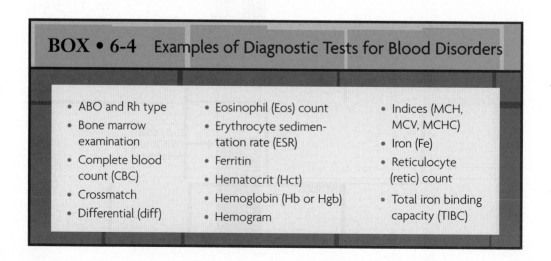

BOX • 6-4   Examples of Diagnostic Tests for Blood Disorders

- ABO and Rh type
- Bone marrow examination
- Complete blood count (CBC)
- Crossmatch
- Differential (diff)
- Eosinophil (Eos) count
- Erythrocyte sedimentation rate (ESR)
- Ferritin
- Hematocrit (Hct)
- Hemoglobin (Hb or Hgb)
- Hemogram
- Indices (MCH, MCV, MCHC)
- Iron (Fe)
- Reticulocyte (retic) count
- Total iron binding capacity (TIBC)

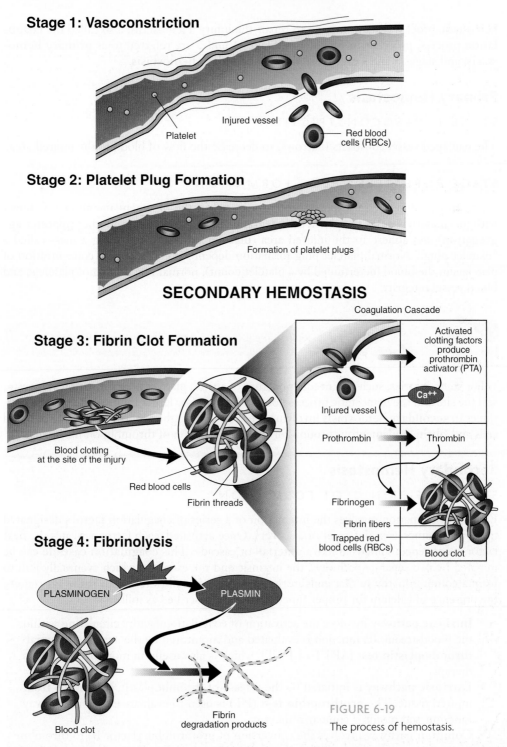

PRIMARY HEMOSTASIS

Stage 1: Vasoconstriction

Injured vessel

Platelet

Red blood
cells (RBCs)

Stage 2: Platelet Plug Formation

Formation of platelet plugs

SECONDARY HEMOSTASIS

Coagulation Cascade

Stage 3: Fibrin Clot Formation

Activated
clotting factors
produce
prothrombin
activator (PTA)

Ca++

Injured vessel

Prothrombin → Thrombin

Blood clotting
at the site of the injury

Red blood cells

Fibrin threads

Fibrinogen

Fibrin fibers

Trapped red
blood cells (RBCs)

Blood clot

Stage 4: Fibrinolysis

PLASMINOGEN → PLASMIN

Blood clot

Fibrin
degradation products

FIGURE 6-19

The process of hemostasis.

207

hemostatic process is set in motion to repair the injury. Hemostasis, also called the **coagulation** process, proceeds in four stages. Stages 1 and 2 are referred to as **primary hemostasis**, and stages 3 and 4 are referred to as **secondary hemostasis**.

Primary Hemostasis

STAGE 1: VASOCONSTRICTION

The damaged vessel constricts (narrows) to decrease the flow of blood to the injured area.

STAGE 2: PLATELET PLUG FORMATION

Injury to the blood vessel exposes protein material in the basement membrane. Contact with this material causes the platelets to degranulate and stick to one another (**platelet aggregation**) and adhere to the injured area (**platelet adhesion**), forming a mass called a "platelet plug." Normal platelet plug formation depends on an adequate concentration of platelets in the blood (determined by a platelet count), normal functioning of platelets, and blood vessel integrity.

> **key · point**   A bleeding time (BT) test assesses platelet plug formation.

For some injuries, such as a needle puncture of a vein, platelet plug formation suffices to seal the site and the hemostatic process goes no further. For larger injuries, the process continues to **secondary hemostasis** involving creation of a tougher "fibrin" clot made of blood cells and **fibrin**, a filamentous protein formed by the action of thrombin on fibrinogen.

Secondary Hemostasis

STAGE 3: FIBRIN CLOT FORMATION

Fibrin clot formation involves the interaction of a series of coagulation **factors** designated by Roman numerals in the order of discovery. Once activated, each factor activates the next factor in sequence, somewhat like a waterfall or cascade. This **coagulation cascade** can be initiated by two separate pathways, the intrinsic and the extrinsic, which eventually join to form a common pathway that ends in the formation of a fibrin clot. All pathways require the presence of calcium for proper function and are described as follows:

- **Intrinsic pathway** involves the activation of coagulation factors circulating within the bloodstream. Its function is evaluated and monitored by the **activated partial thromboplastin test** (APTT or PTT), which is also useful in monitoring heparin therapy.
- **Extrinsic pathway** is initiated by the release of thromboplastin (factor III) from injured tissue. The **prothrombin test** (PT) is used to evaluate extrinsic pathway function and monitor coumarin therapy.
- **Common pathway** involves the conversion of prothrombin (factor II) to thrombin by the action of prothrombin activator (PTA) generated earlier in the coagulation

process as a consequence of vessel injury. Calcium ions are necessary for this reaction to occur. Thrombin splits fibrinogen (factor I) into strands of protein called fibrin. The fibrin creates a netlike structure that traps blood cells and platelets forming a **hemostatic plug** (blood clot), which seals the opening in the injured blood vessel and stops the bleeding.

STAGE 4: FIBRINOLYSIS

Fibrinolysis (fi'brin-ol'i-sis) involves the ultimate removal or dissolution of the blood clot once healing has occurred. This process is possible because activation of the clotting process also releases substances that lead to the conversion of plasminogen (a substance that is normally present in plasma and thus incorporated in the clot) to plasmin. Plasmin is an enzyme that breaks the fibrin into small fragments called **fibrin degradation products** (**fibrin split products**), which are then removed by phagocytic cells.

key • point The coagulation process is kept in check and limited to local sites by the action of natural inhibitors circulating in the plasma along with the coagulation factors. The inhibitors bind with coagulation factors that escape the clotting site and those remaining after clotting is complete.

The Role of the Liver in Hemostasis

The liver plays an important role in the hemostatic process. It is responsible for the synthesis (manufacture) of coagulation factors, such as fibrinogen and prothrombin. It produces the bile salts necessary for the absorption of vitamin K, which is also necessary to the synthesis of the coagulation factors. In addition, mast cells (tissue basophils) in the liver produce heparin. When the liver is diseased, synthesis of coagulation factors is impaired and bleeding may result.

Hemostatic Disorders

- Deep vein thrombosis (DVT): a blood clot that forms in a large vein in the leg.
- Disseminated intravascular coagulation (DIC): a pathologic form of diffuse coagulation in which coagulation factors are consumed to such an extent that bleeding occurs.
- Hemophilia (he'mo-fil'e-a): a hereditary condition characterized by bleeding due to increased coagulation time. The most common type of hemophilia is due to factor VIII deficiency.
- Thrombocytopenia (throm'bo-si'to-pe'ne-a): an abnormal decrease in platelets.

Diagnostic Tests

Examples of diagnostic tests of the hemostatatic process are listed in Box 6-5.

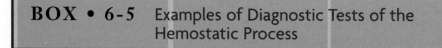

BOX • 6-5 Examples of Diagnostic Tests of the Hemostatic Process

- Bleeding time (BT)
- D-dimer
- Factor assays
- Fibrin degradation products (FDP)
- Platelet function assay (PFA)
- Prothrombin time (PT)
- Partial thromboplastin time (PTT or APTT)

THE LYMPHATIC SYSTEM

Functions

The **lymphatic system** (Fig. 6-20) returns tissue fluid to the bloodstream, protects the body by removing microorganisms and impurities, processes lymphocytes, and delivers fats absorbed from the small intestine to the bloodstream. Lymph vessels spread throughout the entire body much like blood vessels.

Structures

The lymphatic system is made up of fluid called **lymph** and the lymphatic vessels, ducts, and **nodes** (masses of lymph tissue) through which the lymph flows.

Lymph Flow

Body cells are bathed in tissue fluid acquired from the bloodstream. Water, oxygen, and nutrients continually diffuse through the capillary walls into the tissue spaces. Much of the fluid diffuses back into the capillaries along with waste products of metabolism. Excess tissue fluid filters into lymphatic capillaries, where it is called lymph. Lymph fluid is similar to plasma but is 95% water.

Lymphatic capillaries join with larger and larger lymphatic vessels until they empty into one of two terminal vessels, either the right lymphatic duct or the thoracic duct. These ducts then empty into large veins in the upper body. Lymph moves through the vessels primarily owing to skeletal muscle contraction, much like blood moves through the veins. Like veins, lymphatic vessels have valves to keep the lymph flowing in the right direction.

Before reaching the ducts, the lymph passes through a series of structures called **lymph nodes**. Lymphoid tissue, of which nodes are composed, is a special kind of tissue with the ability to remove impurities and process lymphocytes. Thus lymph nodes are able to trap and destroy bacteria and foreign matter and produce lymphocytes. The tonsils, thymus, gastrointestinal tract, and spleen also contain lymphoid tissue.

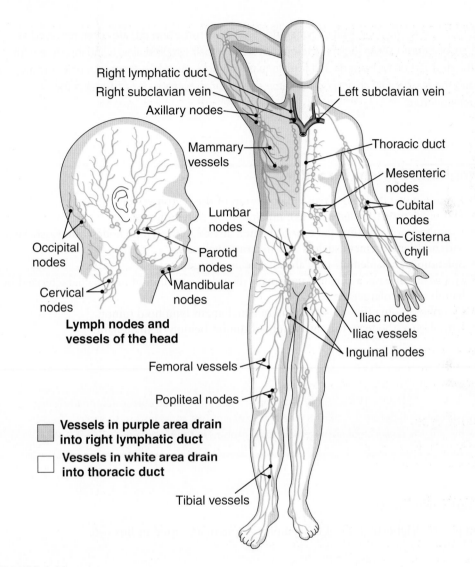

Right lymphatic duct

Right subclavian vein

Axillary nodes

Mammary vessels

Left subclavian vein

Thoracic duct

Mesenteric nodes

Cubital nodes

Cisterna chyli

Lumbar nodes

Occipital nodes

Parotid nodes

Cervical nodes

Mandibular nodes

Lymph nodes and vessels of the head

Iliac nodes

Iliac vessels

Inguinal nodes

Femoral vessels

Popliteal nodes

Vessels in purple area drain into right lymphatic duct

Vessels in white area drain into thoracic duct

Tibial vessels

FIGURE 6-20

Lymphatic system.

caution   Axillary lymph nodes (nodes in the arm pit) are often removed as part of breast cancer surgery. Their removal can impair lymph drainage and interfere with the destruction of bacteria and foreign matter. This is cause for concern in phlebotomy and the reason why an arm on the same side as a mastectomy is not suitable for venipuncture.

Lymphatic System Disorders

- Lymphangitis (lim-fan-ji'tis): inflammation of the lymph vessels.
- Lymphadenitis (lim-fad'e-ni-tis): inflammation of lymph nodes.
- Lymphadenopathy (lim-fad'e-nop'ah-the): disease of the lymph nodes, often associated with node enlargement such as seen in mononucleosis.
- Splenomegaly (splen'no-meg'ah-le): spleen enlargement.
- Hodgkin's disease: a chronic, malignant disorder, common in males, characterized by lymph node enlargement.
- Lymphosarcoma (lim-fo-sar-ko'mah): a malignant lymphoid tumor.
- Lymphoma: the term for any lymphoid tumor, benign or malignant.

key • point   Inflamed lymph nodes may not be able to filter pathogens from the lymph before it returns to the bloodstream. This could lead to septicemia (sep-ti-se'me-ah), the presence of pathogenic microorganisms in the blood.

Diagnostic Tests

Examples of diagnostic tests of the lymphatic system are listed in Box 6-6.

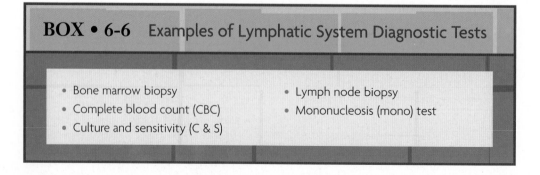

BOX • 6-6 Examples of Lymphatic System Diagnostic Tests

- Bone marrow biopsy
- Complete blood count (CBC)
- Culture and sensitivity (C & S)
- Lymph node biopsy
- Mononucleosis (mono) test

STUDY & REVIEW QUESTIONS

1. **Which of the following is described as an anuclear, biconcave disk?**
   a. Erythrocyte
   b. Granulocyte
   c. Leukocyte
   d. Thrombocyte

2. **The chamber of the heart that receives blood from the systemic circulation is the**
   a. Left atrium
   b. Left ventricle
   c. Right atrium
   d. Right ventricle

3. **The thick muscle layer of the heart is called the**
   a. Endocardium
   b. Epicardium
   c. Myocardium
   d. Pericardium

4. **The ECG shows P waves due to**
   a. Atrial contractions
   b. Delayed contractions
   c. Recovery of the electrical charge
   d. Ventricular contraction

5. **When taking a blood pressure, the systolic pressure is the pressure reading when the**
   a. Artery is compressed and blood flow is cut off
   b. Cuff is completely deflated
   c. First heart sounds are heard as the cuff is deflated
   d. Muffled sound is heard as the cuff is deflated

6. **The purpose of the pulmonary system is to**
   a. Carry blood to and from the lungs
   b. Carry nutrients to the cells
   c. Deliver blood to the systemic system
   d. Remove impurities from the blood

7. **Which of the following blood vessels are listed in the proper order of blood flow?**
   a. Aorta, superior vena cava, vein
   b. Arteriole, venule, capillary
   c. Capillary, venule, vein
   d. Vein, venule, capillary

8. **The internal space of a blood vessel is called the**
   a. Atrium
   b. Lumen
   c. Septum
   d. Valve

9. **The longest vein and the largest artery in the body in that order are**
   a. Cephalic and femoral
   b. Great saphenous and aorta
   c. Inferior vena cava and brachial
   d. Pulmonary and femoral

10. The preferred vein for venipuncture in the "H" pattern is the

    a. Accessory cephalic   c. Cephalic

    b. Basilic   d. Median cubital

11. The major difference between plasma and serum is that plasma

    a. Contains fibrinogen, serum does not

    b. Contains nutrients, plasma does not

    c. Looks clear, serum looks cloudy

    d. Looks dark yellow, serum looks pale yellow

12. An individual's blood type (A, B, AB, or O) is determined by the presence or absence of which of the following on the red blood cells?

    a. Antigens   c. Chemicals

    b. Antibodies   d. Hormones

13. Which is the correct sequence of events after blood vessel injury?

    a. Platelet aggregation, vasoconstriction, fibrin clot formation

    b. Vasoconstriction, platelet aggregation, fibrin clot formation

    c. Vasodilation, platelet adhesion, fibrin clot formation

    d. Fibrinolysis, platelet adhesion, vasoconstriction

14. Lymph originates from

    a. Joint fluid   c. Serum

    b. Plasma   d. Tissue fluid

15. A heart disorder characterized by fluid buildup in the lungs is called

    a. Aortic stenosis   c. Congestive heart failure

    b. Bacterial endocarditis   d. Myocardial infarction

Bibliography and Suggested Readings

Cohen, B. J., & Jason, J. T. (2005). Memmler's the human body in health and disease (10th ed.). Philadelphia: Lippincott Williams & Wilkins.

Fischbach, F. (2003). Laboratory diagnostic tests (7th ed.). Philadelphia: Lippincott Williams & Wilkins.

Herlihy, B., & Maebius, N. K. (2000). The human body in health and illness. Philadelphia: W. B. Saunders.

Mahon, C., Smith, L., & Burns, C. (1998). An introduction to clinical laboratory science. Philadelphia: W. B. Saunders.

Quinley, E. (1998). Immunohematology: principles and practice. Lippincott Williams & Wilkins.

Stedman's (2005) Medical dictionary for the health professions and nursing (5th ed.). Philadelphia: Lippincott Williams & Wilkins.

Stevens, M. L. (1997). Fundamentals of clinical hematology. Philadelphia, W. B. Saunders.

Venes, D. (2005). Taber's cyclopedic medical dictionary (20th ed.). Philadelphia: F. A. Davis.

III

Blood Collection Procedures

BLOOD COLLECTION EQUIPMENT, ADDITIVES, AND ORDER OF DRAW

key•terms

ACD

additive

anticoagulant

antiglycolytic agent

antiseptics

bevel

butterfly needle

clot activator

disinfectant

EDTA

evacuated tube

gauge

glycolysis

heparin

hub

hypodermic needle

lumen

multisample needle

order of draw

potassium oxalate

PST

shaft

sharps container

silica

sodium citrate

sodium fluoride

SPS

SST

thixotropic gel

tube additive

winged infusion set

objectives

Upon successful completion of this chapter, the reader should be able to:

1. Define the key terms and abbreviations listed at the beginning of this chapter.

2. List, describe, and explain the purpose of the equipment and supplies needed to collect blood by venipuncture.

3. Compare and contrast antiseptics and disinfectants and give examples of each.

4. Identify appropriate phlebotomy needles by length, gauge, and any associated color-coding.

5. List and describe evacuated tube system (ETS) and syringe system components, explain how each system works, and tell how to determine which components and system to use.

6. Identify the general categories of additives used in blood collection, list the various additives within each category, and describe how each additive works.

7. Describe the color coding used to identify the presence or absence of additives in blood collection tubes, and name the additive, laboratory departments, and individual tests associated with the various color-coded tubes.

8. List the "order of draw" when collecting multiple tubes and explain why it is important.

The primary duty of the phlebotomist is to collect blood specimens for laboratory testing. Blood is collected by several methods, including arterial puncture, capillary puncture, and venipuncture. This chapter describes general blood collection equipment and supplies commonly needed regardless of the method of collection, as well as blood collection equipment specific to venipuncture. Specific equipment for arterial puncture and skin puncture is described in their respective chapters.

GENERAL BLOOD COLLECTION EQUIPMENT AND SUPPLIES

The following are equipment and supplies commonly needed for all methods of collecting blood specimens.

Blood-Drawing Station

A blood-drawing station is a dedicated area of a medical laboratory or clinic equipped for performing phlebotomy procedures on patients, primarily outpatients sent by their physicians for laboratory testing. A typical blood-drawing station includes a table for supplies, a special chair where the patient sits during the blood collection procedure, and a bed or reclining chair for patients with a history of fainting, persons donating blood, and other special situations. A bed or padded table is also needed if heelsticks or other procedures will be performed on infants and small children.

Phlebotomy Chairs

A phlebotomy chair should be comfortable for the patient and have adjustable armrests to achieve proper positioning of either arm. Special phlebotomy chairs (Fig. 7-1) are available from a number of manufacturers. Most have adjustable armrests that lock in place to prevent the patient from falling should fainting occur.

caution In the absence of a special chair, precautions must be taken to prevent falls and ensure client safety.

Equipment Carriers

Equipment carriers make blood collection equipment portable. This is especially important in a hospital setting and other instances in which the patient cannot come to the laboratory.

HAND-HELD CARRIERS

Hand-held phlebotomy equipment carriers or trays (Fig. 7-2) come in a variety of styles and sizes designed to be easily carried by the phlebotomist and to contain enough equipment for numerous blood draws. They are convenient for "stat" or emergency situations or when relatively few patients need blood work.

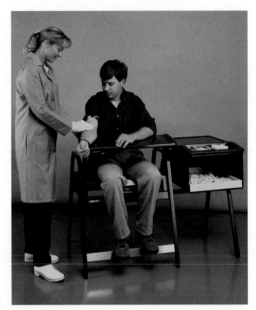

FIGURE 7-1

Phlebotomy chair. (Courtesy Lab Conco, Kansas City, MO.)

PHLEBOTOMY CARTS

Phlebotomy carts (Fig. 7-3) are typically made of stainless steel or strong synthetic material. They have swivel wheels, which glide the carts smoothly and quietly down hospital hallways and in and out of elevators. They normally have several shelves to carry adequate supplies for obtaining blood specimens from many patients. Carts are commonly used for early morning hospital phlebotomy rounds when many patients need lab work and for scheduled "sweeps" (rounds

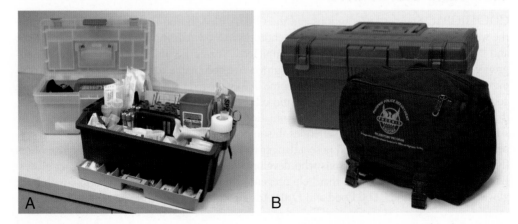

FIGURE 7-2

Several types of phlebotomy equipment carriers. **A.** Covered phlebotomy tray and open tray. **B.** Two types of carriers used by law enforcement officers for DUI blood collections. *Left,* One carried in a car or van. *Right,* A type carried on a motorcycle.

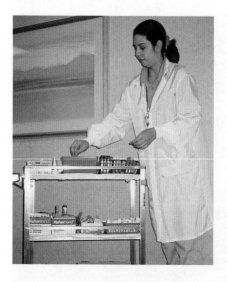

FIGURE 7-3
Phlebotomist with a phlebotomy cart

that occur at regular intervals throughout the day). Carts are bulky and a potential source of nosocomial infections and are not normally brought into patient rooms. Instead, they are parked outside in the hallway. A tray of supplies to be taken into the room is often carried on the cart.

key · point Keeping carts and trays adequately stocked with supplies is an important duty of the phlebotomist.

Gloves and Glove Liners

CDC/HICPAC Standard precautions and the OSHA Bloodborne Pathogen Standard, require the wearing of gloves when performing phlebotomy. A new pair must be used for each patient and be removed when the procedure is completed. Nonsterile, disposable latex, nitrile, neoprene, polyethylene, and vinyl examination gloves are acceptable for most phlebotomy procedures. A good fit is essential. Some gloves come lightly dusted with powder to make them more comfortable to wear and easier to slip on and off. However, the phlebotomist should be aware that glove powder can be a source of contamination for some tests (especially those collected by skin puncture) and can also cause allergies in some users. Powder in latex gloves can help suspend latex particles in the air and pose a danger to those with latex allergy. Special glove liners (Fig. 7-4A) are available for persons who develop allergies or dermatitis from wearing gloves. Barrier hand creams (Fig. 7-4B) that help prevent skin irritation and are compatible with latex gloves are also available. The Food and Drug Administration (FDA) regulates glove quality.

key · point Decontamination of hands after glove removal is essential. Any type of glove may contain defects and some studies suggest that vinyl gloves may not provide an adequate barrier to viruses.

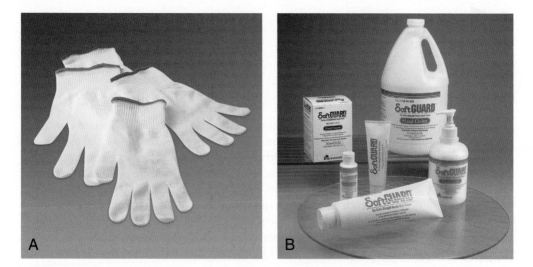

FIGURE 7-4

A. UltraFIT glove liners. **B.** SoftGUARD barrier hand cream.   (Courtesy Erie Scientific Co., Portsmouth, NH.)

Antiseptics

Antiseptics are substances used to prevent sepsis, the presence of microorganisms or their toxic products in the bloodstream. Antiseptics prevent or inhibit the growth and development of microorganisms, but do not necessarily kill them. They are considered safe to use on human skin and are used to clean the site prior to blood collection. The antiseptic most commonly used for routine blood collection is 70% isopropyl alcohol (isopropanol) in individually wrapped prep pads. For a higher degree of antisepsis, the traditional antiseptic has been povidone-iodine in the form of swabsticks or sponge pads for blood culture collection and prep pads for blood gas collection. However, the use of alcohol-based preparations for these procedures is increasing because many patients are allergic to povidone-iodine. A list of antiseptics used in blood collection is shown in Box 7-1.

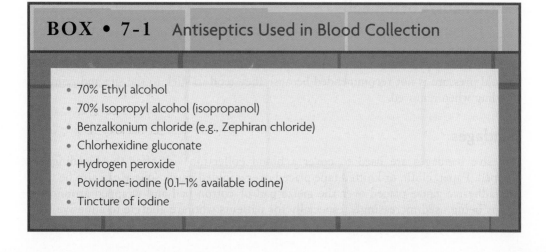

BOX • 7-1   Antiseptics Used in Blood Collection

- 70% Ethyl alcohol
- 70% Isopropyl alcohol (isopropanol)
- Benzalkonium chloride (e.g., Zephiran chloride)
- Chlorhexidine gluconate
- Hydrogen peroxide
- Povidone-iodine (0.1–1% available iodine)
- Tincture of iodine

key • point Cleaning with an antiseptic reduces the number of microorganisms, but does not sterilize the site.

Disinfectants

Disinfectants are EPA-regulated chemical substances or solutions that are used to remove or kill microorganisms on surfaces and instruments. They are typically corrosive and are not safe for use on human skin. According to CDC and HICPAC *Guidelines for Environmental Infection Control in Healthcare Facilities*, use of EPA-registered sodium hypochlorite products is preferred, but solutions made from generic 5.25% sodium hypochlorite (household bleach) may be used. A 1:100 dilution is recommended for decontaminating nonporous surfaces after cleaning up blood or other body fluid spills in patient-care settings. When spills involve large amounts of blood or other body fluids or occur in the laboratory, a 1:10 dilution is applied prior to cleanup. At least 10 minutes of contact time is required for disinfectants to be effective.

key • point Fresh bleach solutions should be made daily or as needed.

Hand Sanitizers

A recent CDC report entitled *Guideline for Hand Hygiene in Health Care Settings* recommends the use of alcohol-based hand sanitizers (Fig. 7-5) for routine decontamination of hands as a substitute for hand washing provided the hands are not visibly soiled. If hands are heavily contaminated with organic material and hand-washing facilities are not available, it is recommended that hands be cleaned with detergent-containing wipes followed by the use of an alcohol-based hand cleaner. Alcohol-based hand cleansers are available in rinses, gels, and foams

Gauze Pads/Cotton Balls

Clean 2 × 2-inch gauze pads folded in fourths are used to hold pressure over the site following blood collection procedures. Special gauze pads with fluid proof backing are also available to help prevent contamination of gloves from blood at the site. Use of cotton balls to hold pressure is not recommended because they tend to stick to the site and reinitiate bleeding when removed.

Bandages

Adhesive bandages are used to cover a blood collection site after the bleeding has stopped. Paper, cloth, or knitted tape placed over a folded gauze square can also be used. Self-adhesive gauze placed over the gauze pad or cotton ball and wrapped around the arm is being used increasingly, especially for patients who are allergic to adhesive ban-

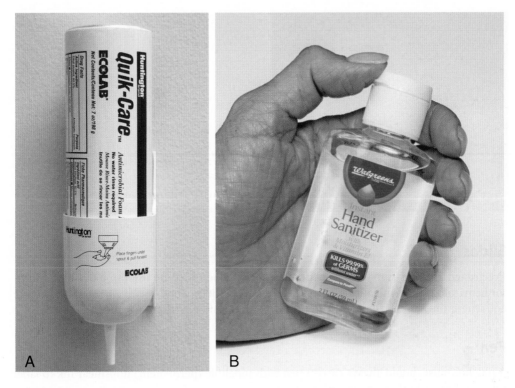

FIGURE 7-5

A. Wall-mounted hand sanitizer dispenser. **B.** Personal size bottle of hand sanitizer.

dages. It is also used to form a pressure bandage following arterial puncture or venipuncture in patients with bleeding problems. Latex-free bandages are available for those with latex allergies.

> **c a u t i o n** Adhesive bandages should not be used on babies younger than 2 years of age because of the danger of aspiration and suffocation.

Needle and Sharps Disposal Containers

Used needles, lancets, and other sharp objects must be disposed of immediately in special containers referred to as **"sharps" containers** (Fig. 7-6), even if they contain safety features. A variety of styles and sizes are available. Most are red for easy identification, but some are clear or opaque to make it easier to tell when they are full. All must be clearly marked with a biohazard symbol and be rigid, puncture resistant, leak proof, and disposable and have locking lids to seal the contents when full, after which they must be properly disposed of as biohazardous waste.

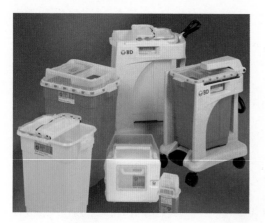

FIGURE 7-6

Several styles of sharps containers. (Courtesy Becton Dickinson, Franklin Lakes, NJ.)

Slides

Precleaned 25 × 75-mm (1 × 3-inch) glass microscope slides are used to make blood films for hematology determinations. Slides are available either plain or with a frosted area at one end where the patient's name or other information can be written in pencil.

Pen

A phlebotomist should always carry a pen with indelible (permanent) nonsmear ink to label tubes and record other patient information.

Watch

A watch, preferably with a sweep second hand or timer, is needed to accurately determine specimen collection times and time certain tests.

ARTERIAL PUNCTURE EQUIPMENT

See Chapter 12.

CAPILLARY PUNCTURE EQUIPMENT

See Chapter 10.

VENIPUNCTURE EQUIPMENT

The following equipment is used for venipuncture procedures in addition to the general blood collection supplies and equipment previously described.

Vein-Locating Devices

There are a number of optional, but useful portable devices on the market to make it easier to locate veins that are difficult to see or feel. Most devices can be used on all ages. Examples include

- Transillumination devices such as the Venoscope II (Fig. 7-7) and Neonatal Transilluminator (Venoscope, L.L.C., Lafayette, LA), and the Transillumination Vein Locator (VL-U) (Promedic, McCordsville, IN). Transillumination means to inspect an organ by passing light through its walls. These devices typically use high-intensity LED lights to shine through the patient's subcutaneous tissue and highlight veins, which absorb the light rather than reflecting it and stand out as dark lines.
- The Vein Entry Indicator device (VEID) by Vascular Technologies (Ness-Ziona, Israel) uses pressure-sensing technology in a device that attaches to a catheter needle insertion unit. When the needle penetrates a blood vessel the device senses the change in pressure and emits a beeping signal that stops when the needle exits the vein.

Tourniquet

A **tourniquet** (Fig. 7-8) is a device that is applied or tied around a patient's arm prior to venipuncture to restrict blood flow. A properly applied tourniquet is tight enough to restrict venous flow out of the area, but not so tight as to restrict arterial flow into the area. Restriction of venous flow distends or inflates the veins, making them larger and easier

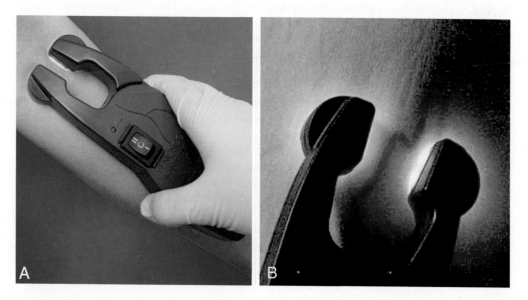

FIGURE 7-7

A. Venoscope II trans-illuminator device. **B.** A vein appears as a dark line between the light-emitting arms of the Venoscope II.   (Venoscope II, LLC, Lafayette, LA.)

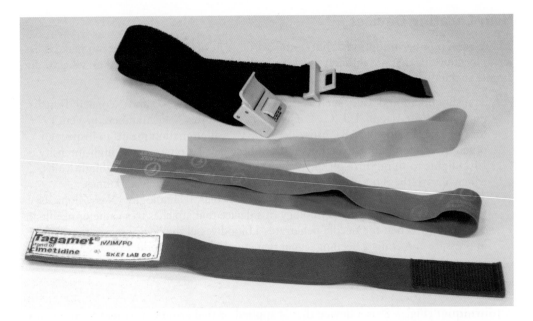

FIGURE 7-8

Several types of tourniquets *(top to bottom):* Buckle closure, latex strap, nonlatex strap, and Velcro closure.

to find, and stretches the vein walls so they are thinner and easier to pierce with a needle. Restriction of blood flow can change blood components if the tourniquet is left in place for more than 1 minute, so a tourniquet must fasten in a way that is easy to release with one hand during blood collection procedures or in emergency situations such as when a patient starts to faint or the needle accidentally backs out of the arm during venipuncture.

There are a number of different types of tourniquets, and most are available in both adult and pediatric sizes. The most common type, a flat strip of stretchable material, such as latex or vinyl, is fairly inexpensive and disposable. It can be used more than once, but is normally thrown away if it gets contaminated with blood.

Reusable tourniquets made of elastic material with a long band of Velcro or similar interlocking material that allows a wide range of adjustment capability are also available. This type may not fit around the arms of extremely obese patients and is not as easy to clean if dirty or contaminated.

Several manufacturers make reusable tourniquets with stretchable webbing and buckle closures. These tourniquets stay on the patient's arm when released and can be tightened again if necessary. They require regular cleaning with disinfectant. Some brands can be autoclaved.

fyi   A blood pressure cuff may be used in place of a tourniquet. The patient's blood pressure is taken and the pressure is then maintained below the patient's diastolic pressure.

Needles

Phlebotomy needles are sterile, disposable, and designed for single use only. They include **multisample needles** (see Evacuated Tube System), **hypodermic needles** (see Syringe System), and **winged infusion (butterfly) needles** used with both the evacuated tube system and the syringe system. Multisample needles are commonly enclosed in sealed twist off shields or covers. Hypodermic needles and butterfly needles are typically sealed in sterile pull-apart packages.

> c a u t i o n   It is important to examine the packaging or seal of a needle before use. If the packaging is open or the seal is broken, the needle is no longer sterile and should not be used.

Specific terminology is used to refer to the parts of a needle. The end that pierces the vein is called the **bevel** because it is "beveled," or cut on a slant. The bevel allows the needle to easily slip into the skin and vein without coring (removal of a portion of the skin or vein). The long cylindrical portion is called the **shaft.** The end that attaches to the blood collection device is called the **hub,** and the internal space of the needle is called the **lumen.** Needles are available in various sizes indicated by length and gauge.

> key • point   It important to visually inspect a needle prior to venipuncture. Needles are mass produced and on rare occasions contain defects such as blocked, blunt, or bent tips or rough bevels or shafts that could injure a patient's vein, cause unnecessary pain, or result in venipuncture failure.

GAUGE

Needle **gauge** is a number that relates to the diameter of the lumen. The needle diameter and the gauge have an inverse (opposite) relationship, that is, the larger the gauge number, the smaller the actual diameter of the needle.

Although blood typically flows more quickly through large-diameter needles, needle gauge is selected according to the size and condition of the patient's vein, the type of procedure, and the equipment being used. Appropriate needles for the collection of most blood specimens for laboratory testing include gauges 20 through 23; however, a 21-gauge needle is considered the standard for most routine phlebotomy situations. Common venipuncture needle gauges with needle type and typical use are shown in Table 7-1.

> key • point   It is important to select the appropriate needle for the situation. A needle that is too large may damage a vein needlessly, and a needle that is too small may hemolyze the specimen.

TABLE 7-1	Common Venipuncture Needle Gauges with Needle Type and Typical Use	
Gauge	**Needle Type**	**Typical Use**
15–17	Special needle attached to collection bag	Collection of donor units, autologous blood donation, and therapeutic phlebotomy
18	Syringe	Used primarily as a transfer needle rather than for blood collection; safety issues have diminished use
20	Multisample syringe	Sometimes used when large-volume tubes are collected or large-volume syringes are used on patients with normal-size veins
21	Multisample syringe	Considered the standard venipuncture needle for routine venipuncture on patients with normal veins or syringe blood culture collection
22	Multisample syringe	Used on older children and adult patients with small veins or syringe draws on difficult veins
23	Butterfly	Veins of infants and children and difficult or hand veins of adults

Manufacturers typically color-code needles by gauge for easy identification. Generally, multisample needles have color-coded caps and hubs (Fig. 7-9), and syringe needles have color-coded hubs. Butterfly needles often have color-coded "wings." Syringe and butterfly needle packaging may also contain color-coding. Needle color-codes vary among manufacturers.

LENGTH

Most multisample needles come in 1-inch or 1.5-inch lengths. Syringe needles come in many lengths; however 1-inch and 1.5-inch ones are most commonly used for venipuncture. Butterfly needles are typically 1/2 to 3/4 of an inch long. Some of the new safety needles come in slightly longer lengths to accommodate resheathing features. Length selection depends primarily upon user preference and the depth of the vein. Many phlebotomists pre-

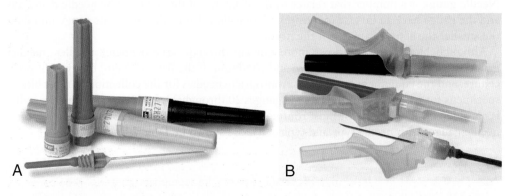

A   B

FIGURE 7-9

Multisample needles with color-coded caps. **A.** Traditional style needles: yellow 20 gauge, green 21 gauge, and black 22 gauge.   (Greiner Bio-One, Kremsmünster, Austria). **B.** BD Eclipse safety needles, black 22 gauge, green 21 gauge.   (Becton Dickinson, Franklin Lakes, NJ.)

fer to use 1-inch needles in routine situations because it is less intimidating to the patient. Others, especially those with larger hands feel that the 1.5-inch needle makes it easier to achieve the proper angle for entering the vein.

SAFETY FEATURES

Needles are available with or without safety features. Safety features must provide immediate permanent containment and be activated using one hand, which must stay behind the needle at all times. Safety features include **resheathing devices** such as shields that cover the needle after use, blunting devices, and equipment with devices that retract the needle after use. The FDA is responsible for clearing medical devices for marketing. Box 7-2 lists desirable characteristics of safety features that the FDA considers important in preventing percutaneous injury.

key • point   According to OSHA regulations, if the needle does not have a safety feature, the equipment it is used with (such as tube holder or syringe) must have a safety feature to minimize the chance of accidental needlesticks.

BOX • 7-2   Desirable Characteristics of Safety Features

- The safety feature is a fixed safety feature that provides a barrier between the hands and the needle after use; the safety feature should allow or require the worker's hands to remain behind the needle at all times.
- The safety feature is an integral part of the device and not an accessory.
- The safety feature is in effect before disassembly and remains in effect after disposal to protect users and trash handlers and for environmental safety.
- The safety feature is as simple as possible, requiring little or no training to use effectively

---

Evacuated Tube System (ETS)

The most common, efficient, and CLSI-preferred system for collecting blood samples is the **evacuated tube system (ETS)** (Fig. 7-10). It is a closed system in which the patient's blood flows through a needle inserted into a vein, directly into a collection tube without being exposed to the air or outside contaminants. The system allows numerous tubes to be collected with a single venipuncture. Evacuated tube systems are available from several manufacturers. Although the design of individual elements may vary slightly by manufacturer, all ETS systems have three basic components, a special blood-drawing needle, a needle and tube holder, and various types of evacuated tubes.

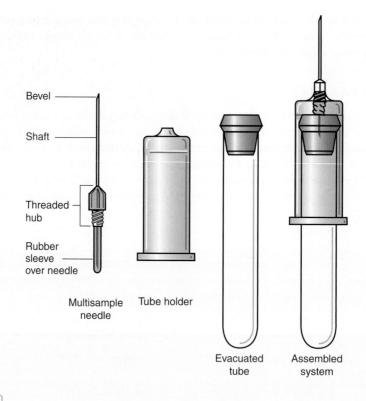

FIGURE 7-10

Traditional components of the evacuated tube system (ETS).

key • point Unless components are specifically designed for use with multiple systems, it is recommended that all ETS components come from the same manufacturer. Mixing components from different manufacturers can lead to problems such as needles coming unscrewed and tubes popping off the needle during venipuncture.

MULTISAMPLE NEEDLES

ETS needles (Fig. 7-9) are called multisample needles because they allow multiple tubes of blood to be collected during a single venipuncture. They are threaded in the middle and have a beveled point on each end. The threaded portion screws into a tube holder. The end of the needle that pierces the vein is longer and has a longer bevel. The shorter end penetrates the tube stopper during specimen collection. It is covered by a sleeve that retracts as the needle goes through the tube stopper so blood can flow into the tube. When the tube is removed, the sleeve slides back over the needle to prevent leakage of blood. ETS needles are available with or without safety features. An ETS needle with a safety feature is shown attached to a tube holder in Figure 7-11.

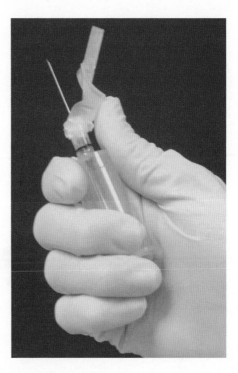

FIGURE 7-11

BD multisample safety needle attached to traditional tube holder.

c a u t i o n ETS needles without safety features must be used with holders that have safety features.

TUBE HOLDERS

A **tube holder** (Fig. 7-12) is a clear, plastic, disposable cylinder with a small threaded opening at one end (often also called a hub) where the needle is screwed into it, and a large opening at the other end where the collection tube is placed. The large end has flanges or extensions on the sides that aid in tube placement and removal.

key • point OSHA regulations require that the tube holder with needle attached be disposed of as a unit after use and never removed from the needle and reused.

Holders are typically available in several sizes to accommodate different-sized tubes, including special sizes for large-diameter blood culture bottles, some of which have adapter inserts to narrow the diameter of the holder and allow collection of evacuated tubes after the blood culture specimens. Adapter inserts are also available so small diameter tubes can be collected in regular-size tube holders. Holders are available with and without safety features.

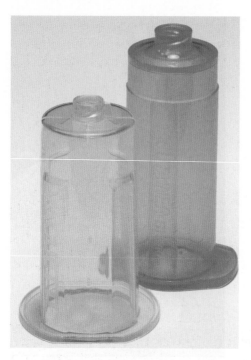

FIGURE 7-12

Traditional needle and tube holder.

c a u t i o n   If the tube holder does not have a safety feature, the needle used with it must have a safety feature.

Safety features include shields that cover the needle and devices that manually or automatically retract the needle into the holder either before or after it is removed from the vein. Several types of holders with safety features are shown in Figure 7-13.

EVACUATED TUBES

Evacuated tubes (Fig. 7-14) are the type of tube used with both the ETS and the syringe method of obtaining blood specimens. (With the syringe method, blood is collected in a syringe and must be immediately transferred into the tubes.) Evacuated tubes come in various sizes and volumes ranging from 1.8 to 15 mL. Tube selection is based on the age of the patient, the amount of blood needed for the test, and the size and condition of the patient's vein. Most laboratories stock several sizes of each type of tube to accommodate various needs. Presently, tubes are available in plastic and glass. For safety reasons, it is strongly recommended that plastic tubes be used if at all possible. Local, state, and federal safety regulatory agencies should be consulted for current applicable regulations.

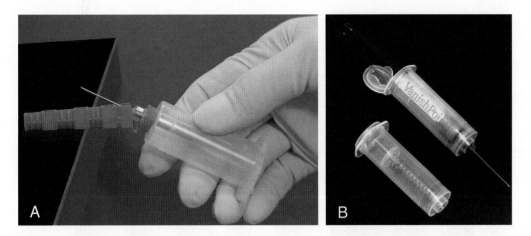

FIGURE 7-13

Safety tube holders. **A.** Venipuncture Needle-Pro with needle resheathing device. **B.** Vanishpoint tube holder with needle-retracting device.   (Courtesy Retractible Technologies, Little Elm, TX.)

Vacuum   Evacuated tubes fill with blood automatically because there is a **vacuum** (negative pressure, or artificially created absence of air) in them. The vacuum is premeasured by the manufacturer so that the tube will draw the precise volume of blood indicated. To reach its stated volume, a tube must be allowed to fill with blood until the normal vacuum is exhausted. A tube that has prematurely lost all or part of its vacuum will fail to properly fill with blood.

> **key • point**   Tubes do not fill with blood all the way to the stopper. When filled properly, there is always a consistent amount of headspace between the level of blood in the tube and the tube stopper.

Premature loss of vacuum can occur from improper storage, opening the tube, dropping the tube, advancing the tube too far onto the needle before venipuncture, or pulling the needle bevel partially out of the skin during venipuncture. Premature loss of vacuum, removing the tube before the vacuum is exhausted, or stoppage of blood flow during the blood draw can result in an underfilled tube called a partial draw or **"short draw"**. Some manufacturers offer special **"short draw" tubes** designed to partially fill without compromising test results. These tubes are used in situations in which it is difficult or inadvisable to draw larger quantities of blood.

> *fyi*   Manufacturer partial draw tubes are often the same size as standard-volume tubes but do not fill to the same level and may fill more slowly.

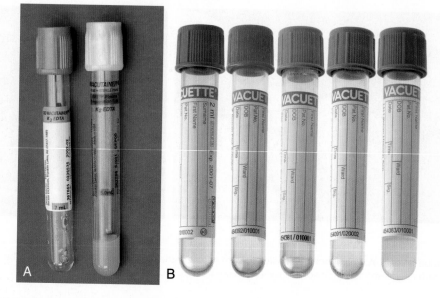

FIGURE 7-14

Evacuated tubes. **A.** Vacutainer Plus Plastic brand evacuated tubes.   (Becton Dickinson, Franklin Lakes, NJ.)
B. Vacuette evacuated tubes.   (Courtesy Greiner Bio-One Kremsmünster, Austria.)

Additive tubes   Most ETS tubes contain some type of **additive.** An additive is any substance placed within a tube other than the tube stopper or the coating of the tube. Blood collected in additive tubes may or may not clot, depending on the additive type. For example, if the additive prevents clotting, the result is a whole blood specimen. Some whole-blood specimens are used directly for testing; others are centrifuged to separate the cells from the fluid portion called plasma. If the additive is a clot activator, the blood will clot and the specimen must be centrifuged to obtain the fluid portion called serum. (See Chapter 6 for a discussion of serum, plasma, and whole blood.)

The amount of additive in a tube will function optimally with the amount of blood it takes to fill the tube to the capacity or volume indicated. Specimen quality can be compromised if the tube is underfilled, so it is important to allow additive tubes to fill with blood until the normal vacuum is exhausted.

c a u t i o n   An underfilled tube that contains an additive will have an incorrect additive-to-blood ratio, which can cause inaccurate test results.

Nonadditive tubes   With the advent of plastic tubes, very few tubes are additive free. (Even serum tubes need an additive to promote clotting if they are plastic.) Any non-additive plastic tubes (Fig. 7-15) that do exist are to be used for clearing or discard

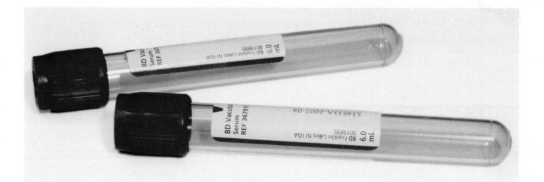

FIGURE 7-15

Nonadditive tubes used as discard or "clear" tubes.

purposes only. A few glass nonadditive red top tubes are still in existence, but most are in the process of being discontinued for safety reasons. Blood collected in a tube will clot when there is nothing in the tube to prevent it. Consequently, nonadditive tubes yield serum samples.

Stoppers   Tube stoppers (tops or closures) are typically made of rubber. Some tubes have a rubber stopper covered by a plastic shield designed to protect lab personnel from blood drops remaining on the stopper after the tube is removed from the needle, and from aerosols (mists) and sprays of specimen when the stopper is removed from the tube. The rigidity of the plastic also prevents removal of the stopper using a "thumb roll," a technique that has been shown to cause aerosol formation.

Color-Coding   Tube stoppers are color-coded. Consequently, it is not unusual for evacuated tubes to be referred to as red tops, green tops, and so forth. For most tubes, the stopper color identifies a type of additive placed in the tube by the manufacturer for a specific purpose. For some tubes, the stopper color indicates a special property of the tube. For example, a royal-blue stopper indicates a trace-element-free tube. Occasionally, there may be more than one stopper color for the same additive. Although color-coding is generally universal, it may vary slightly by manufacturer. Common stopper colors, what they indicate, and what departments use them are shown in Table 7-2. For reference, two manufacturer's tube guides are shown on the last two pages of this book.

EXPIRATION DATES

Manufacturers guarantee reliability of additives and tube vacuum until an expiration date printed on the label, provided the tubes are handled properly and stored between 4 and 25°C. Improper handling or storage can affect additive integrity and tube vacuum, which can lead to compromised test results or improper filling, respectively.

key • point   Always check the expiration date on a tube before using it, and never use a tube that has expired or has been dropped. Discard it instead.

TABLE 7-2   Common Stopper Colors, Additives, and Departments

Stopper Color	Additive	Department(s)
Light blue	Sodium citrate	Coagulation
Red (glass)	None	Chemistry, Blood bank, Serology/ Immunology
Red (plastic)	Clot activator	Chemistry
Red/light gray (plastic)	Nonadditive	NA (Discard tube only)
Red/black (tiger) Gold Red/gold	Clot activator and gel separator	Chemistry
Green/gray Light green	Lithium heparin and gel separator	Chemistry
Green	Lithium heparin Sodium heparin	Chemistry
Lavender Pink	EDTA	Hematology Blood bank
Gray	Sodium fluoride and potassium oxalate Sodium fluoride and EDTA Sodium fluoride	Chemistry
Orange Gray/yellow	Thrombin	Chemistry
Royal blue	None (red label) EDTA (lavender label) Sodium heparin (green label)	Chemistry
Tan (glass tube) Tan (plastic)	Sodium heparin EDTA	Chemistry
Yellow	Sodium polyanethol sulfonate (SPS)	Microbiology
Yellow	Acid citrate dextrose (ACD)	Blood bank/Immunohematology

Syringe System

Although the evacuated tube system is the preferred method of blood collection, a **syringe system** (Fig. 7-16) is sometimes used for patients with small or difficult veins. This system consists of a sterile syringe needle called a hypodermic needle and a sterile plastic syringe with a Luer lock tip (a special tip that allows the needle to attach more securely than a slip tip). A relatively new syringe system component is an OSHA required **syringe transfer device** (Fig.7-17), a piece of equipment used to transfer blood from the syringe into ETS tubes.

SYRINGE NEEDLES

Syringe needles come in a wide range of gauges and lengths for many different uses. Those appropriate for phlebotomy procedures are generally gauges 21 to 23, in 1- or 1.5-inch lengths. When used to draw blood, a syringe needle must have a resheathing feature to allow it to be safely covered and removed so that a transfer device can be attached to the syringe to fill the evacuated tubes. An example of a safety needle attached to a syringe is

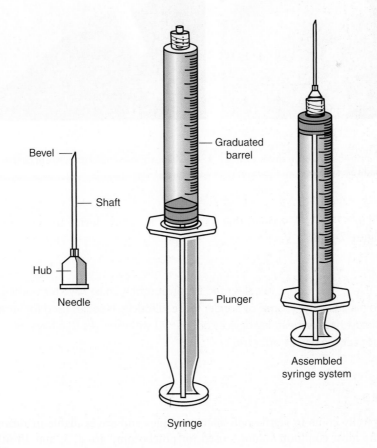

FIGURE 7-16

Traditional syringe system components.

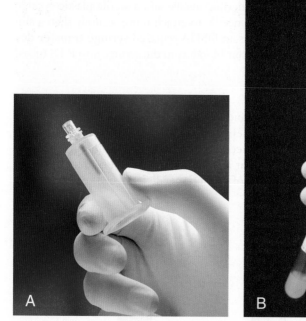
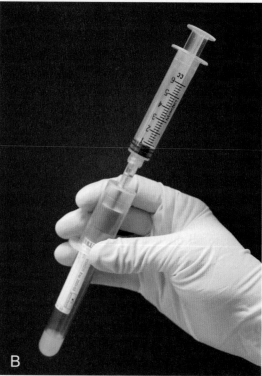

FIGURE 7-17

Syringe transfer devices. **A.** BD transfer device. (Courtesy Becton Dickinson, Franklin Lakes, NJ.). **B.** Greiner transfer device attached to a syringe.

shown in Figure 7-18A. A syringe that has a built in safety device to cover the needle is shown in Figure 7-18B.

c a u t i o n   Syringe needles used for phlebotomy must have resheathing devices to minimize the chance of accidental needlesticks. Needles used for intradermal skin tests must have resheathing devices or be used with syringes that have devices that cover or retract the needle after use.

SYRINGES

Syringes typically come in sterile pull-apart packages and are available in various sizes or volumes. The most common volumes used for phlebotomy are 2, 5, and 10 mL. Syringe volume is selected according to the size and condition of the patient's vein and the amount of blood to be collected. Most syringes come in sterile pull-apart packages.

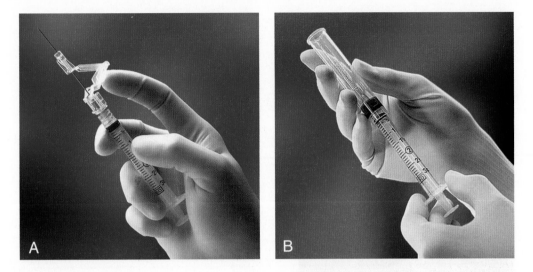

FIGURE 7-18

Syringe safety devices. **A.** Syringe with BD SAFETYGLIDE hypodermic needle attached. **B.** BD SAFETY-LOK syringe. (Courtesy Becton Dickinson, Franklin Lakes, NJ.)

Syringes have two parts: a **barrel,** a cylinder with graduated markings in either milliliters (mL) or cubic centimeters (cc), and a **plunger,** a rodlike device that fits tightly into the barrel (see Fig. 7-15). When drawing venous blood by syringe, the phlebotomist slowly pulls back the plunger, creating a vacuum that causes the barrel to fill with blood.

SYRINGE TRANSFER DEVICE

Blood collected in a syringe must be transferred into ETS tubes. In the past blood was transferred by poking the syringe needle through the tube stopper, or by removing the tube stopper and ejecting blood from the syringe into the tube. Both practices are now considered unsafe. A syringe transfer device allows the safe transfer of blood into the tubes without using the syringe needle or removing the tube stopper. The device is similar to an ETS tube holder, but has a permanently attached needle inside. After completing the draw and exiting the vein, the needle safety device is activated and the needle removed and discarded into the sharps. The transfer device is then attached to the hub of the syringe. An ETS tube is placed inside it and advanced onto the needle until blood flows into the tube. Additional tubes can be filled as long as there is enough blood in the syringe. The transfer device greatly reduces the chance of accidental needlesticks and confines any aerosol or spraying of the specimen that may be generated as tubes are removed from it.

Winged Infusion Set

A **winged infusion blood collection set,** or **butterfly**, is an indispensable tool for collecting blood from small or difficult veins such as hand veins and veins of elderly and pediatric

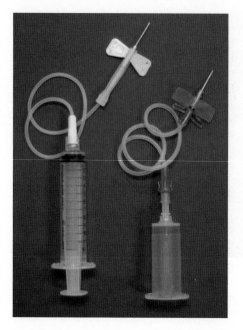

FIGURE 7-19

Winged infusion sets attached to a syringe *(left)* and an evacuated tube holder by means of a Luer adapter.

patients, as it allows much more flexibility and precision than a needle and syringe. It consists of a ½- to ¾-inch stainless steel needle permanently connected to a 5- to 12-inch length of tubing with either a Luer attachment for syringe use or a multisample Luer adapter for use with the evacuated tube system (Fig. 7-19). Multisample Luer adapters are also available separately.

key • point   The first tube collected with a butterfly will underfill because of the air in the tubing. If the tube contains an additive, the blood-to-additive ratio will be affected. If an additive tube is the first tube to be collected, it is important to draw a few milliliters of blood into a nonadditive tube or another additive tube of the same type, and discard it prior to collecting the first tube. This is referred to as collecting a "clear" or discard tube and is especially critical when collecting coagulation tubes using a butterfly.

Plastic extensions that resemble butterfly wings (thus the name butterfly) are attached to the needle where it is joined to the tubing. During use, the needle may be held from above by gripping the "wings" together between the thumb and index finger, allowing the user to achieve the shallow angle of needle insertion required to access small veins.

Butterfly needles come in various gauges, although a 23 gauge is most commonly used for phlebotomy. In rare situations a 25 gauge is used to collect blood from scalp or other tiny veins of premature infants and other neonates.

caution   Using a needle smaller than 23 gauge increases the chance of hemolyzing the specimen.

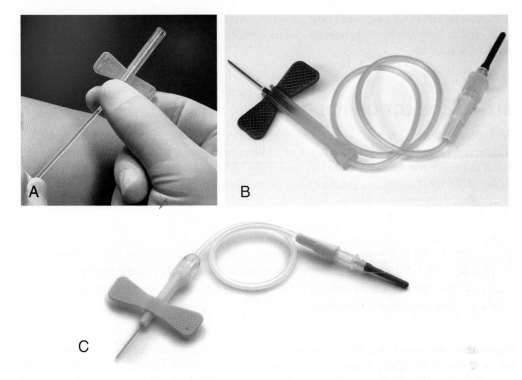

FIGURE 7-20

Examples of safety winged infusion sets. **A.** SAFETY-LOK Blood Collection Set for use with the evacuated tube system.   (Courtesy Becton Dickinson Vacutainer Systems, Franklin Lakes, NJ). **B.** Monoject Angel Wing blood collection set.
(Kendall CO, LP, Mansfield, MA.) **C.** Vacuette safety butterfly blood collection system   (Greiner Bio-One, Kremsmüster, Austria.)

As with other blood collection needles, butterfly needles are required to contain safety devices to reduce the possibility of accidental needlesticks. Butterfly safety devices include locking shields that slide over the needle, blunting devices, and needle retracting devices. See Figure 7-20 for examples of safety butterflies.

Combination Systems

The S-Monovette Blood Collection System (Sarstedt, Inc., Newton, NC) shown in Figure 7-21 is a complete system for blood collection in which the blood collection tube and collection apparatus are combined in a single unit. The unit allows the specimen to be

FIGURE 7-21

S-Monovette Blood Collection System.   (Sarstedt, Inc., Newton, NC.)

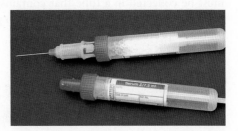

collected by either an evacuated tube or syringe system technique. The units are available with regular or butterfly-style needles. Safety devices are available to contain the needle immediately after use.

BLOOD COLLECTION ADDITIVES

Blood collection tubes and other collection devices often contain one or more additives. There are a number of different types of additives, and each has a specific function. The type required for blood collection generally depends upon the test that has been ordered. In most cases, no substitutions or combining of tubes with different additives is allowed.

> c a u t i o n *Never* transfer blood collected in an additive tube into another additive tube, as different additives may interfere with each other or the testing process. Even if the additives are the same, mixing them together creates an excess of additive and possible interference in testing.

Additives are available in liquid, spray dried, and powder forms. A tube with a powdered additive should be lightly tapped prior to use to settle it to the bottom of the tube. An additive tube must be gently inverted 3 to 8 times, depending on the type, immediately after collection to adequately mix the additive with the specimen. The most common additives are categorized by function.

> c a u t i o n *Never* shake or otherwise vigorously mix a specimen; it can cause hemolysis, which makes most specimens unsuitable for testing.

Anticoagulants

Anticoagulants are substances that prevent blood from clotting (coagulating) by either of two methods: by chelating (binding) or precipitating calcium so it is unavailable to the coagulation process or by inhibiting the formation of thrombin needed to convert fibrinogen to fibrin in the coagulation process. If a test requires whole blood or plasma, the specimen must be collected in a tube that contains an anticoagulant. Anticoagulant specimens must be mixed immediately after collection to prevent microclot formation. Gentle mixing is essential to prevent hemolysis.

> k e y • p o i n t Because the cells are free flowing and not clotted, a specimen collected in anticoagulant will separate through settling or centrifugation and can be resuspended by intentional or inadvertent mixing of the specimen.

TABLE 7-3   Memory Joggers for Anticoagulants

Acronym, Mnemonic, or Acrostic	An Easy Way to Remember:
ECHO	The most common anticoagulants E (EDTA) C (citrate) H (heparin) O (oxalate)
phEDTA *(pronounced like fajita)*	Purple tubes go to hematology and contain EDTA P (purple) h (hematology) EDTA
Spring Creates Colorful Light-Blue Pansies	Sodium citrate tubes go to coagulation, have light blue stoppers, and yield plasma S (sodium) C (citrate) C (coagulation) L (light) B (blue) P (plasma)
HH: Heparin inhibits In-in: Heparin inhibits	Heparin inhibits thrombin formation "H" in heparin and "H" in inhibits Heparin ends with "in," and inhibits starts with "in"
Greenhouses Have Colorful Plants	Green tubes contain heparin for chemistry tests on plasma: G (green) H (heparin) C (chemistry) P (plasma)
GO (gray oxalate)	Gray tubes typically contain oxalate
Gray ox (gray oxalate)	G (gray) O (oxalate)
LL (Lavender last, except for gray)	Lavender is drawn last unless a gray top is ordered Gray tops are rarely ordered, so lavender is often last

There are different types of anticoagulants, each designed for use in certain types of testing. It is important to use the correct anticoagulant for the type of test collected. The most common anticoagulants are **ethylenediaminetetraacetic acid (EDTA), citrates, heparin,** and **oxalates.** Memory joggers to help learn the most common anticoagulants are found in Table 7-3.

EDTA

EDTA, commonly available in a sodium or potassium-based salt, prevents coagulation by binding or chelating calcium. Although it is increasingly being used for blood bank tests also, it is primarily used to provide whole blood specimens for hematology tests because it preserves cell morphology and inhibits platelet aggregation or clumping. EDTA specimens must be mixed immediately after collection to prevent platelet clumping and microclot formation, which can negatively affect test results. Eight inversions are required for proper mixing.

> c a u t i o n   If microclots are detected in a hematology specimen it cannot be used for testing and must be recollected.

CLSI recommends spray-dried EDTA for most hematology tests because liquid EDTA dilutes the specimen and results in lower hemoglobin values, red and white blood cell counts, platelet counts, and packed cell volumes. The dilution effect is even more pronounced if the tubes are not completely filled, so it is important to have the tubes filled until their vacuum is exhausted. Either type of EDTA tube should be properly filled to maintain the correct blood-to-anticoagulant ratio.

> **key • point** Excess EDTA that results when tubes are underfilled causes RBCs to shrink and changes the complete blood count (CBC) results.

EDTA is contained in

- Lavender (purple)-top tubes
- Microcollection containers with lavender tops
- Pink plastic-top tubes with a special blood bank patient ID label
- Pearl-top tubes with thixotropic gel separator
- Royal-blue-top tubes with lavender color-coding on the label

CITRATES

Citrates prevent coagulation by binding or chelating calcium. **Sodium citrate** in light-blue-top tubes is used for coagulation tests because it does the best job of preserving the coagulation factors.

Coagulation tests are performed on plasma, so specimens must first be centrifuged to separate the plasma from the cells. During testing, calcium is added back to the specimen so the clotting process can be initiated and timed.

> **caution** There is a critical 9:1 ratio of blood to anticoagulant in light-blue sodium citrate tubes, so it is important to fill them to the stated capacity. Underfilled tubes cause artificially prolonged clotting times and will not be accepted for testing by most laboratories.

Coagulation specimens require immediate mixing after collection to prevent activation of the coagulation process and microclot formation, which invalidates test results. Three to four gentle inversions are required for proper mixing.

> **caution** Vigorous mixing or an excessive number of inversions can activate platelets and shorten clotting times.

HEPARIN

Heparin prevents clotting by inhibiting **thrombin** formation. (Thrombin is an enzyme needed to convert fibrinogen into the fibrin necessary for clot formation.) Heparinized plasma is often used for stat chemistry tests and other rapid response situations when a fast turn-around time (TAT) for chemistry tests is needed. Faster TAT is possible because time is eliminated that would normally be required for a specimen to clot before serum could be obtained.

key・point Heparinized plasma is preferred over serum for potassium tests because when blood clots, potassium is released from cells into the serum and can falsely elevate results.

Heparinized specimens must be mixed immediately upon collection to prevent clot formation and fibrin generation. Eight inversions are typically required for proper mixing. Gentle mixing is essential to prevent hemolysis. Hemolyzed specimens are unsuitable for many chemistry tests. Heparin is contained in tubes and microcollection containers with green stoppers and in royal blue-top tubes with green on the label. There are three heparin formulations: ammonium, lithium, and sodium heparin. Lithium heparin causes the least interference in chemistry testing and is the most widely used anticoagulant for plasma and whole-blood chemistry tests.

caution It is essential to choose the right heparin formulation for the type of test. Lithium heparin must not be used to collect lithium levels. Sodium heparin must not be used to collect sodium specimens or electrolyte panels because sodium is part of the panel.

OXALATES

Oxalates prevent coagulation by precipitating calcium. **Potassium oxalate** is the most widely used. It is commonly added to tubes containing glucose preservatives (see Antiglycolytic Agents) to provide plasma for glucose testing. Potassium oxalate is most commonly found in evacuated tubes and microcollection containers with gray stoppers. Oxalate specimens must be mixed immediately upon collection to prevent clot formation and fibrin generation. Eight inversions are required for proper mixing.

key・point It is essential to fill oxalate tubes to the stated capacity because excess oxalate causes hemolysis (destruction of red blood cells) and release of hemoglobin into the plasma.

Special-Use Anticoagulants

The following anticoagulants are combined with other additives and have additional properties for special use situations.

ACID CITRATE DEXTROSE (ACD)

ACD solution is available in two formulations (solution A and solution B) for immunohematology tests such as DNA testing and human leukocyte antigen (HLA) phenotyping used in paternity evaluation and to determine transplant compatibility. The acid citrate prevents coagulation by binding calcium, with little effect on cells and platelets. Dextrose acts as a red blood cell nutrient and preservative by maintaining red cell viability. ACD tubes have yellow tops and require eight inversions immediately after collection to prevent clotting.

CITRATE-PHOSPHATE-DEXTROSE (CPD)

CPD is used in collecting units of blood for transfusion. Citrate prevents clotting by chelating calcium, phosphate stabilizes pH, and dextrose provides cells with energy and helps keep them alive.

SODIUM POLYANETHOL SULFONATE (SPS)

SPS prevents coagulation by binding calcium. It is used for blood culture collection because in addition to being an anticoagulant, it reduces the action of a protein called complement that destroys bacteria, slows down phagocytosis (ingestion of bacteria by leukocytes), and reduces the activity of certain antibiotics. SPS tubes have yellow stoppers and require eight inversions to prevent clotting.

Antiglycolytic Agents

An **antiglycolytic agent** is a substance that prevents **glycolysis,** the breakdown or metabolism of glucose (blood sugar) by blood cells. If glycolysis is not prevented, the glucose concentration in a blood specimen decreases at a rate of 10 mg/dL per hour.

key • point Glycolysis occurs faster in newborns, because their metabolism is increased, and in patients with leukemia, because of high metabolic activity of WBCs.

The most common antiglycolytic agent is **sodium fluoride.** It preserves glucose for up to 3 days, and also inhibits the growth of bacteria. Sodium fluoride is commonly used in combination with the anticoagulant potassium oxalate to provide plasma specimens for rapid-response situations. Sodium fluoride tubes have gray stoppers and require eight inversions for proper mixing.

key • point Sodium fluoride tubes are used to collect ethanol specimens to prevent either a decrease in alcohol concentration due to glycolysis, or an increase due to fermentation by bacteria.

Clot Activators

A **clot activator** is a substance that enhances coagulation. Clot activators include substances that provide more surface for platelet activation, such as glass **(silica)** particles and inert clays like **Celite,** and clotting factors such as thrombin. Silica particles are the clot activators in serum separator tubes (SSTs) and plastic red-top tubes. Silica particles cause the blood to clot within 15 to 30 minutes. Blood collected in thrombin tubes generally clots within 5 minutes. Celite tubes are used with some point-of-care coagulation systems. Tubes containing clot activators require five gentle inversions for complete and rapid clotting to occur.

> **key · point** Blood in an SST tube will eventually clot without mixing; however, when it is not mixed, glass particles may become suspended in the serum and interfere in the testing process.

Thixotropic Gel Separator

Thixotropic gel is an inert (nonreacting) synthetic substance initially contained in or near the bottom of certain blood collection tubes. The density of the gel is between that of the cells and the serum or plasma. When a specimen in a gel tube is centrifuged, the gel undergoes a change in viscosity (thickness) and moves to a position between the cells and the serum or plasma, forming a physical barrier between them. This physical separation prevents the cells from continuing to metabolize substances, such as glucose, in the serum or plasma. Becton Dickinson (BD) serum gel tubes have gold plastic or mottled red/gray rubber stoppers and are called serum separator tubes **(SSTs).** Greiner serum gel tubes have red plastic stoppers with yellow tops. BD heparinized gel tubes have light-green plastic or mottled gray/green rubber stoppers and are called plasma separator tubes, or **PSTs.** Greiner heparinized gel tubes have green plastic stoppers with yellow tops. EDTA gel tubes have special pearl-colored stoppers and are called plasma preparation tubes **(PPTs).**

Trace-Element-Free Tubes

Although stopper colors normally indicate a type of additive in a tube, royal-blue stoppers indicate **trace-element-free tubes**. These tubes are made of materials that are as free of trace element contamination as possible and are used for trace element tests, toxicology studies, and nutrient determinations. These tests measure substances present in such small quantities that trace element contamination commonly found in the glass or stopper material of other tubes may leach into the specimen and falsely elevate test results. Royal-blue-top tubes contain EDTA, heparin or no additive, to meet various test requirements. Tube labels are typically color-coded to indicate the type of additive, if any, in the tube.

ORDER OF DRAW

The order in which tubes are collected during a multiple tube draw or are filled from a syringe is important. Filling tubes in the wrong order can lead to interference in testing from contamination of the specimen by additive carryover, tissue thromboplastin, or microorganisms. **Order of draw** is a special sequence of tube collection that is intended to minimize these problems.

fyi Order of draw may vary slightly among institutions. Consult institution protocol before using a specific order of draw.

Carryover/Cross Contamination

Carryover or cross contamination is the transfer of additive from one tube to the next. It can occur when blood in an additive tube touches the needle during ETS blood collection or when blood is transferred from a syringe into ETS tubes. Blood remaining on or within the needle can be transferred to the next tube drawn or filled, contaminating that tube with additive from the previous tube and possibly affecting test results on the specimen. Table 7-4 lists some of the most common tests affected by additive contamination.

TABLE 7-4 Common Tests Affected by Additive Contamination

Contaminating Additive	Tests Potentially Affected
Citrate	Alkaline phosphatase Calcium Phosphorus
EDTA	Alkaline phosphatase Calcium Creatine kinase Partial thromboplastin Potassium Protime Serum iron Sodium
Heparin (all formulations)	Activated clotting time Acid phosphatase Calcium (some test methods) Partial thromboplastin Protime Sodium (sodium formulations) Lithium (lithium formulations)
Oxalates	Acid phosphatase Alkaline phosphatase Amylase Calcium Lactate dehydrogenase Partial thromboplastin Potassium Protime Red cell morphology
Silica (clot activator)	Partial thromboplastin time Protime
Sodium fluoride	Sodium Urea nitrogen

key • point EDTA tubes have been the source of more carryover problems than any other additive. Heparin causes the least interference in tests other than coagulation tests because it also occurs in blood naturally.

Remembering which tests the various additives affect can be difficult. Order of draw eliminates confusion by presenting a sequence of collection that results in the least amount of interference should carryover occur. Chance of carryover can be minimized by making certain that specimen tubes fill from the bottom up during collection and that the contents of the tube do not come in contact with the needle during the draw or when transferring blood into tubes from a syringe.

Tissue Thromboplastin Contamination

Tissue thromboplastin is a substance present in tissue fluid that activates the extrinsic coagulation pathway and can interfere with coagulation tests. It is picked up by the needle during venipuncture and flushed into the first tube filled during ETS collection, or mixed with blood collected in a syringe. Although it is no longer considered a significant problem for prothrombin time (PT) and partial thromboplastin time (PTT) tests unless the draw is difficult and involves a lot of needle manipulation, it may compromise results of other coagulation tests. Therefore, any time a coagulation test other than PT or PTT is the first or only tube collected, a few milliliters of blood should be drawn into a nonadditive tube or another coagulation tube before the coagulation specimen is collected. The extra tube is called a "clear" or "discard" tube because it is used to remove tissue fluid from the needle and is then thrown away. Some institutions still prefer to clear for all coagulation tests, so it is important to follow your institution's policy.

c a u t i o n A discard tube must be drawn to protect the critical 9:1 blood-to-additive ratio of a coagulation tube that is the first or only tube collected using a butterfly, because air in the tubing displaces blood in the tube.

Microbial Contamination

Blood cultures detect microorganisms in the blood and require special site-cleaning measures prior to collection to prevent contamination of the specimen by microorganisms normally found on the skin. Blood culture tubes or bottles are sterile and are collected first in the order of draw to ensure that they are collected when sterility of the site is optimal and to prevent microbial contamination of the needle from the unsterile tops of tubes used to collect other tests. Blood cultures do not often factor into the sequence of collection because they are typically drawn separately.

key・point Contamination of blood culture bottles can lead to false positive results and inappropriate or delayed care for the patient.

CLSI Order of Draw

To minimize the chance of specimen contamination, the CLSI recommends the following order of draw for both ETS collection and when filling tubes from a syringe:

1. Sterile tube (blood culture)
2. Blue-top coagulation tube
3. Serum tube with or without clot activator, with or without gel
4. Heparin tube with or without gel plasma separator
5. EDTA tube
6. Glycolytic inhibitor tube

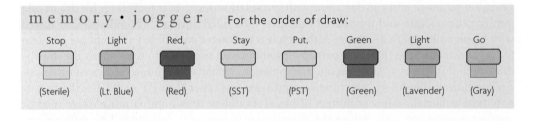

memory・jogger   For the order of draw:

Stop	Light	Red,	Stay	Put,	Green	Light	Go
(Sterile)	(Lt. Blue)	(Red)	(SST)	(PST)	(Green)	(Lavender)	(Gray)

fyi The order of draw memory jogger places the red top before the SST and places the PST before the green top for convenience in memorization.

The CLSI order of draw, with stopper colors, and rationale for collection order, is summarized in Table 7-5.

ALTERNATE SYRINGE ORDER OF DRAW

Because the clotting process is activated the minute blood starts to fill a syringe, some institutions prefer to use a separate order of draw for syringe collections so that tubes most affected by microclot formation are filled as soon as possible. This order of draw assumes that the blood that entered the syringe last is the freshest and least affected by microclot formation. Sterile specimens are still first, followed by light-blue tops, but other anticoagulant tubes come before serum tubes. The alternate syringe order of draw is shown in Box 7-3.

TABLE 7-5 Order of Draw, Stopper Colors, and Rationale for Collection Order

Order of Draw	Tube Stopper Color	Rationale for Collection Order
Blood cultures (sterile collections)	Yellow SPS Sterile media bottles	Minimizes chance of microbial contamination
Coagulation tubes	Light blue	The first additive tube in the order because all other additive tubes affect coagulation tests
Glass nonadditive tubes	Red	Prevents contamination by additives in other tubes
Plastic clot activator tubes Serum separator tubes (SSTs)	Red Red & gray rubber Gold plastic	Filled after coagulation tests because silica particles activate clotting and affect coagulation tests (carryover of silica into subsequent tubes can be overridden by anticoagulant in them)
Plasma separator tubes (PSTs) Heparin tubes	Green & gray rubber Light-green plastic Green	Heparin affects coagulation tests and interferes in collection of serum specimens; causes the least interference in tests other than coagulation tests
EDTA tubes Plasma preparation tubes (PPTs)	Lavender Pink Pearl top	Responsible for more carryover problems than any other additive: elevates Na and K levels,. chelates and decreases calcium and iron levels, elevates PT and PTT results
Oxalate/fluoride tubes	Gray	Sodium fluoride and potassium oxalate affect sodium and potassium levels, respectively. After hematology tubes because oxalate damages cell membranes and causes abnormal RBC morphology. Oxalate interferes in enzyme reactions

BOX • 7-3 Alternate Syringe Order of Draw

1. Sterile specimens (i.e., blood cultures)
2. Light-blue top (i.e., coagulation tubes)
3. Lavender top and plasma preparation tube (PPT)
4. Green top and plasma separator tube (PST)
5. Gray-top oxalate fluoride tube
6. Red top and serum separator tube (SST)

caution To prevent carryover with this order of draw it is important to hold the syringe and transfer device vertical while filling the tubes. This will keep the transfer needle above the fill level of the tube so that it is not contaminated by blood mixed with additive.

memory • jogger For the alternate syringe order of draw:

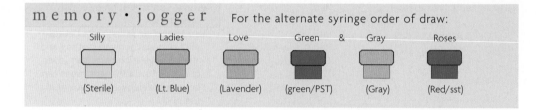

Silly	Ladies	Love	Green	&	Gray	Roses
(Sterile)	(Lt. Blue)	(Lavender)	(green/PST)		(Gray)	(Red/sst)

STUDY & REVIEW QUESTIONS

1. **Which additive prevents glycolysis?**

   a. EDTA

   b. Heparin

   c. Potassium oxalate

   d. Sodium fluoride

2. **All of the following items are typically used to perform routine venipuncture *except***

   a. Disinfectant

   b. Evacuated tubes

   c. Safety needle

   d. Tourniquet

3. **Which of the following tubes can be used to collect a serum specimen?**

   a. Light-blue top

   b. Green top

   c. PST

   d. Red top

4. **A tourniquet is used in venipuncture to**

   a. Concentrate the specimen

   b. Keep the vein from collapsing

   c. Make a vein easier to find and enter

   d. All of the above

5. **You are about to perform routine venipuncture on a patient with no known allergy to antiseptics. Which of the following substances would you use to clean the site?**

   a. 5.25% sodium hypochlorite

   b. 70% isopropyl alcohol

   c. Antibacterial soap and water

   d. Povidone-iodine

6. **Which of the following needles has the largest diameter?**

   a. 18 gauge

   b. 20 gauge

   c. 21 gauge

   d. 23 gauge

7. **What causes evacuated tubes to fill with blood automatically?**

   a. Arterial pressure

   b. Fist pumping by the patient

   c. Pressure created by the tourniquet

   d. Tube vacuum

8. **Lavender-top tubes are most commonly used to collect**

   a. Chemistry tests

   b. Coagulation specimens

   c. Hematology tests

   d. Immunology tests

9. **Of the following tubes or containers, which is filled last in the recommended order of draw?**

   a. Blood culture bottle

   b. Lavender top

   c. Light-blue top

   d. Red top

10. **A butterfly is typically used for**

    a. Coagulation specimens

    b. Difficult and hand veins

    c. Drawing from the basilic vein

    d. All of the above

CASE · STUDY · 7-1

Proper Handling of Anticoagulant Tubes

A mobile blood collector named Chi is collecting an SST and two lavender tops (one for a glycohemoglobin and one for a CBC) on a client named Louise Jones. He fills the SST, lays it down while he places the first lavender top in the tube holder, then picks it up and mixes it as the lavender top is filling. When the lavender top is full, he lays it down while he places the second lavender top in the tube holder. The second lavender top fails to fill with blood so he makes several needle adjustments to try to establish blood flow. Nothing works so he decides to try a new tube. The new tube works fine. While it is filling, he picks up the first lavender top and mixes it. After completing the draw he labels his tubes, putting the hematology label on the lavender top he collected first. He finishes up with the client, delivers the specimens to the laboratory, and goes to lunch. When he returns from break his supervisor tells him to recollect the CBC on Louise Jones because the specimen had a clot in it.

QUESTIONS
1. What can cause clots in EDTA specimens?
2. What most likely caused the clot in this specimen?
3. Did the problem with the second lavender top contribute to the problem?
4. Would the problem with the second lavender top have been an issue if Chi had handled the first lavender top properly? Explain your answer.
5. What can Chi do to prevent this type of thing from happening in the future?

CASE · STUDY · 7-2

Order of Draw

Jake, a phlebotomist, is sent to the ER to collect an EDTA specimen for a stat type and cross-match on an accident victim. He properly identifies the patient and is in the process of filling the lavender-top tube when an ER nurse tells him that the patient's physician wants to add a stat set of electrolytes to the test order. Jake acknowledges her request. He finishes filling the lavender top and grabs a green top. After completing the draw he takes the specimens straight to the laboratory to be processed immediately.

QUESTIONS
1. One of the specimens that Jake drew is compromised. Which one is it?
2. Why is the specimen compromised and how may test results be affected?
3. How could Jake have avoided the problem without drawing blood from the patient twice?

Bibliography and Suggested Readings

Bishop, M., Duben-Engelkirk, J., & Fody, E. (1996). Clinical chemistry, principles, procedures, correlations (3rd ed.). Philadelphia: Lippincott-Raven.

Bishop, M., Fody, E., & Schoeff, L. (2005). Clinical chemistry, principles, procedures, correlations (5th ed.). Philadelphia: Lippincott Williams & Wilkins.

Burtis, C. & Ashwood. E.. (2001). Tietz fundamentals of clinical chemistry (5th ed.). Philadelphia: W. B. Saunders,.

CDC. Guideline for hand hygiene in health care settings, Morbidity and Mortality Weekly Report (MMWR), October 25, 2002;51 (RR-16). Complete report available at http://www.cdc.gov

CDC/HICPAC. Guideline for environmental infection control in health-care facilities. Recommendations of CDC and the Healthcare Infection Control Practices Advisory Committee (HICPAC). Morbidity and Mortality Weekly Report (MMWR), June 2003:52 (RR-10).

College of American Pathologists (CAP). (2005). So you're going to collect a blood specimen (11th ed.) Northfield, IL: CAP.

Gottfried E. L. & Adachi M. M. Prothrombin time (PT) and activated partial thromboplastin time (APTT) can be performed on the first tube. American Journal of Clinical Pathology 1997;107:681–683.

National Committee for Clinical Laboratory Standards, H1–A5. (December 2003). Tubes and additives for blood specimen collection; approved standard (5th ed.).Wayne, PA: NCCLS.

National Committee for Clinical Laboratory Standards, H3–A5. (December 2003). Procedures for the collection of diagnostic blood specimens by venipuncture; approved standard (5th ed.). Wayne, PA: NCCLS.

National Committee for Clinical Laboratory Standards, M29–A2. (2001). Protection of laboratory workers from occupationally acquired infections; approved guideline (2nd ed.). Wayne, PA: NCCLS.

National Committee for Clinical Laboratory Standards, H11–A4. Procedures for the collection of arterial blood specimens; approved standard (4th ed.). Wayne, PA: NCCLS.

OSHA. Bloodborne pathogens standard (29 CFR 1910.1030), the safe practice of phlebotomy and blood tube holder use (CPL2-2.9 at XIII.D.5).

OSHA. Disposal of contaminated needles and blood tube holders used in phlebotomy. Safety and Health Information Bulletin, http://www.osha.gov/dts/shib/shib101503.html, October 15, 2003.

Rodak, B. (2002). Hematology, clinical principles and applications (2nd ed.). Philadelphia: W. B. Saunders.

VENIPUNCTURE PROCEDURES

key·terms

accession	EMLA	NPO
anchor	fasting	palpate
arm/wrist band	hospice	patency
ASAP	ID band/bracelet	patient ID
bar code	ID card	pre-op/post-op
bedside manner	MR number	reflux
concentric circles	needle phobia	requisition
DNR/DNAR	needle sheath	STAT/stat

objectives

Upon successful completion of this chapter, the reader should be able to:

1. Define the key terms and abbreviations listed at the beginning of this chapter.
2. Describe the test request process, identify the types of requisitions used, and list the required requisition information.
3. List and define test status designations, identify status priorities, and describe the procedure to follow for each status designation.
4. Describe proper bedside manner and how to handle special situations associated with patient contact.
5. Explain the importance of proper patient identification and describe what information is verified, how to handle discrepancies, and what to do if a patient's ID band is missing.
6. Describe how to prepare patients for testing, how to answer inquiries concerning tests, and what to do if a patient objects to the test.
7. Describe how to verify fasting and other diet requirements and what to do when diet requirements have not been met.
8. Describe each step in the venipuncture procedure, list necessary information found on specimen tube labels, and list the acceptable reasons for inability to collect a specimen.
9. Describe collection procedures when using a butterfly or syringe and the proper way to safely dispense blood into tubes following syringe collection.
10. Describe unique requirements associated with drawing from special populations including pediatric, geriatric, and long-term-care patients.

Venipuncture is the term used to describe the process of collecting or "drawing" blood from a vein. It is the most common way to collect blood specimens for laboratory testing. Although steps may vary slightly, venipuncture procedures in this chapter were written to conform to CLSI Standard H3-A5, *Procedures for the Collection of Diagnostic Blood Specimens by Venipuncture* and include the steps necessary to obtain an appropriately identified quality blood specimen from a patient's arm, wrist, or hand veins. Venipuncture techniques illustrated in this chapter include ETS, butterfly, and syringe procedures, which have the following steps in common.

VENIPUNCTURE STEPS

Step 1: Review and Accession Test Request

Blood collection procedures legally begin with the test request. Typically, a physician or other qualified healthcare professional requests laboratory testing, with the exception of certain rapid tests that can be purchased and performed at home by consumers and blood specimens requested by law enforcement officials and used for evidence. Some states have legalized "Direct Access Testing (DAT)" in which patients are allowed to order some of their own blood tests.

THE TEST REQUISITION

The form on which test orders are entered is called a **requisition**. Test requisitions become part of a patient's medical record and require specific information to ensure that the right patient is tested, the physician's orders are met, the correct tests are performed at the proper time under the required conditions, and the patient is billed properly. Required requisition information is listed in Box 8-1. Requisitions come in manual and computer-generated forms.

> **key • point** Verbal test requests are sometimes used in emergencies; however, the request is usually documented on standard request forms or entered in the computer by the time the phlebotomist arrives to collect the specimen.

Manual Requisitions   Manual requisitions (Fig. 8-1) come in many different styles and types. Some are a three-part form that serves as a request, report, and billing form. With increased use of computer systems, use of manual requisitions is declining. However, they are typically used as a backup when computer systems fail.

Computer Requisitions   Computer requisitions (Fig. 8-2) normally contain the actual labels that are placed on the specimen tubes immediately after collection. In addition to patient identification and test status information, many indicate the type of tube needed for

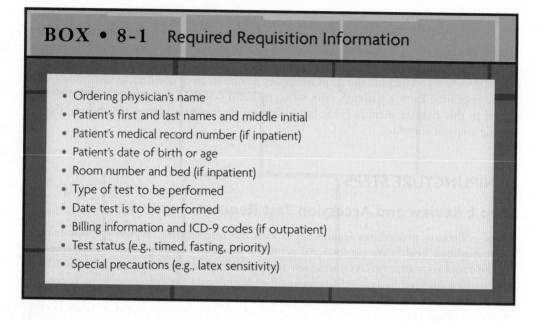

BOX • 8-1   Required Requisition Information

- Ordering physician's name
- Patient's first and last names and middle initial
- Patient's medical record number (if inpatient)
- Patient's date of birth or age
- Room number and bed (if inpatient)
- Type of test to be performed
- Date test is to be performed
- Billing information and ICD-9 codes (if outpatient)
- Test status (e.g., timed, fasting, priority)
- Special precautions (e.g., latex sensitivity)

the specimen, and some indicate additional patient information such as "potential bleeder" or "no venipuncture right arm."

key • point   When a computer-generated label is used, the phlebotomist is typically required to write the time of collection and his or her initials on the label after collecting the specimen.

Bar Code Requisitions   Either type of requisition may contain a **bar code**, a series of black stripes and white spaces of varying widths that correspond to letters and numbers (see Fig. 8-2). The stripes and spaces are grouped together to represent patient names, identification numbers, or laboratory tests. Manual requisitions that have bar codes normally contain copies of the bar code that can be peeled off and placed on the specimens. Computer requisitions typically have the bar code printed on each label. Bar code information can be scanned into a computer using a special light or laser to identify the information represented. Bar code systems allow fast, accurate processing, and their use has been shown to decrease laboratory errors associated with clerical mistakes.

RECEIPT OF THE TEST REQUEST

Computer requisitions for inpatients usually print out at a special computer terminal (Fig. 8-3) at the phlebotomist station in the laboratory. Typically, outpatients are given

Quest Diagnostics — SmithKline Beecham Clinical Laboratories, Now a Part of Quest Diagnostics

SelecTest® HOSPITAL

85351402-2   6606516-8

BOSWELL MEMORIAL HOSPITAL
10401 W THUNDERBIRD BLVD
SUN CITY, AZ 85351-3004

PXPBR00   623-876-5381

PATIENT INFORMATION - PLEASE PRINT
PRINT NAME (LAST, FIRST, MIDDLE) OR REGISTRATION NO

DID YOU REMEMBER...
TO REQUEST OR MARK TEST(S)?
TO PROVIDE ORDER CODE(S) FOR HANDWRITTEN TESTS?

ROOM #   REGISTRATION #   LAB REFERENCE #

DOB (MM/DD/YYYY)   SEX   M☐ F☐   PATIENT I.D. #

☐ Call Results to:( )   ☐ Fax Results to:( )

Report Comments:

Internal Comments:

☐ STAT
☐ STAT PICK UP

REFERRING PHYSICIAN   REF. PHYSICIAN PROVIDER #

DATE COLLECTED   TIME   ☐ AM ☐ PM   ☐ Fasting (Hours)

☐ Serum ☐ Plasma ☐ Blood ☐ Urine ☐ Frozen ☐ Other

Referred (side): F=FROZEN, P=PLASMA, B=LIGHT BLUE TOP TUBE, L=LAVENDER TOP TUBE, G=GRAY TOP TUBE, R=RED TOP TUBE, Y=YELLOW CAP URINE BOTTLE, U=SCREW CAP URINE BOTTLE, S=SERUM SEPARATOR TUBE

PANELS

Code	Test	
7352	☐ CARDIOLIPIN ANTIBODIES (IgG, IgA, IgM)	S
4451	☐ CK ISOENZYME PANEL (Total + Isoenzymes)	FS
7940	☐ EBV AB EVAL, COMP (anti-VCA IgM, anti-VCA IgG, anti-EA(D), anti-EA(R), anti-EBNA)	S
10306	☐ HEPATITIS PANEL, ACUTE W/REFLEX (HbsAg w/reflex confirm, HC Ab, HA Ab IgM, HbcAb, IgM)	S
7083	☐ IMMUNOGLOBULINS (IgG,IgA,IgM)	S
4411	☐ LDH ISOENZYME PANEL (Total + Isoenzymes)	S
7260	☐ THYROID AUTOANTIBODIES (Thyroglobulin + Peroxidase)	S
7065	☐ VITAMIN B12/FOLIC ACID	1

TESTS

Code	Test	
237	☐ AFP TUMOR MARKER	S
227	☐ ALDOLASE	FS
230	☐ ALDOSTERONE	S
249	☐ ANA W/REFLEX TITER	S
8431	☐ ANCA	S
683	☐ ANGIOTENSIN CONVERT ENZYME	S
4420	☐ C-REACTIVE PROTEIN	S
29256	☐ CA 125	S
5819	☐ CA 15-3	S
4698	☐ CA 19-9	FS
29493	☐ CA 27.29	S
329	☐ CARBAMAZEPINE	1
4661	☐ CARDIOLIPIN IGA AB	S
4662	☐ CARDIOLIPIN IGG AB	S
4663	☐ CARDIOLIPIN IGM AB	S
978	☐ CEA	S
377	☐ CK ISOENZYMES	FS
374	☐ CK, TOTAL	S
351	☐ COMPLEMENT C3	FS
353	☐ COMPLEMENT C4	FS
618	☐ COMPLEMENT, TOTAL (CH50)	FS
367	☐ CORTISOL	S
402	☐ DHEA SULFATE	S
255	☐ DNA AB, NATIVE	S
7849	☐ EBV ANTI-EA (D+R)	S
8564	☐ EBV ANTI-EBNA	S
8474	☐ EBV ANTI-VCA IGG	S

Code	Test	
8426	☐ EBV ANTI-VCA IGM	S
427	☐ ERYTHROPOIETIN	S
429	☐ ESTRADIOL	S
457	☐ FERRITIN	S
467	☐ FOLIC ACID, RBC	1
466	☐ FOLIC ACID, SERUM	1
470	☐ FSH	S
4112	☐ FTA-ABS	S
478	☐ GASTRIN	FS
29407	☐ H. PYLORI IGG, QUAL	S
29408	☐ H. PYLORI IGG, QUANT	S
502	☐ HAPTOGLOBIN	S
496	☐ HEMOGLOBIN A1C	L
517	☐ HEMOGLOBIN ELECTROPHORESIS	L
508	☐ HEP A AB - TOTAL	S
512	☐ HEP A IGM AB	S
501	☐ HEP B CORE AB, TOTAL	S
4848	☐ HEP B CORE IGM AB	S
499	☐ HEP B SURFACE AB QUAL	S
8475	☐ HEP B SURFACE AB QUANT	S
498	☐ HEP B SURFACE AG W/REFLEX CONFIRM	S
8472	☐ HEP C VIRUS AB	S
6449	☐ HIV SCR-WB CONF	S
31789	☐ HOMOCYSTEINE	1
539	☐ IMMUNOGLOBULIN A	S
542	☐ IMMUNOGLOBULIN E	S
545	☐ IMMUNOGLOBULIN G	S
561	☐ IMMUNOGLOBULIN M	S
597	☐ INSULIN	FS
593	☐ LDH ISOENZYMES	S
599	☐ LDH, TOTAL	S
6687	☐ LEAD (B)	1
615	☐ LEGIONELLA PNEUMO AB 1-6	S
606	☐ LH	S
613	☐ LIPASE	1
7079	☐ LITHIUM	1
6646	☐ LUPUS ANTICOAGULANT	S
4555	☐ LYME DISEASE AB-WB CONF	S
6517	☐ MICROALBUMIN (U)	1
259	☐ MICROALB/CREAT RATIO	U
8624	☐ MITOCHONDRIAL AB	S
659	☐ MUMPS VIRUS IGG	S
272	☐ MYCO PNEUMONIAE IGG AB	S
4847	☐ NORTRIPTYLINE	1
745	☐ PREALBUMIN	S
746	☐ PROGESTERONE	S
747	☐ PROLACTIN	S
	☐ PROTEIN ELECTROPHORESIS	S

Code	Test	
754	☐ PROTEIN, TOTAL	S
5363	☐ PSA	S
8847	☐ PT WITH INR	1
8446	☐ PTH, INTACT W/CALCIUM	FS
8837	☐ PTH, INTACT(IRMA) W/CALCIUM	FS
787	☐ RENIN ACTIVITY	1
4418	☐ RHEUMATOID FACTOR	S
799	☐ RPR (MONITORING) W/REFLEX TITER	S
36125	☐ RPR (DX) W/REFLEX CONFIRM TP-PA	S
802	☐ RUBELLA IGG AB	S
964	☐ RUBEOLA IGG AB	S
30261	☐ STONE ANALYSIS, KIDNEY	1
30260	☐ STONE ANALYSIS, OTHER	1
34429	☐ T-3, FREE	S
859	☐ T-3, TOTAL	S
861	☐ T-3, UPTAKE	S
867	☐ T-4 (THYROXINE)	S
866	☐ T-4, FREE	S
7924	☐ T-HELPER/SUPPRESSOR RATIO	1
30741	☐ TESTOSTERONE, FREE AND TOTAL	S
873	☐ TESTOSTERONE, TOTAL	S
267	☐ THYROGLOBULIN AB	S
5081	☐ THYROID PEROXIDASE AB	S
891	☐ TRANSFERRIN	S
899	☐ TSH	S
36127	☐ TSH W/REFLEX T-4, FREE	S
916	☐ VALPROIC ACID	1
4439	☐ VARICELLA-ZOSTER IGG AB	S
4128	☐ VDRL, CSF	1
927	☐ VITAMIN B12	S
934	☐ VMA (U)	1

MICROBIOLOGY

SOURCE: _____

Code	Test	
8756	☐ C DIFFICILE TOXIN A	1
389	☐ CULTURE, BLOOD	1
690	☐ CULTURE, CHLAMYDIA TRACH	1
4553	☐ CULTURE, FUNGUS	1
2692	☐ CULTURE, HSV (RAPID)	1
2649	☐ CULTURE, HSV WITH TYPING	1
4554	☐ CULTURE, MYCOBACTERIUM	1
395	☐ CULTURE, URINE, RTN	1
689	☐ CULTURE, VIRUS, COMP	1
6919	☐ DNA PROBE, CHL & GC	1
8502	☐ DNA PROBE, CHLAMYDIA	1
8501	☐ DNA PROBE, GC	1
30264	☐ E. COLI SHIGA TOXINS, EIA STOOL	1
681	☐ OVA & PARASITES	1

ADDITIONAL TESTS: (MUST INCLUDE COMPLETE TEST NAME AND ORDER CODE. REFER TO SBCL DIRECTORY OF SERVICES.)

TOTAL TESTS ORDERED

85351402 6606516	85351402 6606516
REQHPLA	
85351402 6606516	85351402 6606516

FIGURE 8-1

Manual requisition. (Courtesy Sun Health Systems, Sun City AZ.)

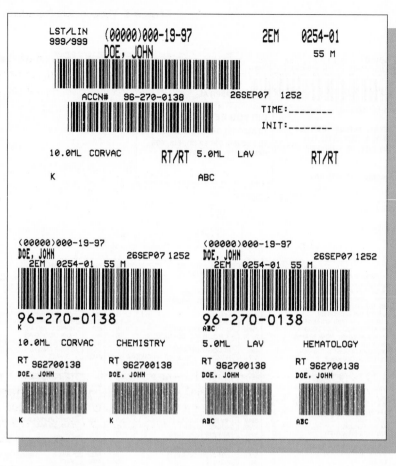

FIGURE 8-2

Computer requisition with bar code.

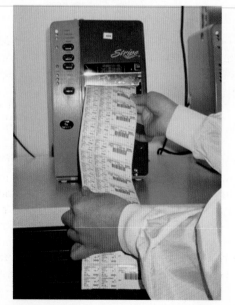

FIGURE 8-3

Computer requisitions printing at a terminal in the laboratory.

laboratory requisitions or prescription slips with test orders written on them by their physicians and are responsible for taking them to a blood collection site. It is up to personnel of the blood collection site to make certain required information is on the requisition provided by the patient or fill out a requisition from the physician's prescription slip.

REVIEWING THE REQUISITION

A thorough review of the test requisition helps to avoid duplication of orders, ensures that the specimen is collected at the right time and under the proper conditions, and identifies special equipment that may be required. When reviewing a requisition the phlebotomist must:

- Check to see that all required information is present and complete.
- Verify the tests to be collected and time and date of collection.
- Identify diet restrictions or other special circumstances that must be met prior to collection.
- Determine test status or collection priority (Table 8-1).

ACCESSIONING THE TEST REQUEST

The definition of **accession** is to record in the order received. To accession a specimen means to take steps to unmistakably connect the specimen and the accompanying paperwork with a specific individual. When a test request is accessioned it is assigned a unique number that is used to identify the specimen and all associated processes and paperwork and connect them to the patient. This helps to ensure prompt and accurate processing from receipt of the order to reporting of test results.

Step 2: Approach, Identify, and Prepare Patient

APPROACHING THE PATIENT

Being organized and efficient plays a role in a positive and productive collection experience. Before collecting the specimens, the phlebotomist should arrange the requisitions according to priority and review them to see that needed equipment is on the blood-collecting tray or cart before proceeding to the patient's room. Outpatients are typically summoned into the drawing area from the waiting room in order of arrival and check in. As with inpatients, STAT requests take priority over all others.

Looking for Signs   Looking for signs containing information concerning the patient is an important part of the approach to an inpatient. Signs are typically posted on the door to the patient's room or on the wall beside or behind the head of the patient's bed. Of particular importance to phlebotomists are signs that indicate infection control precautions to be followed when entering the room and signs that prohibit blood pressures or blood draws (Fig. 8-4A) from a particular arm. Other commonly encountered signs may identify limits to the number of visitors allowed in the room at one time, indicate that "fall" precautions are to be observed for the patient, or warn that the patient has a severe allergy (*e.g.*, to latex

TABLE 8-1 Common Test Status Designations

Status	Meaning	When Used	Collection Conditions	Test Examples	Priority
STAT (stat)	Immediately (from Latin *statim*)	Test results are urgently needed on critical patients	Immediately collect, test, and report results. Alert lab staff when delivered. ER stats typically have priority over other stats	Glucose H & H Electrolytes Cardiac enzymes	First
Med Emerg	Medical Emergency (Replaces STAT)	Same as STAT	Same as STAT	Same as STAT	Same as STAT
Timed	Collect at a specific time	Tests for which timing is critical for accurate results	Collect as close as possible to requested time. Record actual time collected	2-hour PP GTT, Cortisol Cardiac Enzymes TDM Blood cultures	Second
ASAP	As soon as possible	Test results are needed soon to respond to a serious situation, but patient is not critical	Follow hospital protocol for type of test	Electrolytes Glucose H & H	Second or third depending on test
Fasting	No food or drink except water for 8–12 hours prior to specimen collection	To eliminate diet effects on test results	Verify patient has fasted. If patient has not fasted, check to see if specimen should still be collected	Glucose Cholesterol Triglycerides	Fourth
NPO	Nothing by mouth (from Latin *nulla per os*)	Prior to surgery or other anesthesia procedures	Do not give patient food or water. Refer requests to physician or nurse	N/A	N/A
Pre-op	Before an operation	To determine patient suitability for surgery	Collect before the patient goes to surgery	CBC PTT Platelet function studies	Same as ASAP
Post-op	After an operation	Assess patient condition after surgery	Collect when patient is out of surgery	H & H	Same as ASAP
Routine	Relating to established procedure	Used to establish a diagnosis or monitor a patient's progress	Collect in a timely manner, but no urgency involved. Typically collected on morning sweeps or the next scheduled sweep	CBC Chem profile	None

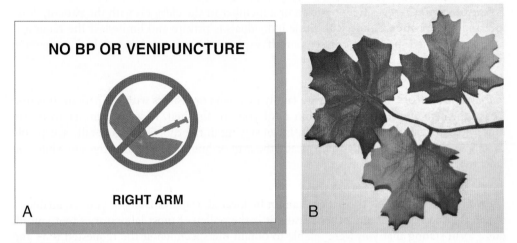

FIGURE 8-4

Two examples of warning signs. **A.** No blood pressures or venipuncture in right arm. (Courtesy Brevis Corp, Salt Lake City, UT.) **B.** Fall-colored leaves symbolizing fall precautions.

or flowers). A sign with the letters **DNR** (do not resuscitate) or **DNAR** (do not attempt resuscitation) means that there is an order (also called a no code order) stating that the patient should not be revived if he or she stops breathing. A physician at the request of the patient or the patient's guardian typically writes the order.

fyi   A *code* is a way to transmit a message, normally understood by healthcare personnel only, over the facility's public address system. A code uses numbers or words to convey information needed by healthcare personnel to respond to certain situations.

Pictures are sometimes used in place of written warnings. For example, a sign with a picture of fall leaves (Fig. 8-4B) is sometimes used to indicate fall precautions. A picture of a fallen leaf with a teardrop on it is sometimes used on obstetric wards to indicate that a patient has lost a baby.

Entering a Patient's Room   Doors to patients' rooms are usually open. If the door is closed, knock lightly, open the door slowly, and say something like "good morning" before proceeding into the room. Even if the door is open, it is a good idea to knock lightly to make occupants aware that you are about to enter. Curtains are often pulled closed when nurses are working with patients or when patients are using bedpans or urinals. Make your presence known before proceeding or opening the curtain to protect the patient's privacy and avoid embarrassment.

Physicians and Clergy   If a physician or a member of the clergy is with the patient, don't interrupt. The patient's time with these individuals is private and limited. If the request is for a stat or timed specimen, excuse yourself, explain why you are there, and ask permission to proceed.

Family and Visitors   Often there are family members or visitors with the patient. It is best to ask them to step outside the room until you are finished. Most will prefer to do so; however, some family members will insist on staying in the room. It is generally acceptable to let a willing family member help steady the arm or hold pressure over the site while you label tubes.

Unavailable Patient   If the patient cannot be located, is unavailable, or you are unable to obtain the specimen for any other reason, it is the policy of most laboratories that you fill out a form stating that you were unable to obtain the specimen at the requested time and the reason why. The original copy of this form is left at the nurses' station and a copy goes to the lab.

Identifying Yourself   Identify yourself to the patient by stating your name, your title and why you are there (e.g., "Good morning. I am Joe Smith, a phlebotomist. I'm here to collect a blood specimen if it is all right with you."). If you are a student, let the patient know this and ask permission to do the blood draw. This is a part of informed consent and patient rights. The patient has a right to refuse to have blood drawn by a student or anyone else. A phlebotomist must never collect a blood specimen against a patient's will. Objections should be reported to the appropriate personnel.

c a u t i o n   Be aware of conflicting permission statements. This often happens with student phlebotomists. For example, when a student asks permission to collect the specimen, a patient may say "Yes, but I would rather not." The patient has given permission and taken back that permission in the same statement. In this case it is best if someone else collects the specimen.

Bedside Manner   The behavior of a healthcare provider toward, or as perceived by, a patient is called **bedside manner**. Approaching a patient is more than simply calling an outpatient into the drawing room or finding an inpatient's room and proceeding to collect the specimen. The manner in which you approach and interact with the patient sets the stage for whether or not the patient perceives you as a professional. Gaining the patient's trust and confidence and putting the patient at ease are important aspects of a successful encounter and an important part of professional bedside manner. A phlebotomist with a professional bedside manner and appearance will more easily gain a patient's trust. A confident phlebotomist will convey that confidence to patients and help them feel at ease.

> **key · point** A cheerful, pleasant manner and an exchange of small talk will help to put a patient at ease as well as divert attention from any discomfort associated with the procedure.

PATIENT IDENTIFICATION

Patient identification (ID), the process of verifying a patient's identity, is the most important step in specimen collection. Obtaining a specimen from the wrong patient can have serious, even fatal, consequences, especially specimens for type and crossmatch prior to blood transfusion. Misidentifying a patient or specimen can be grounds for dismissal of the person responsible and can even lead to a malpractice lawsuit against that person.

Verifying Name and Date of Birth When identifying a patient, ask the patient to state his or her full name and identification number and/or date of birth. For example, *never* say, "Are you Mrs. Smith?" A person who is very ill, hard of hearing, or sedated may say "Yes" to anything. Use a "memory jogger," such as having a patient spell an unusual name, or comment in some positive way about a name, to help remember that you verified it. The patient's response must match the information on the requisition.

Checking Identification Bracelets If the patient's response matches the information on the requisition, proceed to check the patient's **ID band** or **bracelet** (Fig. 8-5A) (also called an **arm band** or **wrist band**) if applicable. Inpatients are normally required to wear an ID band, usually on the wrist. The typical ID band (Fig. 8-5B) lists the patient's name and hospital identification number or **medical record (MR) number**. Additional information includes the patient's birth date or age, room number and bed designation, and physician's name

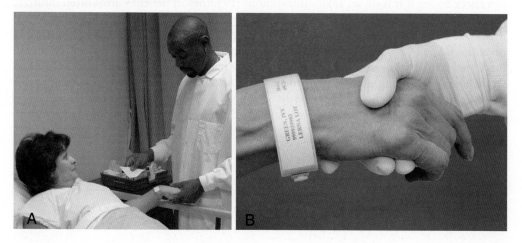

FIGURE 8-5

A. Phlebotomist at bedside checking patient identification band. **B.** Close-up of a typical identification bracelet.

The patient name, MR number, and date of birth (DOB) or age on the ID band must match the information on the requisition *exactly*. It is not unusual to have patients with the same or similar names in the hospital at the same time. (Examples are patients with common last names, fathers and sons that have been in accidents, multiple-birth babies, and relatives involved in tissue transplant procedures.) There have even been instances when two unrelated patients shared the same full name and birth date. Two patients will not, however, have the same hospital or medical record number, although they may be similar.

Identification protocol may vary slightly from one healthcare institution to another. Generally, ID information such as room number, bed number, and physician name are allowed to differ. For instance, occasionally a room number will differ because the patient has been moved. The name of the ordering physician may be different since it is not unusual for a patient to be under the care of several different physicians at the same time.

3-Way ID   To avoid identification and mislabeling errors some inpatient facilities require what is referred to as 3-Way ID in which the patient is identified by three means; the patient's verbal ID statement, a check of the ID band, and a visual comparison of the labeled specimen with the patient's ID band before leaving the bedside.

ID Discrepancies   If there is a discrepancy between the name, MR number, or date of birth on the ID band and the information on the requisition, the patient's nurse should be notified. The specimen should not be obtained until the discrepancy is addressed and the patient's identity is verified.

Missing ID   If there is no ID band on either of an inpatient's wrists, ask the patient if you can check to see if it is on an ankle. Intravenous (IV) lines in patient's arms often infiltrate the surrounding tissues and cause swelling that necessitates removal of the ID band. When this occurs, especially on a patient with IV lines in both arms, nursing personnel sometimes place the ID band around an ankle. In some instances, an ID band is removed from an IV-infiltrated arm or while other procedures are being performed on the patient and placed on an IV pole or the night table by the patient's bed. An ID band on an IV pole or night table could belong to a patient who previously occupied that bed and should not be used. It is also not unusual for a new patient to occupy a bed before the nursing staff has a chance to attach his or her ID band.

c a u t i o n   *Never* verify information from an ID band that is not attached to the patient or collect a specimen from a inpatient who is not wearing an ID band.

If a patient is not wearing an ID band it is usually acceptable to ask the patient's nurse to attach an ID band before collecting the specimen. Some sites require the phlebotomist to fill out a special form stating that the specimen was not collected because the patient did not have an ID band. The form is left at the nurse's station. It is then up to the patient's nurse to attach an ID band and inform the lab when it has been done so that the specimen can be collected. In rare emergency situations in which there is no time to wait for attachment of an ID band, the patient's nurse is allowed to verify the patient's ID. In such cases the nurse must sign or initial the requisition. Follow institution protocol.

Sleeping Patients   Obviously, proper identification and informed consent cannot take place if the patient is asleep. If you encounter a sleeping patient, as is often the case in hospitals and nursing homes, wake the person gently. Try not to startle the patient, as this can affect test results. Speak softly but distinctly. If the room is darkened, avoid turning on bright overhead lighting, at least until the patient's eyes have adjusted to being open, and warn the patient first.

> **c a u t i o n**   *Never* attempt to collect a blood specimen from a sleeping patient. Such an attempt may startle the patient and cause injury to the patient or the phlebotomist.

Unconscious Patients   Unconscious patients are often encountered in emergency rooms and intensive care units. Ask a relative or the nurse to identify the patient. Speak to the patient as you would to someone who is alert. Identify yourself and inform the patient of your intent. Unconscious patients can often hear what is going on around them even though they are unresponsive.

> **c a u t i o n**   An unconscious patient may be able to feel pain and move when you insert the needle, so it may be necessary to have someone assist you in holding the arm during the blood draw.

Emergency Room ID Procedures   It is not uncommon for an emergency room (ER) to receive an unconscious patient with no identification. In many institutions, the phlebotomist is allowed to attach a special three-part identification band (Fig 8-6) such as a Typenex Blood Recipient ID band (Fenwal Laboratories, a division of Travenol Laboratories, Deerfield, IL) to an unidentified ER patient's wrist. All three parts contain the same number. The first part becomes the patient's ID band. The second part is attached to the specimen. The third part is used if the patient needs a transfusion, and it is attached to the unit of blood. Follow your institution's protocol for unidentified patients.

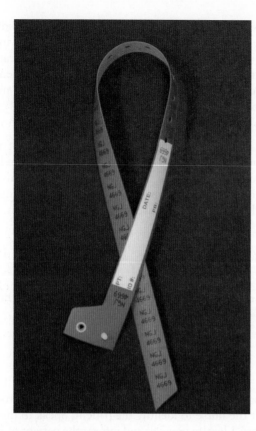

FIGURE 8-6

Example of special 3-part ID band used for unidentified ER patients.

> c a u t i o n　*Never* collect a specimen without some way to positively connect that specimen to the patient.

Identification of Young, Mentally Incompetent, or Non-English-Speaking Patients　If the patient is young, mentally incompetent, or non-English-speaking, ask the patient's nurse, attendant, relative, or friend to identify the patient by name, address, and identification number or birth date. This information must match the information on the test requisition and the patient's ID band if applicable.

Outpatient ID　Typically, the outpatient collection site receptionist verifies the patient's identity and fills out the proper lab requisition or generates one via computer. Some labs supply requisition forms to physicians who use their services, so some outpatients arrive at the collection site with lab requisitions that are already filled out. Information must still be verified, and patients may be required to show proof of identification such as a driver's license or other picture ID. Outpatients do not normally have ID bands. However, they may have a clinic-issued **ID card** that contains their name and other information identifying them as a clinic patient. ID cards are sometimes used to imprint specimen requisitions or labels using an address-o-graph type of machine. Even if a receptionist has identified the patient, a phlebotomist must still personally verify the patient's ID after calling him or her into the blood-drawing area from the waiting room. Simply calling a person's name and having someone respond is not verification enough. Anxious or hard-of-hearing patients may think their name has been called, when in fact a similar name was called. Always ask an outpatient to state his or her name and date of birth and compare it with the requisition before obtaining the specimen.

PREPARING THE PATIENT

Explaining the Procedure   Most patients have had a blood test before. A statement of your intent to perform a blood test is usually sufficient for them to understand what is about to occur. A patient who has never had a blood test may require a more detailed explanation. Special procedures may require additional information. If a patient does not speak or understand English, you may have to use sign language or other nonverbal means to demonstrate what is to occur. If this fails, an interpreter must be located. Speaking slowly and distinctly, using sign language, or writing down information may be necessary for patients with hearing problems.

key • point   Regardless of difficulties involved, you must always determine that the patient understands what is about to take place and obtain permission before proceeding. This is part of informed consent.

Addressing Patient Inquiries   Some healthcare facilities will allow the phlebotomist to tell the patient the name of the test or tests to be performed. Others prefer that all inquiries be directed to the patient's physician. Never attempt to explain the purpose of a test to a patient. Because a particular test can be ordered to rule out a number of different problems, any attempt to explain its purpose could mislead or unduly alarm the patient. Handle such inquiries by stating that it is best to have the doctor or nurse explain them.

When bedside testing is being performed (such as glucose monitoring), the patient is often aware of the type of test being performed and may ask about results. Follow facility protocol for addressing such requests or check with patient's nurse or physician to see if it is acceptable to tell the patient the results.

Handling Patient Objections   Although most patients understand that blood tests are needed in the course of treatment, occasionally a patient will object to the procedure. Outpatients rarely object because typically they have been personally directed by their physician to obtain testing and in most cases given a test requisition. Inpatients on the other hand, may not be aware of all the tests that have been ordered or the frequency with which some tests must be repeated. Some may have difficult veins and just get tired of the ordeal. A reminder that the doctor ordered the test and needs the results to provide proper care will sometimes convince the patient to cooperate.

key • point   Do not attempt to badger the patient into cooperating or to restrain a conscious, mentally alert adult patient to obtain a specimen. Remember, a patient *does* have the right to refuse testing.

Sometimes a patient objects at first, but is not really serious. However, if a patient truly objects and refuses to let you collect the specimen, write on the requisition that the patient has refused to have blood drawn and notify the appropriate personnel that the specimen was not obtained because of patient refusal. Depending upon institution policy, you may be required to fill out a special form stating why you were unable to collect the specimen.

Handling Difficult Patients   The patient may not echo your cheerful, pleasant manner. Hospitalization or illness is typically a stressful situation. The patient may be lonely, scared, fearful, or just plain disagreeable and may react in a negative manner toward you. It is important to remain calm and professional and treat the patient in a caring manner under all circumstances.

Addressing Needle Phobia   An admission of **needle phobia** (intense fear of needles) by a patient or signs that suggest it, such as extreme fear or apprehension in advance of venipuncture, should not be taken lightly. Needle phobic individuals can experience a shock type reflex during or immediately following venipuncture. Symptoms include pallor (paleness), profuse sweating, lightheadedness, nausea, and fainting. In severe cases, patients have been known to suffer arrhythmia and even cardiac arrest. Needle phobia is estimated to affect more than 10% of the population to such a degree that they avoid medical care. It is important that those who do have the courage to submit to blood tests are treated with empathy and special attention and that steps be taken to minimize any trauma associated with the venipuncture. Basic steps that can be taken include:

- Have the patient lie down during the procedure, with legs elevated.
- Apply an ice pack to the site for 10 to 15 minutes to numb it before venipuncture.
- Have only the most experienced and skilled phlebotomist perform the venipuncture.

It is recommended that anyone who has suffered a severe reaction as a result of needle phobia have future procedures involving needles performed at sites where personnel are trained in CPR and a defibrillator is readily accessible.

Addressing Objects in the Patient's Mouth   Do not allow a patient to eat, drink, chew gum, or have a thermometer, toothpick, or any other foreign object in the mouth during blood collection. Objects in the mouth can cause choking. A bite reflex could break a thermometer and injure a patient. Politely ask patients to stop eating or drinking and remove objects from their mouths until you are finished with the venipuncture.

Step 3: Verify Diet Restrictions and Latex Sensitivity

DIET RESTRICTIONS

It is important to verify that any special diet instructions or restrictions have been followed. The most common diet requirement is for the patient to fast (refrain from eating) for a certain period of time, typically overnight such as after the last meal of the day or after midnight, until the specimen is collected the following morning. If the patient did not fast or follow other diet instructions, the patient's physician or nurse must be notified so that a decision can be made as to whether or not to proceed with the test.

key • point   If told to proceed with specimen collection, it is important to write "nonfasting" on the requisition and the specimen label.

LATEX SENSITIVITY

Exposure to latex can trigger life-threatening reactions in those allergic to it. If a patient is allergic to latex it is extremely important to verify that all equipment used on him or her is latex free and that no latex items are brought into the room, even if they are for use on another patient in the same room.

Step 4: Sanitize Hands

Proper hand hygiene plays a major role in preventing the spread of infection and is an important step in the venipuncture procedure that should not be forgotten or performed poorly. Depending on the degree of contamination, hands can be decontaminated by washing or use of alcohol-based hand sanitizers (Fig. 8-7), normally available in the form of gels or foams. When using hand sanitizers it is important to use a generous amount and allow the alcohol to evaporate to achieve proper antisepsis. If hands are visibly dirty or contaminated with blood or other body fluids, they must be washed with soap and water. If hand-washing facilities are not available, visibly contaminated hands should be cleaned with detergent-containing wipes followed by the use of an alcohol-based hand cleaner. Gloves are sometimes put on at this point. Follow facility protocol.

fyi   Some phlebotomists prefer to put gloves on at this point; others prefer to wait until after vein selection and equipment assembly. Follow facility protocol.

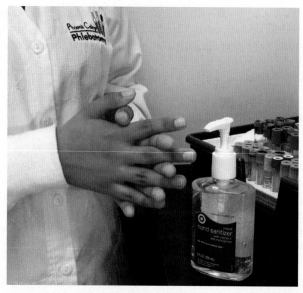

FIGURE 8-7

Phlebotomist applying hand sanitizer.

Step 5: Position Patient, Apply Tourniquet, and Ask Patient to Make a Fist

POSITIONING THE PATIENT

Inpatients normally have blood drawn while lying down in their beds. Outpatients at most facilities are drawn while sitting up in special blood-drawing chairs (Fig. 8-8A). If a special chair is not available, the patient should be seated in one that is sturdy and comfortable and has armrests in case the patient faints (Fig. 8-8B). If a suitable chair is not available or an outpatient is in a weakened condition or known to have fainting tendencies, the blood can be drawn with the patient in a reclining chair or lying on a sofa or bed. With all blood draws, be prepared to react in case the patient feels faint or loses consciousness.

> caution Because of the possibility of fainting, a patient should *never* be standing or seated on a high or backless stool during blood collection.

When venipuncture is performed on a hand or wrist vein, the patient's hand must be well supported on a bed, rolled towel, or armrest. For venipuncture in the antecubital area, the patient's arm should be extended downward in a straight line from the shoulder to wrist and *not* bent at the elbow (In some cases a slight bend may be necessary to avoid hyperextension of the elbow). This position helps "fix" the veins so they are less apt to roll and makes them easier to locate because gravity causes them to enlarge and become

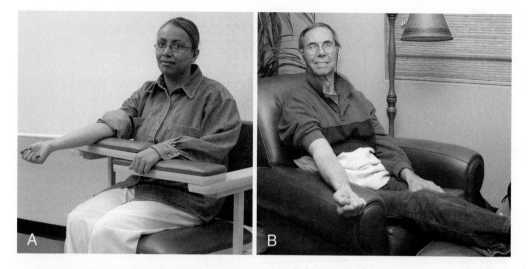

FIGURE 8-8
A. Patient seated in a special blood-drawing chair. **B.** Home draw patient seated in a reclining chair.

more prominent. In addition, a downward position is necessary to ensure that blood collection tubes fill from the bottom up. This prevents reflux or backflow of tube contents into the patient's vein (see Chapter 9) and additive carryover between tubes if multiple tubes are collected.

Proper positioning is somewhat harder to achieve with patients who are lying down, especially if the head of the bed cannot be raised. If necessary, a pillow or rolled towel can be used to support and position the arm so at least the hand is lower than the elbow. Bed rails may be let down, but be careful not to catch IV lines, catheter bags and tubing, or other patient apparatus. Bed rails *must* be raised again when the procedure is finished. Many phlebotomists have learned to collect specimens with bed rails in place so they don't have to worry about forgetting to put them back up when they are finished.

△ c a u t i o n   A phlebotomist who lowers a bed rail and forgets to raise it can be held liable if the patient falls out of bed and is injured.

TOURNIQUET APPLICATION AND FIST CLENCHING

A tourniquet is applied 3 to 4 inches above the intended venipuncture site to restrict venous blood flow and make the veins more prominent. If it is closer to the site, the vein may collapse as blood is removed. If it is too far above the site, it may be ineffective. When drawing blood from a hand vein the tourniquet is applied proximal to the wrist bone.

key • point   If a patient has prominent visible veins, tourniquet application can wait until after the site is cleaned and you are ready to insert the needle.

The tourniquet should be tight enough to slow venous flow without affecting arterial flow. This allows more blood to flow into the area than out. As a result, blood backs up in the veins, enlarging them so they are easier to see and distending or stretching them so the walls are thinner and easier to pierce with a needle. A tourniquet that is too tight may prevent arterial blood flow into the area and result in failure to obtain blood. One that is too loose will be useless. The tourniquet should feel snug or slightly tight to the patient. It should lie flat around the circumference of the arm and not be rolled, twisted, or so tight that it pinches, hurts, or causes the arm to turn red or purple.

fyi   A tourniquet has a greater tendency to roll or twist on arms of obese patients. Two tourniquets placed one on top of the other and used together will sometimes be sturdy enough to prevent the problem.

If a patient has sensitive skin or dermatitis, apply the tourniquet over a dry washcloth or gauze wrapped around the arm or a hospital gown sleeve if facility policy allows. A tourniquet is sometimes applied over an outpatient's sleeve if the sleeve is tight and cannot be pushed or rolled up far enough above the site. Ask the outpatient for permission before doing so, however, as some patients may object. *Never* apply a tourniquet over an open sore. Choose another site. Instructions for tying a latex or vinyl strip tourniquet are shown in Procedure 8-1.

When the tourniquet is in place, ask the patient to clench or make a fist. When a patient makes a fist, the veins in that arm become more prominent, making them easier to locate and enter with a needle. Pumping (repeatedly opening and closing the fist) should be discouraged as it causes muscle movement that can make vein location more difficult and cause changes in blood components that could affect test results.

key • point   Fist pumping most notably affects potassium and ionized calcium levels.

Step 6: Select Vein, Release Tourniquet, and Ask Patient to Open Fist

The preferred venipuncture site is the antecubital area of the arm where a number of veins lie fairly close to the surface. Typically, the most prominent of these are the median cubital, cephalic, and basilic veins in the "H" pattern, and the median, median cephalic, and median basilic veins in the "M" pattern (see Chapter 6). The median cubital and median veins are normally closer to the surface, more stationary, and in an area where nerve injury is least likely.

Tourniquet Application

Purpose: Properly apply a tourniquet to a patient's arm as an aid to venipuncture

Equipment: Vinyl or latex strap tourniquet

Note: Steps listed are for a right-handed individual. If you are left handed, substitute dominant and nondominant, respectively, for right and left references.

Step	Explanation/Rationale
1. Place the tourniquet around the arm 3-4 inches above the intended venipuncture site 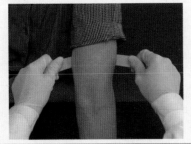	If closer to the site, the vein may collapse as blood is withdrawn. If too far above the site, it may be ineffective
2. Grasp one side of the tourniquet in each hand a few inches from the end	Allows sufficient length for fastening the tourniquet and creating the loop in step 7
3. Apply a small amount of tension and maintain it throughout the process	Tension is needed so the tourniquet will be snug when tied. If too much tension is applied it will be too tight and it will roll up on itself or twist and cause discomfort
4. Bring the two sides together and grasp them both between the thumb and forefinger of the right hand 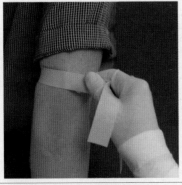	This is preparation for crossing the sides over each other
5. Reach over the right hand and grasp the right side of the tourniquet between the thumb and forefinger of the left hand and release it from the grip of the right hand	The tourniquet ends will now be held in opposite hands, with the sides crossed over each other

(Continued)

PROCEDURE 8-1 *(Continued)*

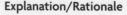

Step	Explanation/Rationale
6. Cross the left end over the right end near the left index finger, grasping both sides together between the thumb and forefinger of the left hand, close to the patient's arm	If it there is too much space between the left index finger and the patient's arm, the tourniquet will be too loose

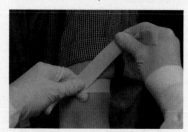

| 7. While securely grasping both sides, use either the left middle finger or the right index finger to tuck a portion of the left side under the right side, and pull it into a loop. | The loop allows the tourniquet to be released quickly by a slight tug on the end that forms it |

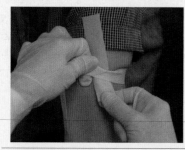

| 8. A properly tied tourniquet with the ends pointing toward the shoulder | The tourniquet ends should point toward the shoulder to prevent them from contaminating the blood collection site |

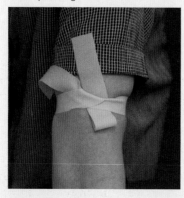

Consequently, they are the first choices for venipuncture, followed by the cephalic and median cephalic veins. The basilic and median basilic veins are last choice veins because they are near the median nerve and brachial artery, which could be punctured accidentally.

> **c a u t i o n**   According to CLSI Standard H3-A5, an attempt must have been made to locate the median cubital vein on both arms before considering an alternate vein, and due to the possibility of nerve injury and damage to the brachial artery, the basilic vein should not be chosen unless no other vein is more prominent.

A patient will generally have the most prominent veins in the dominant arm. It should be examined first, unless there is a reason that it should not be used. Some veins may be easily visible; others will have to be located entirely by feel. To locate a vein, **palpate** (examine by touch or feel) the area by pushing down on the skin with the tip of the index finger (Fig. 8-9). In addition to locating veins, palpating helps determine their **patency** (state of being freely open), size and depth, and the direction or the path they follow. Consequently, even visible veins must be palpated to judge suitability for venipuncture.

When you have found a vein, roll your finger from one side to the other while pressing against it to help judge its size. Trace its path to determine a proper entry point by palpating above and below where you first feel it. Press and release it several times to determine depth and patency. Depth is indicated by the degree of pressure required to feel it. A patent (open) vein is turgid (distended from being filled with blood), giving it a bounce or resilience, and has a tubelike feel. An artery has a pulse and must be avoided. (Do not use the thumb to palpate as it has a pulse that could lead you to think that a vein is an artery.)

> **c a u t i o n**   To avoid inadvertently puncturing an artery, *never* select a vein that overlies or is close to where you feel a pulse.

Do not select a vein that feels hard and cordlike or lacks resilience, as it is probably sclerosed or thrombosed (see Chapter 9). Such veins roll easily, are hard to penetrate, and may not have adequate blood flow to yield a representative blood sample. Tendons are also hard and lack resilience. Rotating the patient's arm slightly helps locate veins and differentiate them from other structures. Dimming the lights and using a transilluminator device or halogen flashlight can help locate veins, especially in infants and children. Wiping the site with alcohol often makes surface veins such as hand veins appear more visible. (This step *does not* take the place of cleaning after vein selection.) If no suitable antecubital vein can be found, check the other arm. If no suitable antecubital vein can be found in either arm, check for veins on the back of the hand or wrist.

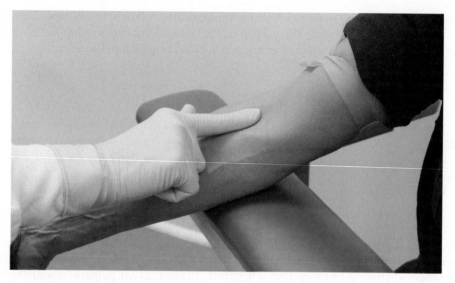

FIGURE 8-9

Phlebotomist palpating the antecubital area for a vein.

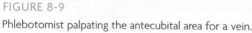

caution   *Do not* use veins on the underside of the wrist because nerves lie close to the veins in this area and can easily be injured.

If a suitable vein still cannot be found, massage the arm from wrist to elbow to force blood into the area or wrap a warm, wet towel around the arm or hand for a few minutes. Warming the site increases blood flow and makes veins easier to feel. The site should not be manipulated excessively, however, as this may change the composition of blood in the area and cause erroneous test results. In the absence of a suitable vein, a capillary puncture may have to be considered if the test can be performed on capillary blood.

After you have selected a suitable vein, mentally visualize its location if it is not obvious. Making a mental note of the position of the vein in reference to landmarks such as a freckle, mole, hair, skin crease, superficial surface vein, or imperfection makes relocation easier after the delay while the site is cleaned. Do not mark the site with a pen. This contaminates the site and the pen. The pen can become a source of infection transmission if it is used on other patients. An acceptable way to mark the site using an alcohol pad is shown in Figure 8-10. This, of course, is done before the site is cleaned, so the pad must be placed far enough away from the site so it is not disturbed in the cleaning process.

If the tourniquet was applied during vein selection, release it and ask the patient to open the fist. This allows the vein to return to normal and minimizes the effects of stasis from blockage of blood flow on specimen composition.

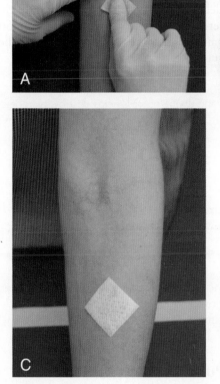

FIGURE 8-10

Marking the site with an alcohol pad.
A. Align the corner of a clean alcohol pad over the vein located by the index finger. **B.** Slide the pad away from the site, paralleling the direction of the vein and keeping the corner of the pad pointing in the direction of the vein. **C.** Alcohol pad pointing in the direction of the vein.

key · point   According to CLSI, when a tourniquet is used during preliminary vein selection, it should be released and reapplied after 2 minutes.

Step 7: Clean and Air-Dry Site

The venipuncture site must be cleaned with an antiseptic prior to venipuncture. Otherwise, microorganisms from the skin could be picked up by the needle and carried into the vein, creating the possibility of infection, or flushed into the collection tube on blood flow, contaminating the specimen. The recommended antiseptic for cleaning a venipuncture site is 70% isopropyl alcohol typically available in sterile, prepackaged pads referred to as alcohol prep pads.

fyi An antiseptic does *not* sterilize the site; however, it does inhibit microbial growth.

Clean the site with a circular motion, starting at the point where you expect to insert the needle, and moving outward in ever-widening **concentric circles** (circles with a common center) until you have cleaned an area approximately 2 to 3 inches in diameter. Use sufficient pressure to remove surface dirt and debris but do not rub so vigorously that you abrade the skin, especially on infants and elderly patients whose skin is thin and more delicate. If the site is especially dirty, clean it again with another alcohol prep pad. Allow the area to dry naturally for 30 seconds to 1 minute.

key · point The evaporation and drying process helps destroy microbes, prevents specimen hemolysis from alcohol contamination, and avoids a burning sensation when the needle is inserted.

To prevent contamination of the site

- *Do not* dry the alcohol with unsterile gauze
- *Do not* fan the site with your hand or blow on it to hasten drying time
- *Do not* touch the site after cleaning it

key · point If it is necessary to repalpate the vein after the site has been cleaned, clean it again or decontaminate the gloved finger used to palpate and touch only above or below the expected needle entry point.

Step 8: Prepare Equipment and Put on Gloves

Assemble blood collection system components and supplies if you have not already done so. Choose the collection system, needle size, and tube volume according to the age of the patient, size and location of the vein, and amount of blood to be collected. Select tubes according to the tests that have been ordered. Select and attach the needle to the collection device but *do not* remove the **needle sheath** (cap or cover) at this time. Put on a clean pair of gloves if you have not already done so.

caution Either the needle, tube holder, or syringe selected must have an OSHA required safety feature to help protect the user from accidental needlesticks.

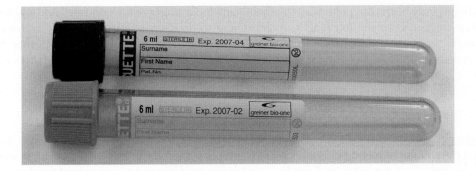

FIGURE 8-11

Expiration dates on ETS tubes.

ETS EQUIPMENT PREPARATION

Select the appropriate ETS tubes. Check the expiration date (Fig. 8-11) on each one to make certain it has not expired. (Discard any tube that is beyond its expiration date.) Tap additive tubes lightly to dislodge any additive that may be adhering to the tube stopper. Inspect the seal of the needle. If it is broken, discard it and select a new one. Twist the needle cover apart to expose the short or back end of the needle that is covered by a retractable sleeve. Screw this end of the needle into the threaded hub of an ETS tube holder. Place the first tube in the holder and use a slight clockwise twist to push it onto the needle just far enough to secure it and keep it from falling out, but not far enough to release the tube vacuum. It is acceptable to delay positioning the tube in the holder until the needle is inserted in the patient's vein.

WINGED INFUSION SET (BUTTERFLY) PREPARATION

Although they are available in various gauges, a 23-gauge butterfly is most commonly used for small and difficult veins. Butterfly needles are also available in two basic types. One type has a hub that can be attached to a syringe. The second type has a hub with a multisample Luer adapter that can be threaded onto an ETS tube holder. Select the type according to the method you have chosen to collect the specimen. The method chosen (ETS or syringe) typically depends on the size, condition, and location of the vein as well as the skill and personal preference of the user. In some cases a syringe and butterfly are used after a failed attempt at blood collection using a butterfly and ETS holder. For either method, the butterfly needle typically contains the safety feature.

Verify sterility of the butterfly packaging before aseptically opening it and removing the butterfly. To help preserve needle sterility (a butterfly needle cover is typically an open-ended tubular sheath), it is a good idea to retain the package so you can put the needle back in it temporarily while retying the tourniquet. Attach the butterfly to the evacuated tube holder or syringe. Butterfly tubing may be coiled somewhat because it was coiled in the package. To help straighten it and keep it from coiling back up, use the thumb and index finger of one hand to grasp the tubing just beyond the point where it attaches to the needle. Gently grasp the tubing a little below this point with the thumb and index finger of the opposite hand and slide these fingers down the full length of the tubing while stretching it slightly. Be extremely careful not to loosen the tubing from the needle at the one end or the hub at the other. Select the appropriate small-volume tubes for the tests ordered. (The vacuum of large tubes may collapse the vein or hemolyze the specimen).

SYRINGE EQUIPMENT PREPARATION

Select a syringe and needle size compatible with the size and condition of the patient's veins and the amount of blood to be collected. To comply with OSHA regulations you must select a needle-locking syringe (e.g., Luer lock) to use for the draw, and a syringe transfer device to transfer blood from the syringe to the ETS tubes. Syringes and syringe needles designed for blood collection are normally available in sterile pull-apart packages. The syringe plunger is typically already pulled back slightly. To ensure that the plunger moves freely but still maintain syringe sterility, move the plunger back and forth a few times and advance it to the end of the syringe before opening the sterile package. Open the needle packages in an aseptic manner and securely attach the needle to the syringe. A blood specimen collected in a syringe will have to be transferred to ETS tubes. Small-volume tubes are typically chosen because the amount of blood that can be collected in a syringe is limited. Partially open the transfer device package to make removal easy when it comes time to use it.

POSITIONING EQUIPMENT FOR USE

Place collection equipment and other supplies, such as gauze and alcohol pads, within easy reach, typically on the same side of the patient's arm as your free hand during venipuncture. Make certain that extra supplies, ETS tubes for example, are within easy reach. If using a phlebotomy tray, place it within easy reach.

> c a u t i o n   *Do not* place the phlebotomy tray on a patient's bed or any other place that could be contaminated by it.

Step 9: Reapply Tourniquet, Uncap and Inspect Needle

Reapply the tourniquet, being careful not to touch the cleaned area. Be aware that there are a few tests (i.e., lactic acid) that must be collected without using a tourniquet.

Pick up collection equipment with your dominant hand. Both an ETS tube holder and a syringe are held close to the needle hub with the thumb on top and two or three fingers underneath and slightly to the side. Turn your wrist upward slightly so the opening of the tube holder remains accessible. Hold the wing portion of the butterfly between your thumb and index finger or fold the wings upright and grasp them together. Cradle the butterfly tubing and holder or syringe in the palm of your dominant hand or lay it next to the patient's hand.

Remove the needle cover and visually inspect the needle. Although rare, a needle can have obstructions that could impair blood flow or imperfections such as roughness or barbs that could hurt the patient or damage the vein. If any are noted, discard the needle and select a new one.

> c a u t i o n   Once the cap is removed, *do not* let the needle touch anything prior to venipuncture. If it does, remove it and replace it with a new one.

Step 10: Ask Patient to Remake a Fist, Anchor Vein, and Insert Needle

At this time the patient is asked to again make a fist. The nondominant hand is used to **anchor** (secure firmly) the vein while the collection equipment is held and the needle inserted using the dominant hand.

ANCHORING

To anchor antecubital veins, grasp the patient's arm with your free hand, using your fingers to support the back of the arm just below the elbow. Place your thumb a minimum of 1 to 2 inches below and slightly to the side of the intended venipuncture site, and pull the skin toward the wrist (Fig. 8-12). This stretches the skin taut (tight), anchoring the vein and helping

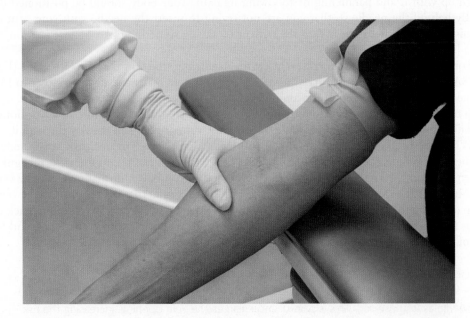

FIGURE 8-12

Proper placement of thumb and fingers when anchoring a vein.

to keep it from moving or rolling to the side upon needle entry. (If the vein rolls, the needle may slip beside the vein, not into it.) In addition, a needle passes through taut skin more easily and with less pain. Even so, it is not uncommon for an apprehensive patient to suddenly pull back the arm as the needle is inserted. Because your fingers are wrapped around the arm, the patient is less likely to pull away from your grasp, and the needle is more likely to stay in the vein. This is known as the "L" hold technique for anchoring the vein.

caution For safety reasons, *do not* use a two-finger technique (also called "C" hold) in which the entry point of the vein is straddled by the index finger above and the thumb below. If the patient pulls the arm back when the needle is inserted, there is a possibility that the needle may recoil as it comes out of the arm and spring back into your index finger.

One way to anchor a hand vein is to use your free hand to hold the patient's hand just below the knuckles, and use your thumb to pull the skin taut over the knuckles while bending the patient's fingers. Another way is to have the patient make a tight fist. Encircle the fist with your fingers, and use your thumb to pull the skin over the knuckles.

NEEDLE INSERTION

Hold the collection device or butterfly needle in your dominant hand as described in step 9. The bevel of the needle should be facing up. Position the needle above the vein so it is lined up with it and paralleling or following its path. Your body should be positioned directly behind the needle so that you are not trying to insert the needle with your arm or hands at an awkward angle. Warn the patient by saying something like "There is going to be a little poke (or stick) now."

For antecubital site venipunctures, insert the needle into the skin at a 15 to 30° angle (Fig. 8-13A), depending on the depth of the vein. (A shallow vein may need an angle closer to 15°, while a deeper vein may require an angle closer to 30°.) Use one smooth, steady forward motion to penetrate first the skin and then the vein. Advancing the needle too slowly prolongs any discomfort. A rapid jab can result in missing the vein or going all the way through it.

When the needle enters the vein, you will feel a slight "give" or decrease in resistance. Some phlebotomists describe this as a "pop." (This is especially important to recognize when using an ETS needle and tube holder, as there is no visual confirmation when the vein is entered.) When you sense the "pop" or are otherwise certain that the needle is in the vein, stop advancing it, and securely anchor the tube holder or syringe by pressing the back of your fingers or knuckles against the arm. Discontinue anchoring with your thumb and let go of the arm with that hand.

caution Do not deeply depress the skin by forcefully pushing down on the needle as it is inserted. This is painful and enlarges the vein opening, increasing the risk of blood leakage at the site.

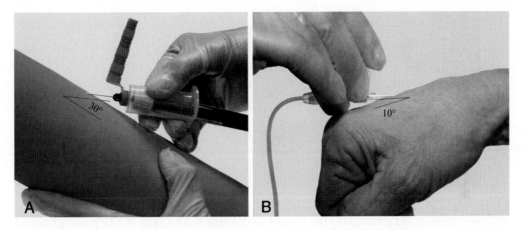

FIGURE 8-13

A. Illustration of a 30° angle of needle insertion. **B.** Illustration of a 10° angle of needle insertion.

When using a butterfly needle on a hand vein, insert it into the vein at a shallow angle between 10 and 15° (see Fig. 8-13B), being careful not to push it through the back wall of the vein. You may need to slightly increase the angle of the needle bevel at first to get it to slip into the vein. A "flash" or small amount of blood will appear in the tubing when the needle is in the vein. "Seat" the needle by slightly threading it within the lumen (central area of the vein). This helps keep the needle from twisting back out of the vein if you let go of it. If the needle does start to come out of the vein, secure it with the thumb of the opposite hand.

At this point, some phlebotomists switch to holding the blood collection device in their nondominant hand so that tube changes can be made with the dominant hand. This is accomplished by gently slipping the fingers of the opposite hand under the holder and placing the thumb atop the holder as the other hand lets go. Many phlebotomists, particularly those who are left handed, do not change hands but continue to steady the holder in the same hand and change tubes with the opposite. Whatever the method, it is important to hold the blood collection device steady so there is minimal needle movement.

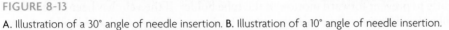 **key · point** If the tube holder or syringe is not securely anchored, the needle can push through the back of the vein or pull out of the vein when tubes are changed or the syringe is filled.

Step 11: Establish Blood Flow, Release Tourniquet, and Ask Patient to Open Fist

To establish blood flow when using the ETS system, the collection tube must be advanced into the tube holder until the stopper is completely penetrated by the needle. This is accomplished most efficiently by pushing the tube with your thumb while your index and

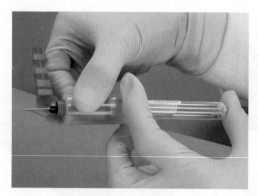

FIGURE 8-14

Proper placement of fingers and thumb when advancing a tube in an ETS holder.

middle fingers straddle and grasp the flanges of the tube holder (Fig. 8-14); pulling back on them slightly to prevent forward motion of the tube holder. If the vein has been successfully entered, blood will begin to flow into the tube. If using a syringe, a flash of blood in the syringe hub indicates that the vein has been successfully entered. Blood flow into the syringe is achieved by slowly pulling back on the plunger with your free hand.

Release the tourniquet and ask the patient to release the fist as soon as blood flows freely into the first ETS tube or is established in the syringe. Blood should continue to flow until multiple tubes have been collected or the syringe filled. On elderly patients and others with fragile veins that might collapse or in other difficult draw situations where release of the tourniquet might cause blood flow to stop, the tourniquet is sometimes left on until the last tube is filled. *Do not*, however, leave the tourniquet on for more than 1 minute or test results may be affected.

fyi Typically, several tubes can be filled in less than a minute.

Step 12: Fill, Remove, and Mix Tubes in Order of Draw or Fill Syringe

Following the order of draw, place ETS tubes in the holder and advance them onto the needle.

ETS tubes fill automatically until the tube vacuum is exhausted or lost. A syringe is filled manually by slowly and steadily pulling back on the plunger until the barrel is filled to the appropriate level.

key • point According to CLSI, if a coagulation tube is the first tube to be drawn when using a butterfly, a discard tube should be drawn first to fill the tubing dead space and ensure a correct blood-to-anticoagulant ratio when the coagulation tube is filled. The discard tube can be a nonadditive tube or another coagulation tube and does not have to be filled completely.

Maintain needle position while the tubes or syringe are filling. Try not to pull up, press down, or move the needle back and forth or sideways in the vein. These actions can be painful to the patient and enlarge the hole in the vein, resulting in leakage of blood and hematoma formation.

Keep the arm in a downward position so that blood fills ETS tubes from the bottom up and does not contact the needle in the tube holder. Under certain conditions, **reflux** (flow of blood from the tube back into the vein) and a possible adverse patient reaction from additives can occur if tube blood is in contract with the needle. Additive-containing blood on or in the needle could also contaminate subsequent tubes when multiple tubes are collected. Do not change position of the tube or allow back and forth movement of the blood in the tube, as this too can cause reflux. A downward arm position also helps maintain blood flow.

> c a u t i o n   If the stopper end of the tube fills first, blood in the tube is in contact with the needle and reflux can occur if there is a change in pressure in the patient' vein.

To ensure a proper ratio of additive to blood, allow ETS tubes to fill until the normal vacuum is exhausted and blood ceases to flow. Tubes do not fill completely to the top. When blood flow stops, remove the tube, using a reverse twist and pulling motion while bracing the thumb or index finger against the flange of the holder. The rubber sleeve will cover the needle and prevent leakage of blood into the tube holder. If the tube contains an additive, mix it by gently inverting it 3 to 8 times (depending upon the type of additive and manufacturer's recommendations) as soon as it is removed from the tube holder and before putting it down (Fig. 8-15). Lack of, delayed, or inadequate mixing can lead to clot formation and necessitate recollection of the specimen. Nonadditive tubes do not require mixing.

> c a u t i o n   *Do not* shake or vigorously mix blood specimens as this can cause hemolysis (breakage of red blood cells and release of hemoglobin into the serum or plasma.).

FIGURE 8-15

Phlebotomist mixing a heparin tube.

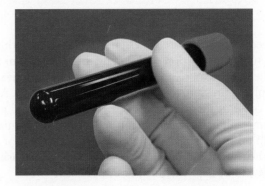

If other ETS tubes are to be drawn, place them in the holder, use a clockwise twist to engage them with the needle, and push them the rest of the way onto the needle until blood flow is established. Steady the tube holder so that the needle does not pull out of or penetrate through the vein as tubes are placed and removed. If the needle backs out of the skin even slightly, the vacuum of the tube will be lost (evidenced by a hissing sound) and the tube will stop filling. Unless the tube already has an adequate amount of blood for the test, a new one will have to be filled. Remember to follow the proper order of draw (see Chapter 7).

When the last ETS tube has been filled, remove it from the holder and mix it, if applicable, before removing the needle from the arm. If the tube is still engaged when the needle is removed from the arm, the needle may drip blood and cause needless contamination.

key • point   The practice of releasing the tube from the needle, but leaving it in the holder during needle removal is awkward and increases the chance of needlesticks. It also delays proper mixing of tube contents, which can lead to microclot formation in anticoagulant tubes.

If the tourniquet is still on, release it before removing the needle. If the needle is removed with the tourniquet in place, blood may run down the arm and alarm the patient.

Step 13: Place Gauze, Remove Needle, Activate Safety Feature, and Apply Pressure

After the last tube has been removed from the holder or an adequate amount of blood has been collected if using a syringe, fold a clean gauze square into fourths and place it directly over the site where the needle enters the skin. Hold the gauze lightly in place but do not press down on it until the needle is removed.

caution   *Do not* press down on the gauze while the needle is in the vein. It puts pressure on the needle during removal causing pain, and the needle may slit the vein and the skin as it is withdrawn.

If the needle safety feature is designed to function within the vein, activate it according to manufacturer's instructions. Withdraw the needle from the vein in one smooth motion. If the needle safety feature operates outside the vein, activate it immediately while simultaneously applying pressure to the site with your free hand. Apply pressure to the site for 3 to 5 minutes or until the bleeding stops. Failure to apply pressure or applying inadequate pressure can result in leakage of blood and hematoma formation. It is acceptable to have the patient hold pressure while you proceed to label tubes (or fill them if a syringe was used), providing the patient is fully alert and able to so. *Do not* ask the patient to bend the arm up. The arm should be kept extended or even raised.

key · point Studies show that folding the arm back at the elbow to hold pressure or keep the gauze in place after a blood draw actually increases the chance of bruising by keeping the wound open (especially if it is to the side of the arm) or disrupting the platelet plug when the arm is lowered.

If the sharps container has been moved out of reach (as sometimes happens in emergencies when others are working on the patient at the same time) and the patient is not able to hold pressure, it is generally acceptable to bend the patient's arm up temporarily while locating the sharps container and disposing of the collection device.

Step 14: Discard Collection Unit, Syringe Needle, or Transfer Device

caution OSHA regulations prohibit cutting, bending, breaking, or recapping blood collection needles or removing them from tube holders after use.

A needle and tube holder must be promptly discarded in a sharps container as a single unit. A syringe safety needle, however, may be removed and discarded separately so the syringe can be attached to a syringe transfer device and tubes filled at this point. A transfer device is similar to an ETS holder but has a permanently attached needle inside. After the device is attached to the syringe, an ETS tube is placed inside it and advanced onto the needle until blood flows into the tube. Additional tubes can be filled as long as there is enough blood left in the syringe. When the transfer is complete, the syringe and transfer device unit is discarded in a sharps container.

Step 15: Label Tubes

Tubes must be labeled immediately after blood collection, never before, and the label must be permanently attached to the tube before leaving an inpatient's bedside or dismissing an outpatient.

If using a preprinted computer or bar code label, you will need to write the date, time, your initials, and other pertinent information on the label immediately before or after attaching it to the tube. If you do not have a preprinted label, you will have to hand print the required information on the tube yourself. Any handwritten labeling must be done with a permanent ink pen. Labels should include the following information as a minimum:

- Patient's first and last names
- Patient's identification number (if applicable) or date of birth
- Date and time of collection
- Phlebotomist's initials
- Pertinent additional information such as "fasting"

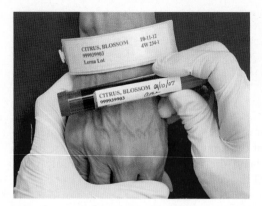

FIGURE 8-16

Phlebotomist comparing labeled tube with patient's ID band.

Before leaving an inpatient, compare the information on each labeled tube with the patient's ID band (Fig. 8-16) and the requisition. Both inpatient and outpatient tubes must be placed in a biohazard bag or other suitable container for transport to the laboratory.

Step 16: Observe Special Handling Instructions

Follow special specimen handling requirements, if applicable. Place specimens that to need to be cooled (e.g., ammonia) in crushed ice slurry. Put specimens that must be kept at body temperature (e.g., cold agglutinin) in a 37°C heat block or other suitable warming device. Wrap specimens that require protection from light (e.g., bilirubin) in aluminum foil or other light-blocking material or place them in a light-blocking container.

Step 17: Check Patient's Arm and Apply Bandage

Examine the venipuncture site to determine if bleeding has stopped. (Bleeding can continue from the vein even though it has stopped at the surface of the skin). If you are certain it has stopped, apply an adhesive bandage (or tape and folded gauze square) over the site. If the patient is allergic to adhesive bandages, apply paper tape over a clean folded gauze square. If the patient has sensitive skin or is allergic to adhesives, place a folded gauze square over the site and wrap gauze around it and fasten the gauze with paper tape, or wrap the site with self-adhering gauzelike material such as Coban. Instruct the patient to leave the bandage on for a minimum of 15 minutes, after which it should be removed to avoid irritation. Instruct an outpatient not to carry a purse or other heavy object or lift heavy objects with that arm for a minimum of 1 hour.

> **caution** If bleeding has not stopped, the phlebotomist must apply pressure until it does. If the patient continues to bleed beyond 5 minutes, the appropriate personnel such as the patient's physician or nurse should be notified.

Step 18: Dispose of Contaminated Materials

Dispose of contaminated materials in the proper biohazard containers or according to facility protocol and other materials such as needle caps and wrappers in the trash receptacle. Make sure that you have your tourniquet and that other equipment is returned to the proper place.

Step 19: Thank Patient, Remove Gloves, and Sanitize Hands

Thank the patient for his or her cooperation. This is courteous and lets the patient know that the procedure is complete. Remove gloves aseptically as described in Chapter 3, discard them in the manner required by your institution, and sanitize your hands before leaving the area.

Step 20: Transport Specimen to the Lab

Transport specimens to the laboratory or designated pickup site in a timely fashion. Prompt delivery to the laboratory protects specimen integrity and is typically achieved by personal delivery, transportation through a pneumatic tube system, or arranged pickup by a courier service. The phlebotomist is typically responsible for verifying and documenting collection by computer entry or manual entry in a logbook.

ROUTINE ETS VENIPUNCTURE

Most venipunctures are routine and can be performed on antecubital veins using an ETS system. This system is preferred because it is direct, efficient, relatively safe for the patient and the blood drawer, and allows multiple tubes to be easily collected. Routine ETS venipuncture is illustrated in Procedure 8-2.

PROCEDURE 8-2

Routine ETS Venipuncture

Purpose: To obtain a blood specimen for patient diagnostic or monitoring purposes from an antecubital vein using the evacuated tube system (ETS)

Equipment: Tourniquet; gloves; antiseptic prep pad; ETS needle*, tube holder* and tubes; gauze pads; sharps container; permanent ink pen; bandage

*Either the needle or tube holder must have a safety feature to prevent needlesticks.

Step	Explanation/Rationale
1. Review and accession test request	A test request is reviewed for completeness, date and time of collection, status, and priority. The accession process records the request and assigns it a unique number used to identify the specimen and related processes and paperwork

(Continued)

Step	Explanation/Rationale
2. Approach, identify, and prepare patient 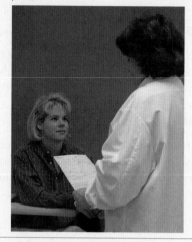	The right approach for a successful patient encounter includes a professional bedside manner, being organized and efficient, and looking for signs that convey important inpatient information or infection control precautions. Correct ID is vital to patient safety and meaningful test results. Name and DOB must be verified and matched to the test order and inpatient's ID band. Preparing the patient by explaining procedures and addressing inquiries helps reduce patient anxiety.
3. Verify diet restrictions and latex sensitivity 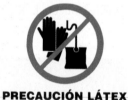 **LATEX PRECAUTIONS** **PRECAUCIÓN LÁTEX**	Test results can be meaningless or misinterpreted and patient care compromised if diet requirements have not been met. In such cases, consult the physician or nurse before proceeding. Exposure to latex can trigger a life-threatening reaction in those allergic to it, so it is vital that no latex items be used on a latex sensitive patient or even brought into the room
4. Sanitize hands 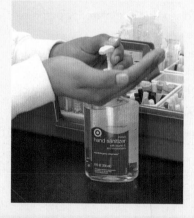	Proper hand hygiene plays a major role in infection control by protecting the phlebotomist, patient, and others from contamination. Gloves are sometimes put on at this point. Follow facility protocol

Step	Explanation/Rationale
5. Position patient, apply tourniquet, and ask patient to make a fist 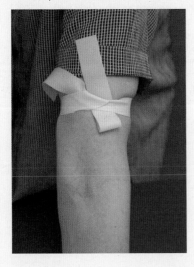	Proper positioning is important to patient comfort and venipuncture success. Place the patient's arm downward in a straight line from shoulder to wrist to aid in vein selection and avoid reflux as tubes are filled. A tourniquet placed 3-4 inches above the antecubital area enlarges veins and makes them easier to see, feel, and enter with a needle A clenched fist makes the veins easier to see and feel and helps keep them from rolling
6. Select vein, release tourniquet, ask patient to open fist 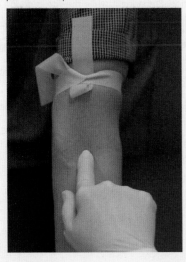	Select a large, well-anchored vein. The median cubital is the first choice, followed by the cephalic. The basilic should not be chosen unless no other vein is more prominent in either arm. Releasing the tourniquet and opening the fist helps prevent hemoconcentration

(Continued)

PROCEDURE 8-2 *(Continued)*

Step	Explanation/Rationale
7. Clean and air-dry site 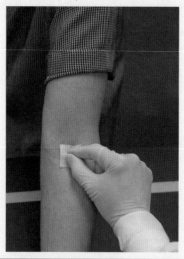	Cleaning the site with an antiseptic such as 70% isopropyl alcohol helps avoid contaminating the specimen or patient with skin surface bacteria picked up by the needle during venipuncture. Letting the site dry naturally permits maximum antiseptic action, prevents contamination caused by wiping, and avoids stinging on needle entry and specimen hemolysis from residual alcohol.
8. Prepare equipment and put on gloves 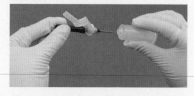	Selecting appropriate equipment for the size, condition, and location of the vein, is easier after vein selection. Preparing it while the site is drying saves time. Attach a needle to an ETS holder. Put the first tube in the holder now (See step 10) or wait until after needle entry. According to the OSHA BBP Standard, gloves must be worn during phlebotomy procedures
9. Reapply tourniquet, uncap and inspect needle 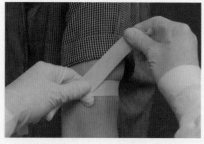	The tourniquet aids needle entry. Pick up the tube holder with your dominant hand, placing your thumb on top near the needle end, and fingers underneath. Uncap and inspect the needle for defects, and discard it if flawed

Step	Explanation/Rationale
10. Ask patient to remake a fist, anchor vein, and insert needle 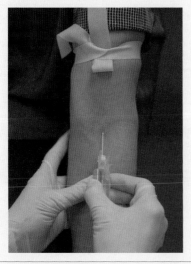	The fist aids needle entry. Anchoring stretches the skin so the needle enters easily and with less pain, and keeps the vein from rolling. Anchor by grasping the arm just below the elbow, supporting the back of it with your fingers. Place your thumb 1 to 2 inches below and slightly beside the vein, and pull the skin toward the wrist. Warn the patient. Line the needle up with the vein and insert it into the skin using a smooth forward motion. Stop when you feel a decrease in resistance, often described as a "pop," and press your fingers into the arm to anchor the holder
11. Establish blood flow, release tourniquet, ask patient to open fist 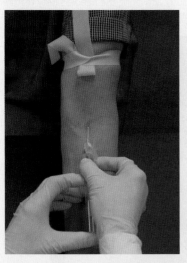 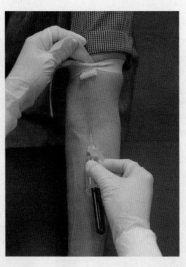	Blood will not flow until the needle pierces the tube stopper. Place a tube in the holder and push it part way onto the needle with a clockwise twist. Grasp the holder flanges with your middle and index fingers, pulling back slightly to keep the holder from moving, and push the tube onto the needle with your thumb.

(Continued)

PROCEDURE 8-2 *(Continued)*

Step	Explanation/Rationale
	Releasing the tourniquet and opening the fist allows blood flow to normalize (See step 6). According to CLSI standards, the tourniquet should be released as soon as possible after blood begins to flow, and should not be left on longer than 1 minute
12. Fill, remove, and mix tubes in order of draw 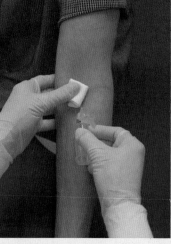	Fill additive tubes until the vacuum is exhausted to ensure correct blood to additive ratio, and mix them immediately upon removal from the holder using 3 to 8 gentle inversions (depending on type and manufacturer) to prevent clot formation. Follow CLSI Order of Draw to prevent additive carryover between tubes
13. Place gauze, remove needle, activate safety feature and apply pressure	A clean folded gauze square is placed over the site so pressure can be applied immediately after needle removal. Remove the needle in one smooth motion without lifting up or pressing down on it. Immediately apply pressure to the site with your free hand while simultaneously activating the needle safety feature with the other to prevent the chance of a needlestick

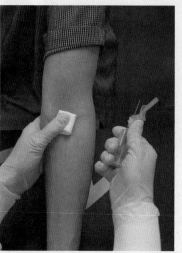

Step	Explanation/Rationale

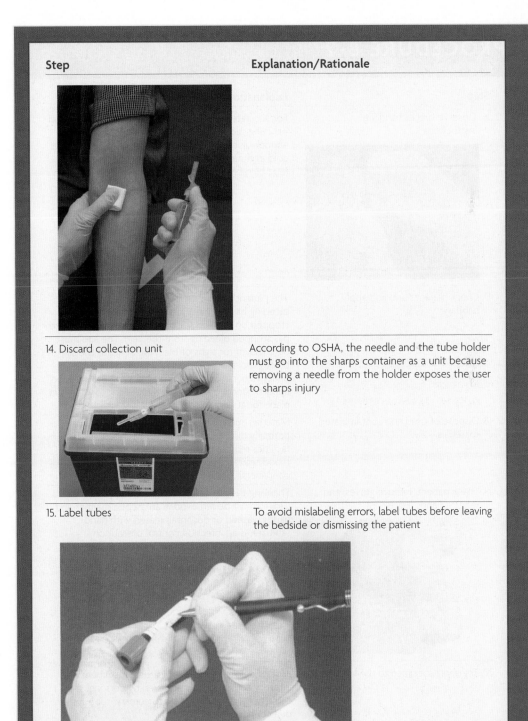

14. Discard collection unit

According to OSHA, the needle and the tube holder must go into the sharps container as a unit because removing a needle from the holder exposes the user to sharps injury

15. Label tubes

To avoid mislabeling errors, label tubes before leaving the bedside or dismissing the patient

(Continued)

PROCEDURE 8-2 *(Continued)*

Step	Explanation/Rationale
16. Observe special handling instructions 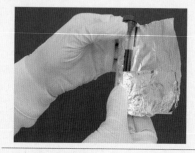	For accurate results, some specimens require special handling such as cooling in crushed ice (e.g., ammonia), transportation at body temperature (e.g., cold agglutinin), or protection from light (e.g., bilirubin)
17. Check patient's arm and apply bandage	The patient's arm must be examined to verify that bleeding has stopped. Just because bleeding has stopped on the skin surface does not mean the site has stopped bleeding from the vein. The site must be checked for signs of bleeding beneath the skin. If bleeding persists beyond 5 minutes, notify the patient's nurse or physician. If bleeding has stopped, apply a bandage and advise the patient to keep it in place for at least 15 minutes
18. Dispose of used and contaminated materials	Materials such as needle caps and wrappers are normally discarded in the regular trash. Some facilities require that contaminated items such as blood soaked gauze be discarded in biohazard containers
19. Thank patient, remove gloves, and sanitize hands (Fig. 8-18S) 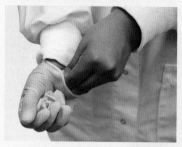	Thanking the patient is courteous and professional. Gloves must be removed in an aseptic manner and hands washed or decontaminated with hand sanitizer as an infection control precaution
20. Transport specimen to the lab	Prompt delivery to the lab protects specimen integrity and is typically achieved by personal delivery, transportation via a pneumatic tube system, or a courier service

BUTTERFLY PROCEDURE

A phlebotomist may elect to use a winged infusion set (butterfly) when attempting to draw blood from antecubital veins of infants and small children or from difficult adult veins, such as small antecubital veins or wrist and hand veins. A butterfly needle (i.e., 23 gauge) is appropriate in these situations because it is less likely to collapse or "blow" (rupture) the vein. A butterfly can be used with an ETS tube holder or a syringe (see Syringe Venipuncture Procedure). Small-volume tubes should be chosen when a butterfly is used with an ETS holder because the vacuum of large tubes may collapse the vein or hemolyze the specimen. Venipuncture of a hand vein using a butterfly and ETS holder is illustrated in Procedure 8-3.

PROCEDURE 8-3

Venipuncture of a Hand Vein Using a Butterfly and ETS Holder

Purpose: To obtain a blood specimen for patient diagnostic or monitoring purposes from a hand vein using a butterfly and ETS holder

Equipment: Tourniquet; gloves; antiseptic prep pad; butterfly needle with safety feature; ETS tube holder and tubes; gauze pads; sharps container; permanent ink pen; bandage

Step	Explanation/Rationale
1–4. (Same as routine ETS venipuncture)	See Procedure 8-2: steps 1 through 4
5. Position hand, apply tourniquet, ask patient to close the hand	Proper arm position is important to the comfort of the patient and the success of venipuncture. Support the hand on the bed or armrest. Have the patient bend the fingers slightly or make a fist. A tourniquet is necessary to increase venous filling and aid in vein selection. Apply it proximal to the wrist bone A closed hand or clenched fist sometimes makes the veins easier to see and feel
6. Select vein, release tourniquet, relax hand	Select a vein that has bounce or resilience and can be easily anchored. Wiping the hand with alcohol sometimes makes the veins more visible. Finding a suitable vein can take a while. Releasing the tourniquet and opening the fist allows blood flow to return to normal and minimizes effects of hemoconcentration
7. Clean and air-dry site	Same as routine ETS venipuncture (See Procedure 8-2: step 7)
8. Prepare equipment and put on gloves	It is easier to select appropriate equipment after the vein has been chosen. Preparing it while the site is drying saves time.

(Continued)

PROCEDURE 8-3   *(Continued)*

Step	Explanation/Rationale
	Attach the butterfly to an ETS holder. Grasp the tubing near the needle end and run your fingers down its length, stretching it slightly to help keep it from coiling back up. Position the first tube in the holder now or wait until after needle entry. According to the OSHA BBP Standard, gloves must be worn during phlebotomy procedures
9. Reapply tourniquet, uncap and inspect needle	The tourniquet aids needle entry. Hold the wing portion of the butterfly between your thumb and index finger or fold the wings upright and grasp them together. Cradle the tubing and holder in the palm of your dominant hand or lay it next to the patient's hand. Uncap and inspect the needle for defects, and discard it if flawed
10. Anchor vein, and insert needle	Anchoring stretches the skin so the needle enters easily and with less pain, and keeps the vein from rolling. To anchor, use your nondominant hand to hold the patient's hand just below the knuckles and pull the skin taut over the knuckles with your thumb while bending the patient's fingers. Another way is to have the patient make a tight fist, encircle the fist with your fingers, and use your thumb to pull the skin over the knuckles. Insert the needle into the vein at a shallow angle between 10 and 15°. A "flash" or small amount of blood will appear in the tubing when the needle is in the vein. "Seat" the needle by slightly threading it within the lumen of the vein to keep it from twisting back out of the vein if you let go of it
11. Establish blood flow and release tourniquet	The flash of blood in the tubing indicates vein entry. Blood will not flow until the needle pierces a tube stopper. Place a tube in the holder and push it part way onto the needle with a clockwise twist. Grasp the holder flanges with your middle and index fingers, pulling back slightly to keep the holder from moving, and push the tube onto the needle with your thumb. Releasing the tourniquet allows blood flow to normalize (See step 6)

Step	Explanation/Rationale
12. Fill, remove and mix tubes in order of draw	Maintain tubing and holder below the site and positioned so that the tubes fill from the bottom up to prevent reflux. Fill additive tubes until the vacuum is exhausted to ensure the correct blood- to-additive ratio, and mix them immediately upon removal from the holder using 3 to 8 gentle inversions (depending on type and manufacturer) to prevent clot formation. Follow CLSI Order of Draw to prevent additive carryover between tubes. If a coagulation tube is the first or only tube collected, draw a discard tube first to remove air in the tubing and assure proper filling of the coagulation tube
13. Place gauze, remove needle, activate safety device, and apply pressure	A clean folded gauze square is placed over the site so pressure can be applied immediately after needle removal. Remove the needle in one smooth motion without lifting up or pressing down on it. Immediately apply pressure to the site with your free hand, while simultaneously activating the needle safety device with the other to prevent the chance of a needlestick
14. Discard collection unit	According to OSHA, the needle and tube holder must go into the sharps container as a unit because removing a needle from the holder exposes the user to sharps injury
15–20. (Same as routine ETS venipuncture)	See Procedure 8-2: steps 15 through 20

SYRINGE VENIPUNCTURE PROCEDURE

The preferred method of obtaining venipuncture specimens is the evacuated tube method. In fact, according to CLSI Standard H3-A5, blood collection with a needle and syringe should be avoided for safety reasons. Even so, a needle or butterfly and syringe are sometimes used when the patient has extremely small, fragile, or weak veins. The vacuum pressure of an evacuated tube may be too great for such veins and cause them to collapse easily. This is often the case with elderly patients and newborn infants. When a syringe is used, the amount of pressure can be reduced somewhat over that of a tube by pulling the plunger back slowly. If the syringe fills too slowly, however, there is the possibility that the specimen will begin to clot either before enough blood is collected or before it can be transferred to the appropriate tubes. A special syringe transfer device is required to safely transfer blood from the syringe into the ETS tubes. Venipuncture with a needle and syringe is illustrated in Procedure 8-4. Steps to follow when using a transfer device to fill tubes with blood from a syringe are shown in Procedure 8–5.

PROCEDURE 8-4

Needle and Syringe Venipuncture

Purpose: To obtain a blood specimen for patient diagnostic or monitoring purposes from an antecubital vein using a needle and syringe

Equipment: Tourniquet; gloves; antiseptic prep pad; syringe needle*; syringe*, ETS tubes; gauze pads; sharps container; permanent ink pen; bandage

*Either the needle or tube holder must have a safety feature to prevent needlesticks.

Step	Rationale/Explanation
1–7. (Same as routine ETS venipuncture)	See Procedure 8-2: steps 1 through 7
8. Prepare equipment and put on gloves	It is easier to select appropriate equipment after the vein has been chosen. Preparing it while the site is drying saves time. Select the syringe needle according to the size and location of the vein, and select the syringe and tube size according to the volume of blood required for the tests. Attach the needle to the syringe but do not remove the cap at this time. Hold the syringe as you would an ETS tube holder. According to the OSHA BBP Standard, gloves must be worn during phlebotomy procedures

Step	Explanation/Rationale
9. Reapply tourniquet, uncap and inspect needle	The tourniquet aids in venipuncture. Hold the syringe in your dominant hand as you would an ETS holder. Place your thumb on top near the needle end, and fingers underneath. Uncap and inspect the needle for defects and discard it if flawed. Although it is rare, a needle can have defects. Discard one that is flawed
10. Ask patient to make a fist, anchor vein, and insert needle 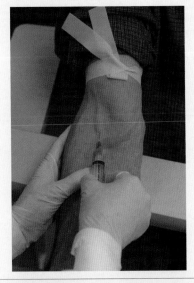	The fist aids needle entry. Anchoring stretches the skin so the needle enters easily and with less pain and keeps the vein from rolling. Anchor by grasping the arm just below the elbow, supporting the back of it with your fingers. Place your thumb 1 to 2 inches below and slightly beside the vein and pull the skin toward the wrist. Warn the patient. Line the needle up with the vein and insert it into the skin using a smooth forward motion. Stop when you feel a decrease in resistance, often described as a "pop," and press your fingers into the arm to anchor the holder
11. Establish blood flow, release tourniquet, ask patient to open fist 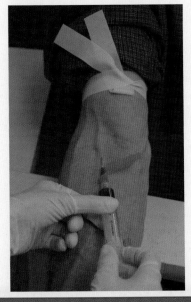	Establishment of blood flow is normally indicated by blood in the hub of the syringe. In some cases blood will not flow until the syringe plunger is pulled back. Releasing the tourniquet and opening the fist allows blood flow to return to normal and helps prevent hemoconcentration. According to CLSI Standard H3-A5, the tourniquet should be released as soon as possible after blood begins to flow and should not be left on longer than 1 minute

(Continued)

Step	Explanation/Rationale
12. Fill syringe	Venous blood will not automatically flow into a syringe. It must be filled by slowly pulling back on the plunger with your free hand. Steady the syringe as you would an ETS holder during routine venipuncture
13. Place gauze, withdraw needle, activate safety device, apply pressure 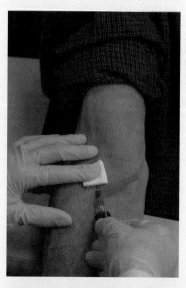 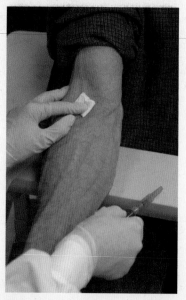	A clean, folded gauze square is placed over the site so pressure can be applied immediately after needle removal. Remove the needle without lifting up or pressing down on it. Immediately apply pressure to the site with your free hand and simultaneously activate the needle safety device with the other

Step	Explanation/Rationale
14. Discard needle, fill tubes, discard syringe and transfer device 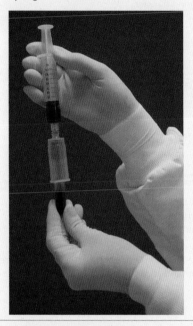	The needle must be removed and discarded in the sharps container so that a transfer device for filling the tubes can be attached to the syringe. A transfer device greatly reduces the chance of accidental needlesticks and confines any aerosol or spraying that may be generated as the tube is removed. An ETS tube is placed in the transfer device in the order of draw and pushed onto the internal needle until the stopper is pierced. Blood from the syringe is then safely drawn into the tube. Several tubes can be filled as long as there is enough blood in the syringe. After use, the syringe and transfer device unit is discarded in the sharps container
15–20. (Same as routine ETS venipuncture)	See Procedure 8-2, steps 15 through 20

PROCEDURE 8-5

Using A Syringe Transfer Device

Purpose: To safely transfer blood from a syringe into ETS tubes

Equipment: Syringe transfer device

Step	Explanation/Rationale
1. Remove the needle from the syringe and discard it in a sharps container	The needle must be removed to attach the transfer device

(Continued)

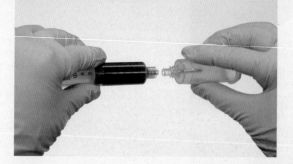

PROCEDURE 8-5   *(Continued)*

Step	Explanation/Rationale
2. Attach the syringe hub to the transfer device hub, rotating it to ensure secure attachment	Secure attachment is necessary to prevent blood leakage during transfer

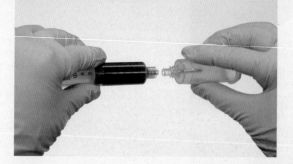

Step	Explanation/Rationale
3. Hold the syringe vertically with the tip down and the transfer device at the bottom	Ensures vertical placement of tubes to prevent additive carryover
4. Place an ETS tube in the barrel of the transfer device and push it all the way to the end	The device has an internal needle that will puncture the stopper and allow blood to flow into the tube

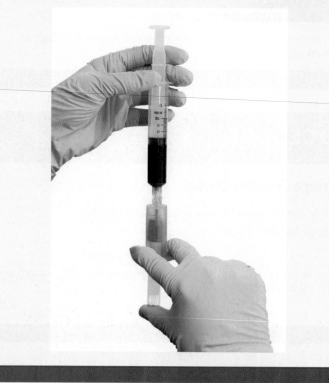

Step	Explanation/Rationale
5. Follow the order of draw if multiple tubes are filled	The order of draw is designed to prevent additive carryover between tubes
6. Keep the tubes and transfer device vertical	Ensures that tubes fill from bottom to top, preventing additive contact with the needle and cross contamination of subsequent tubes
7. Let tubes fill using the vacuum draw of the tube. Do not push on the syringe plunger	Forcing blood into a tube by pushing the plunger can hemolyze the specimen or cause the tube stopper to pop off, splashing tube contents

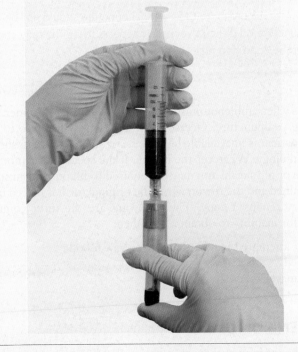

Step	Explanation/Rationale
8. If you must underfill a tube, hold back the plunger to stop blood flow before removing it	Tubes quickly fill until the vacuum is gone. Holding back the plunger stops the tube from filling
9. Mix additive tubes as soon as they are removed	Additive tubes must be mixed immediately for proper function, including preventing clot formation in anticoagulant tubes
10. When finished, discard the syringe and transfer device unit in a sharps container	Removing the transfer device from the syringe would expose the user to blood in the hubs of both units. The transfer device must go into the sharps container because of the internal needle

Procedure for Inability to Collect Specimen

If you are unable to obtain a specimen on the first try, evaluate the problem and try again below the first site, on the opposite arm, or on a hand or wrist vein. If the patient's veins are small or fragile, it may be necessary to use a butterfly or syringe on the second attempt.

If the second attempt is unsuccessful, ask another phlebotomist to take over. Unsuccessful venipuncture attempts are frustrating to the patient and the phlebotomist. Should the second phlebotomist be unsuccessful after two attempts, it is a good idea to give the patient a rest if the request is not stat or timed and try again at a later time.

> **caution** According to CLSI, arterial puncture should not be used as an alternative to venipuncture on difficult veins. If it appears to be the only choice, the patient's physician should be consulted first.

There are times when a phlebotomist is not able to collect a specimen from a patient even before attempting venipuncture. Occasionally, a patient will refuse to have blood drawn. Other times, the patient is unavailable because he or she has gone to surgery or for another test, such as in radiology. Whatever the reason, if the specimen cannot be obtained, notify the patient's nurse or physician. You may be required to fill out a form stating that the specimen was not obtained and the reason why. The original form is placed in the patient's chart and the laboratory retains a copy. The following are the most common and generally accepted reasons for inability to obtain a specimen:

- Phlebotomist attempted but was unable to draw blood
- Patient refused
- Patient was unavailable

PEDIATRIC VENIPUNCTURE

Collecting blood by venipuncture from infants and children may be necessary for tests that require large amounts of blood (i.e., cross-matching and blood cultures) and tests that cannot normally be performed by skin puncture (i.e., ammonia levels, and most coagulation studies). Venipuncture in children under the age of two should be limited to superficial veins and not deep, hard-to-find veins. Normally, the most accessible veins of infants and toddlers are the veins of the antecubital fossa and forearm. Other potential venipuncture sites include the medial wrist, the dorsum of the foot, the scalp, and the medial ankle. Venipuncture of these sites, however, requires special training and the permission of the patient's physician.

Challenges

Capillary collection is normally recommended for pediatric patients, especially newborns and infants up to 12 months, because their veins are small and not well developed, and there is a considerable risk of permanent damage. There are, however, times when capillary collection is not feasible or possible due to type or volume requirements of tests ordered, and a venipuncture is necessary. Performing venipuncture on pediatric patients presents special challenges and requires the expertise and skill of an experienced phlebotomist. In addition, every attempt should be made to collect the minimum amount of blood required for testing, because infants and young children have much smaller blood volumes than older children and adults. Removal of large quantities of blood at once or even small quantities on a regular basis, as is often the case when an infant or child is in intensive care, can lead to anemia. Removing more than 10% of an infant's blood volume at one time can lead to shock and cardiac arrest. Consequently, most facilities have limits on the amount of blood that can be removed per draw and for various time periods from 24 hours up to a month. For example, many facilities do not allow more than 3% of a child's blood volume to be collected at any one time and allow no more than 10% in an entire month.

fyi   CLSI recommends that procedures be in place to monitor amounts of blood drawn from pediatric, geriatric, and other vulnerable patients to avoid phlebotomy-induced anemia.

No one would intentionally put a patient's life at risk by drawing too much blood. However, a phlebotomist who fails to keep track of amounts of blood collected or who is unable to judge how much blood can be collected safely could do just that. Consequently, for safe practice, a competent phlebotomist should be able to calculate blood volume. The formula for calculating blood volume is shown in Appendix D.

Dealing with Parents or Guardians

If parents or guardians are present, it is important for the phlebotomist to earn their trust before attempting the procedure. A phlebotomist who behaves in a warm and friendly manner and displays a calm, confident, and caring attitude will more easily earn that trust and limit his or her own anxiety as well. Parents or guardians may give the best prediction of how cooperative the child will be. Ask them about the child's past experiences with blood collection to gain insight into how the child may behave and approaches that might work. Give them the option of staying in the room during the procedure or waiting outside until you are finished. Their presence and involvement should be encouraged, however, as studies show that it reduces a child's anxiety and has a positive effect on the child's behavior.

Dealing with the Child

With older children, it is important to gain their trust as with adults. However, children typically have a wider zone of comfort, which means that you cannot get as close to them as an adult without them feeling threatened. Approach them slowly and determine their degree of anxiety or fear before handling equipment or touching their arms to look for a vein. An adult towering over a child is intimidating. Physically lower yourself to the patient's level. Explain what you are going to do in terms the child can understand and answer questions honestly.

key · point *Never* tell a child that it won't hurt. Instead say it may hurt just a little bit, but it will be over quickly.

Help the child to understand the importance of remaining still. Give the child a job to do such as holding the gauze or adhesive bandage. Offer the child a reward for being brave. However, *do not* put conditions on receiving the reward, such as "you can have sticker if you don't cry." Some crying is to be anticipated, and it is important to let the child know that it is all right to cry.

key · point Calm a crying child as soon as possible, because the stress of crying and struggling can alter blood components and lead to erroneous test results.

Pain Interventions

Interventions to ease pain include the use of a **eutectic** (easily melted) **mixture of local anesthetic (EMLA)** for newborns through adults and oral sucrose and pacifiers for infants and toddlers.

EMLA is a topical anesthetic containing lidocaine and prilocaine that can be applied to intact skin by a nurse or physician. It is available in a cream that must be covered with a clear dressing after application or a patch. It takes approximately 1 hour (a major drawback to its use) for it to anesthetize the area to a depth of approximately 5 mm. It cannot be used on patients who are allergic to local anesthetics.

Use of a 12 to 24% solution of oral sucrose has been shown to reduce the pain of procedures such as heel puncture and venipuncture in infants up to 6 months of age. A 24% solution of sucrose (prepared by mixing 4 teaspoons of water with 1 teaspoon of sugar) can be administered by dropper, nipple, oral syringe, or on a pacifier, provided it will not interfere with the tests to be collected. Sucrose nipples or pacifiers are available commercially. The sucrose must be given to the infant 2 minutes before the procedure, and its pain relieving-benefits last for approximately 5 minutes. Studies have shown that infants given sucrose or even a regular pacifier by itself cry for a shorter time and are more alert and less fussy after the procedure.

Selecting a Method of Restraint

Immobilization of the patient is a critical aspect in obtaining an adequate specimen from infants and children while ensuring their safety. A newborn or young infant can be wrapped in a blanket but physical restraint is often required for older infants, toddlers, and younger children. Older children may be able to sit by themselves in the blood drawing chair, but a parent or another phlebotomist should help steady the arm.

Toddlers are most easily restrained by having them sit upright on a parent's lap (Fig. 8–17). The arm to be used for venipuncture is extended to the front and downward. The

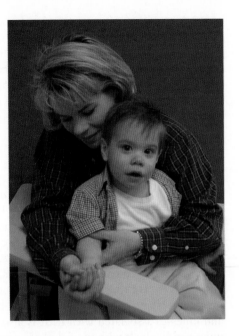

FIGURE 8-17
Seated adult restraining a toddler.

parent places an arm around the toddler and over the arm that is not being used. The other arm supports the venipuncture arm from behind, at the bend of the elbow. This helps steady the child's arm and prevents the child from twisting the arm during the draw.

If the child is lying down, the parent or another phlebotomist typically leans over the child from the opposite side of the bed. One arm reaches around and holds the venipuncture arm from behind, the other reaches across the child's body, holding the child's other arm secure against his or her torso.

Equipment Selection

Venipuncture of an antecubital vein is most easily accomplished using a 23-gauge butterfly needle attached to an evacuated tube holder or syringe. The tubing of the butterfly allows flexibility if the child struggles or twists during the draw. Using the evacuated tube method of collection is preferred because it minimizes chances of clotted specimens and inadequately filled tubes. However, the smallest tubes available should be used to reduce the risk of creating too much vacuum draw on the vein and causing it to collapse. In difficult draw situations a small amount of blood can be drawn into a syringe and the blood placed in microcollection tubes (capillary tubes or bullets) rather than ETS tubes.

c a u t i o n   Laboratory personnel will assume blood in capillary tubes is capillary blood. If venous blood is placed in a capillary tube it is important to label the specimen as venous blood because reference ranges for some tests differ depending on the source of the specimen.

Procedures

Regardless of the collection method, every attempt should be made to collect the minimum amount of blood required for testing because of the small blood volume of the patient. Follow proper identification requirements outlined earlier in the chapter. You may be required to wear a mask, gown, and gloves in the newborn nursery or neonatal ICU.

GERIATRIC VENIPUNCTURE

According to the National Institute on Aging (NIA), life expectancy has doubled over the last century and there are now over 35 million Americans age 65 or older. This segment of the population is expected to grow by 137 % over the next 50 years and become the major focus in healthcare. Already a major portion of laboratory testing is performed on the elderly. (See Table 8-2 for a list of tests commonly ordered on geriatric patients.)

Although aging is a normal process, it involves physical, psychological, and social changes leading to conditions, behaviors, and habits that may seem unusual to those unaccustomed to working with elderly patients. To feel comfortable working with them one must understand the aging process and be familiar with the physical limitations, diseases, and illnesses associated with it. It is also important to remember that elderly patients are unique individuals with special needs who deserve to be treated with compassion, kindness, patience, and respect.

Challenges

Physical effects of aging, such as skin changes and hearing and vision problems; mobility issues often related to arthritis and osteoporosis; diseases such as diabetes; and mental and emotional conditions, present challenges not only to the patient, but to a phlebotomist's technical expertise and interpersonal skills as well.

TABLE 8-2 Tests Commonly Ordered on Geriatric Patients	
Test	**Typical Indications for Ordering**
ANA, RA, or RF	Diagnose lupus and rheumatoid arthritis, which can affect nervous system function
CBC	Determine hemoglobin levels, detect infection, and identify blood disorders
BUN/creatinine	Diagnose kidney function disorders that may be responsible for problems such as confusion, coma, seizures, and tremors
Calcium/magnesium	Identify abnormal levels associated with seizures and muscle problems
Electrolytes	Determine sodium & potassium levels, critical to proper nervous system function
ESR	Detect inflammation; identify collagen vascular diseases
Glucose	Detect and monitor diabetes; abnormal levels can cause confusion, seizures, or coma or lead to peripheral neuropathy
PT/PTT	Monitor blood-thinning medications; important in heart conditions, coagulation problems, and stroke management
SPEP, IPEP	Identify protein or immune globulin disorders that lead to nerve damage
VDRL/FTA	Diagnose or rule out syphilis, which can cause nerve damage and dementia

SKIN CHANGES

Skin changes include loss of collagen and subcutaneous fat, resulting in wrinkled, sagging, thin skin with a decreased ability to stay adequately hydrated. Lack of hydration along with impaired peripheral circulation caused by age-related narrowing of blood vessels make it harder to obtain adequate blood flow, especially during skin puncture. In addition, aging skin cells are replaced more slowly, causing the skin to lose elasticity and increasing the likelihood of injury. Blood vessels also lose elasticity, becoming more fragile and more likely to collapse, resulting in an increased chance of bruising and failure to obtain blood, respectively.

key • point   Skin changes make veins in the elderly easier to see; however, sagging skin combined with loss of muscle tone may make it harder to anchor veins and keep them from rolling.

HEARING IMPAIRMENT

Effects of aging include loss of auditory hair cells resulting in a hearing loss in upper frequencies and trouble distinguishing sounds such as ch, s, sh, and z. Hearing-impaired patients may strain to hear and have difficulty answering questions and understanding instructions. If you know or have reason to suspect that a patient has a hearing impairment, move closer and face the patient when you speak. Speak clearly and distinctly, but use your normal tone of voice. Never shout; shouting raises the pitch of your voice and makes it harder to understand. Allow the patient enough time to answer questions and confirm patient responses to avoid misunderstanding. Repeat information if necessary. Watch for nonverbal verification that the patient understands. Be mindful of nonverbal messages you may be inadvertently sending. Use pencil and paper to communicate if necessary. A relative or attendant often accompanies a patient with a hearing or other communication problem. If this person is included in the conversation, do not speak to him or her directly as if the patient were not present.

key • point   Although hearing loss is common in the elderly, never assume that an elderly person is hard of hearing.

VISUAL IMPAIRMENT

Effects of aging on the eyes include a diminished ability of the lens to adjust, causing farsightedness; clouding of the lens or cataract formation resulting in dim vision; and other changes that lead to light intolerance and poor night vision. The phlebotomy area should have adequate lighting without glare. Be aware that you may need to guide elderly patients to the drawing chair or escort them to the restroom if a urine specimen is requested. Provide written instructions in large print, avoid using gestures when speaking, and use a normal tone of voice.

key • point A common mistake and one that is irritating to the visually impaired is to raise your voice when speaking to them.

MENTAL IMPAIRMENT

Slower nerve conduction associated with aging leads to slower learning, slower reaction times, and a diminished perception of pain that leads to an increase in injuries. Reduced cerebral circulation can lead to loss of balance and frequent falls. The effects of some medications can make problems worse. Speak clearly and slowly and give the patient plenty of time to respond. You may need to repeat your statement or question more than once. Be especially careful in obtaining patient identification information and verifying compliance with diet instructions. If a relative or attendant is with the patient, verify information with him or her.

Alzheimer's disease and other forms of dementia can render a patient unable to communicate meaningfully, requiring you to communicate through a relative or other caregiver. Some Alzheimer's patients will act absolutely normal, and others will exhibit anger and hostility that should not be taken personally. Always approach patients in a calm, professional manner. Use short, simple statements and explain things slowly. You may require assistance to keep the patient's arm in place during the draw.

key • point Although mental confusion and dementia are common in elderly patients, always assume an elderly person is of sound mind unless you have information to the contrary.

EFFECTS OF DISEASE

Although most elderly persons are generally healthy, many are not. Some of the diseases that affect the elderly and the challenges they present to the patient and the phlebotomist include the following:

Arthritis　The two basic types of arthritis are osteoarthritis and rheumatoid arthritis. Osteoarthritis occurs with aging and also results from joint injury. The hips and knees are most commonly affected and can cause difficulty getting in and out of a blood-drawing chair. Rheumatoid arthritis affects connective tissue throughout the body and can occur at any age. Although it primarily affects the joints, connective tissue in the heart, lungs, eyes, kidneys, and skin may also be affected. Inflammation associated with both types of arthritis may leave joints swollen and painful and cause the patient to restrict movement. It may result in the patient being unable or unwilling to straighten an arm or open a hand. Use the other arm if it is unaffected. If that is not an option, let the patient decide what position is comfortable. A butterfly needle with 12-inch tubing helps provide the flexibility needed to access veins from awkward angles.

⚠ **c a u t i o n**   Never use force to extend a patient's arm or open a hand, as it can cause pain and injury.

Coagulation Problems   Patients who have coagulation disorders or who take blood-thinning medications as a result of heart problems or strokes are at risk of hematoma formation or uncontrolled bleeding at the blood collection site. Make certain adequate pressure is held over the site until bleeding is stopped. You must hold pressure if the patient is unable to do so. However, do not hold pressure so tightly that the patient is injured or bruised and do not apply a pressure bandage in lieu of holding pressure. If bleeding persists, notify the patient's physician or follow your facility's policy.

Diabetes   Many elderly patients have diabetes. Diabetes affects circulation and healing, particularly in the lower extremities, and generally makes venipuncture of leg, ankle, and foot veins off limits. Peripheral circulation problems and scarring from numerous skin punctures to check glucose can make skin puncture collections difficult. Warming the site before blood collection can help encourage blood flow.

Parkinson's Disease and Stroke   Stroke and Parkinson's disease can affect speech. The frustration it can cause both the patient and the phlebotomist can present a barrier to effective communication. Allow these patients time to speak and do not try to finish their sentences. Keep in mind that difficulty speaking does not imply problems in comprehension. Tremors and movement of the hands of Parkinson's patients can make blood collection difficult, and the patient may require help to hold still.

Pulmonary Function Problems   The effects of colds and influenza are more severe in the elderly. Age-related changes in pulmonary function reduce elasticity of airway tissues and decrease effectiveness of respiratory defense systems. Weakened chest muscles reduce the ability to clear secretions and increase the chance of developing pneumonia. If you have a cold, refrain from drawing blood from elderly patients if possible or wear a mask.

OTHER PROBLEMS

Disease and loss of immune function in the elderly increase the chance of infection. Lack of appetite due to disease or decreased sense of smell and taste can result in emaciation. Poor nutrition can intensify the affects of aging on the skin, affect clotting ability, and contribute to anemia.

Safety Issues

While all patients require an unencumbered traffic pattern, geriatric patients may need wider open areas to accommodate wheelchairs and walkers. Some patients tend to shuffle when they walk, so floors should have nonslip surfaces and be free of clutter. Dispose of equipment packaging properly and look out for items inadvertently dropped on the floor. Floor mats should stay snug against the floor so that they do not become a tripping hazard for any age patient and employees as well.

Patients in Wheelchairs

Many geriatric patients are wheelchair bound or are so weak they are transported to the laboratory in wheelchairs. Be careful moving wheelchair patients (Fig. 8-18) from the waiting room to the blood drawing room. Remember to lock wheels when drawing patients in wheelchairs, assisting them to and from the drawing chair, or after returning them to waiting areas. Never attempt to lift patients to transfer them from a wheelchair to a drawing chair. Attempting to do so can result in injury to the patient, the phlebotomist, or both.

> **key · point** It is generally safest and easiest to draw blood with the patient in the wheelchair, supporting the arm on a pillow or on a special padded board placed across the arms of the chair.

Blood Collection Procedures

Although the venipuncture steps are basically the same for all patients, extra care must be taken in the following areas when drawing elderly patients.

PATIENT IDENTIFICATION

Be extra careful identifying patients with mental or hearing impairments. Never rely on nods of agreement or other nonverbal responses. Verify patient information with a relative or attendant, if possible.

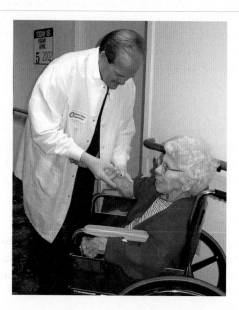

FIGURE 8-18
Elderly patient in a wheelchair.

EQUIPMENT SELECTION

It is often best to use butterfly needles and pediatric or short-draw tubes for venipuncture on the elderly. Although veins may appear prominent, they are apt to roll or collapse easily, making blood collection difficult. It is best to select equipment after you have selected the venipuncture site so you can choose the best equipment for the size, condition, and location of the vein. If the veins are extremely fragile, you may have to collect the specimen by syringe or finger puncture.

TOURNIQUET APPLICATION

Apply the tourniquet snugly, but loose enough to avoid damaging the patient's skin. A tourniquet that is too tight can cause the vein to collapse when it is released or the tube is engaged. It can also distend the vein so much that it "blows" or splits open on needle entry, resulting in hematoma formation. It is acceptable to apply the tourniquet over the patient's sleeve or a clean dry washcloth wrapped around the arm.

key • point   Geriatric patients in the 90s and 100s are seen more often lately, and their veins are very sensitive to tourniquet pressure.

SELECT THE VENIPUNCTURE SITE

Elderly patients, especially inpatients, often have bruising in the antecubital (AC) area from previous blood draws. Venipuncture in a bruised site should be avoided as it can be painful to the patient and the hemostatic process occurring in the area can lead to erroneous test results. If both AC areas are bruised, select a needle entry point below the bruising. Be aware that some elderly patients may not be able to make a fist because of muscle weakness.

If no suitable vein can be found, gently massage the arm from wrist to elbow to force blood into the area or wrap a warm, wet towel around the arm or hand for a few minutes to increase blood flow. Avoid heavy manipulation of the arm as it can cause bruising and affect test results. Have the patient hold the arm down at the side for a few minutes to let gravity help back up blood flow. When a suitable vein has been selected, release the tourniquet to allow blood flow to return to normal while you clean the site and ready your equipment.

CLEAN THE SITE

Clean the site in the same manner as routine venipuncture, being careful not to rub too vigorously as that may abrade or otherwise damage the skin. The site may need to be cleaned a second time on some elderly patients who are unable to bathe regularly.

PERFORM THE VENIPUNCTURE

Although actually quite fragile, an elderly patient's veins often feel tough and have a tendency to roll. Anchoring them firmly and entering quickly increases the chance of successful venipuncture. If the skin is loose and the vein is poorly fixed in the tissue, it sometimes helps to wrap your hand around the arm from behind and pull the skin taut from both sides rather than anchoring with your thumb. Because veins in the elderly tend to be close to the surface of the skin, a shallow angle of needle insertion may be required.

HOLD PRESSURE

As discussed earlier under Coagulation Problems, it may take longer for bleeding to stop in elderly patients, especially if they are on anticoagulant therapy. Bleeding must have stopped before the bandage is applied. If bleeding is excessively prolonged, the patient's nurse or physician must be notified and laboratory facility procedures followed.

DIALYSIS PATIENTS

Dialysis is a procedure in which patients whose kidneys do not function adequately have their blood artificially filtered to remove waste products. The most common reason for dialysis is end- stage renal disease (ESRD), a serious condition in which the kidneys have so deteriorated that they fail to function. The most common cause of ESRD is diabetes. The second most common cause is high blood pressure. Patients with ERSD require ongoing dialysis treatments or a kidney transplant.

In one type of dialysis called hemodialysis, the patient's blood is filtered through a special machine often referred to as an artificial kidney. Access for hemodialysis is commonly provided by permanently fusing an artery and vein in the forearm creating an arteriovenous (AV) shunt or fistula (see Chapter 9). During dialysis a special needle and tubing set is inserted into the fistula to provide blood flow to the dialysis machine. A typical AV fistula appears as a loop just under the skin in the forearm above the wrist and has a buzzing sensation called a "thrill" when palpated. The fistula arm must not be used to take blood pressures or perform venipuncture.

key • point   A phlebotomist must be able to recognize a fistula to avoid damaging the area as it is the dialysis patient's lifeline.

LONG-TERM-CARE PATIENTS

Long-term care includes a variety of healthcare and social services required by certain patients with functional disabilities who cannot care for themselves but do not require hospitalization. Although long-term care serves the needs of patients of all ages, primary recipients are the elderly. Long-term care is delivered in adult daycare facilities, nursing homes, assisted living facilities, rehabilitation facilities (Fig. 8-19), and even in private homes.

HOME CARE PATIENTS

Care for the sick at home plays an important role in today's healthcare delivery system. Many individuals who in the past would have been confined to a healthcare institution are now able to remain at home where numerous studies show they are happier and get better sooner or survive longer. Home care services are provided through numerous agencies and

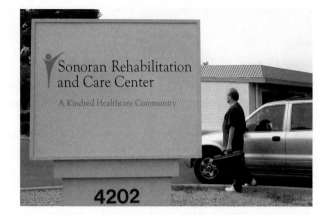

FIGURE 8-19

A phlebotomist making a visit to a rehabilitation center.

include professional nursing; home health aid; physical, occupational, and respiratory therapy; and laboratory services. Laboratory services are often provided by mobile phlebotomists who go to the patient's home to collect specimens and then deliver them to the laboratory for testing. A home care phlebotomist must have exceptional phlebotomy, interpersonal, and organizational skills; be able to function independently; and be comfortable working in varied situations and under unusual circumstances. Mobile phlebotomists must carry all necessary phlebotomy supplies including sharps containers and biohazard bags for disposal of contaminated items and containers for properly protecting specimens during transportation with them, typically in their own private vehicles (Fig. 8-20).

HOSPICE PATIENTS

Hospice is a type of care for patients who are terminally ill. Hospice care allows them to spend their last days in a peaceful, supportive atmosphere that emphasizes pain management to help keep them comfortable. Some individuals are uncomfortable with the subject of death or being around patients who are dying and react with indifference out of ignorance. Phlebotomists who deal with hospice patients must understand the situation and be able to approach them with care, kindness, and respect.

FIGURE 8-20

A traveling phlebotomist getting supplies from the back of his vehicle.

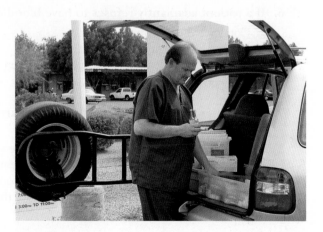

STUDY & REVIEW QUESTIONS

1. **NPO means**
   a. New patient orders
   b. Needed post operative
   c. Nothing by mouth
   d. Nutrition post operative

2. **Which of the following is required requisition information?**
   a. Ordering physician's name
   b. Patient's first and last name
   c. Type of test to be performed
   d. All of the above

3. **The following test orders for different patients have been received at the same time. Which test would you collect first?**
   a. Fasting glucose
   b. STAT glucose in the ER
   c. STAT hemoglobin in ICU
   d. ASAP CBC in ICU

4. **A member of the clergy is with the patient when you arrive to collect a routine specimen. What should you do?**
   a. Ask the patient's nurse what to do
   b. Come back later after the clergy member has gone
   c. Fill out a form saying you were unable to collect the specimen
   d. Say "Excuse me, I need to collect a specimen from this patient"

5. **You are asked to collect a specimen from an inpatient. The patient is not wearing an ID band. What do you do?**
   a. Ask the patient's name and collect the specimen if it matches the requisition
   b. Ask the patient's nurse to put an ID band on the patient before you draw the specimen
   c. Identify the patient by the name card on the door
   d. Refuse to draw the specimen and cancel the request

6. **If a patient adamantly refuses to have blood drawn, you should**
   a. Convince the patient to cooperate
   b. Notify the patient's nurse or physician
   c. Restrain the patient and collect the specimen
   d. Write a note to the physician

7. **An inpatient is eating breakfast when you arrive to collect a fasting glucose. What is the best thing to do?**
   a. Consult with the patient's nurse to see if the specimen should be collected
   b. Draw the specimen quickly before the patient finishes eating
   c. Draw the specimen and write "nonfasting" on the requisition
   d. Fill out form stating that you didn't collect the specimen because the patient wasn't fasting

8. **After cleaning the venipuncture site with alcohol, the phlebotomist should**

   a. Allow the alcohol to dry completely
   b. Fan the site to help the alcohol dry
   c. Dry the site with a regular gauze pad or cotton ball
   d. Insert the needle quickly before the alcohol has a chance to dry

9. **The tourniquet should be released**

   a. As soon as blood flow is established
   b. Before the needle is removed from the arm
   c. Within 1 minute of application
   d. All of the above

10. **Which statement is true of syringe venipuncture?**

    a. A syringe is sometimes used for veins that collapse easily
    b. A syringe is the recommended way to collect most blood specimens
    c. The best way to fill a syringe is to pull the plunger all the way back when you see the "flash"
    d. There is no way to tell when the needle is in the vein when using a syringe

11. **After inserting a butterfly needle, the phlebotomist needs to "seat" it, meaning**

    a. Have the patient make a tight fist to keep the needle in place
    b. Keep the skin taut during the entire procedure
    c. Push the needle up against the back wall of the vein
    d. Slightly thread the needle within the lumen of the vein

12. **Blood collection tubes are labeled**

    a. As soon as the test order is received
    b. Before the specimen is collected
    c. Immediately after specimen collection
    d. Whenever it is most convenient

13. **What is the best approach to use on an 8-year-old child who needs to have blood drawn?**

    a. Explain what you are going to do in simple terms and ask the child to cooperate
    b. Have someone restrain the child to avoid resistance and collect the specimen
    c. Offer the child a treat or toy, but only if he or she doesn't cry
    d. Tell the child that it won't hurt and that it will only take a few seconds

14. **Which type of patient is most likely to have an arteriovenous fistula or graft?**

    a. Arthritic   c. Hospice
    b. Dialysis   d. Wheelchair bound

15. **Which of the following is proper procedure when dealing with an elderly patient?**
    a. Address your questions to an attendant if the patient has a hearing problem
    b. Speak very loudly so that the patient can hear you
    c. Tie the tourniquet extra tightly to make the veins more prominent
    d. Make certain adequate pressure is held over the site until bleeding is stopped

CASE · STUDY · 8-1

Patient Identification

Jenny works with several other phlebotomists in a busy outpatient lab. This day has been particularly hectic, with many patients filling the waiting room. Jenny is working as fast as she can to draw patients. Toward the end of the day, after Jenny finishes drawing what seems like the millionth patient, she mentions how extra busy it has been to a coworker. The coworker says, "Yes it has, but it looks like there is only one patient left." Jenny grabs the paperwork and heads for the door of the waiting room. As her coworker has said, there is only one patient, an elderly woman, sitting there reading a book. The paperwork is for a patient named Jane Rogers. "You must be Jane," she says, glancing at the name on the paperwork. The patient looks up and smiles. "Have you been waiting long?" Jenny asks. The patient replies, "Not really," and Jenny escorts her to a drawing chair. The patient is a difficult draw, and Jenny makes two attempts to collect the specimen. The second one is successful. Jenny places the labels on the tubes, dates and initials them, bandages the patient, and sends her on her way. About 5 minutes later a somewhat younger woman appears at the reception window and says, "My name is Jane Rogers. I just stepped outside to make a phone call and was wondering if you called my name while I was gone." The receptionist notices that the patient's name is checked off the registration log. The receptionist turns around and asks if anyone had called a patient named Jane Rogers. "I already drew her," Jenny says as she walks over to the receptionist window. The woman at the window is not the one Jenny just drew; however, her information matches information on the requisition used to draw that patient.

QUESTIONS
1. What error did Jenny make in identifying the patient?
2. What assumptions did Jenny make that contributed to her drawing the wrong patient?
3. Who might the other patient that Jenny mistakenly drew have been?
4. How can the error be corrected?

CASE · STUDY · 8-2

Blood Draw Refusal

Two phlebotomists went to a pediatric ward to collect a blood specimen from a young boy whom they had drawn many times before. The child told them to go away and that he was not supposed to have any more blood tests. The boy's parents were not present, but in the past they had always given permission for blood draws over the child's objections. The phlebotomists ignored the child, and one of them collected the specimen while the other restrained him. It was later determined that the boy's parents had earlier filed a written request that the child was to have no more blood drawn.

QUESTIONS
1. What error did the phlebotomists make in drawing the child?
2. What assumptions were made in deciding to draw the child over his objections?
3. What might be the consequences of the phlebotomists' actions?

Bibliography and Suggested Readings

Bishop, M. L., Duben-Engelkirk, J. L., & Fody, E. P. (2001). Clinical chemistry: principles, procedures, correlations (4th ed). Philadelphia: Lippincott Williams & Wilkins.

BD™ Blood Transfer Device product literature. Franklin Lakes, NJ: BD Vacutainer Systems.

College of American Pathologists (CAP) Publications Committee Phlebotomy Subgroup. (2005). So you're going to collect a blood specimen: an introduction to phlebotomy (11th ed). Northfield, IL.

Food and Drug Administration (FDA). Allergic reactions to latex-containing medical devices. FDA Med Alert, March 29, 1991.

Graden, M., et al. Pain reduction at venipuncture in newborns: oral glucose compared with local anesthetic cream. Pediatrics 2002;110:1053–1057.

Lindh, V., Wiklund, U., & Hakanssom, S. Assessment of the effect of EMLA during venipuncture in newborn by analysis of heart rate variability. Pain 2000;86:247–254.

Mitchell, A. & Waltman, PA. Oral sucrose and pain relief for preterm infants. Pain Management Nursing 2003;4(2):62–69.

Molle E., Kronberger J., & West-stack C. (2005). Clinical medical assisting (2nd ed). Philadelphia: Lippincott Williams & Wilkins.

National Committee for Clinical Laboratory Standards, H3–A5. (December 2003). Procedures for the collection of diagnostic blood specimens by venipuncture (5th ed). Wayne, PA: CLSI.

Warren, M., Eason, C., Burch, P., & Pfeiffer-Ewens, J. (2002). Medical assisting, a commitment to service. St. Paul: EMC Paradigm.

PREANALYTICAL CONSIDERATIONS

key•terms

A-line

AV shunt/fistula/graft

basal state

bilirubin

CVAD

CVC

diurnal/circadian

edema

exsanguination

hematoma

hemoconcentration

hemolysis

hemolyzed

heparin/saline lock

iatrogenic

icteric

implanted port

IV

jaundice

lipemia

lipemic

lymphostasis

mastectomy

petechiae

PICC

preanalytical

reference ranges

sclerosed

syncope

thrombosed

vasovagal syncope

venous stasis

objectives

Upon successful completion of this chapter, the reader should be able to:

1. Define the key terms and abbreviations listed at the beginning of this chapter.

2. List and describe the physiologic variables that influence laboratory test results and identify the tests most affected by each one.

3. List problem areas to avoid in site selection, identify causes for concern, and describe procedures to follow when encountering each.

4. Identify and describe various vascular access sites and devices and explain what to do when they are encountered.

5. Identify, describe, and explain how to handle patient complications associated with blood collection.

6. Identify, describe, and explain how to avoid or handle procedural error risks, specimen quality concerns, and reasons for failure to draw blood.

The **preanalytical** (before analysis) phase of the testing process begins when a test is ordered and ends when testing begins. Numerous factors associated with this phase of the testing process if not properly addressed can lead to errors that can affect specimen quality, jeopardize the health and safety of the patient, and ultimately increase the cost of medical care. Since each patient situation is unique, in addition to possessing the technical skills needed to perform a blood draw, a phlebotomist must have knowledge of the many patient variables, complications, and procedural errors associated with blood collection to avoid or reduce any negative impact.

BASAL STATE

Basal state refers to the resting metabolic state of the body early in the morning after fasting for a minimum of 12 hours. A basal state specimen is ideal for establishing **reference ranges** (normal laboratory test values for healthy individuals) on inpatients, because the effects of diet, exercise, and other controllable factors on test results are minimized or eliminated. Basal state is influenced by a number of physiologic patient variables such as age, gender, and conditions of the body that cannot be eliminated.

fyi Outpatient specimens are not basal state specimens and may have slightly different normal values.

PHYSIOLOGIC VARIABLES

Age

Values for some blood components vary considerably depending upon the age of the patient. For example, red blood cell (RBC) and white blood cell (WBC) values are normally higher in newborns than in adults. Some physiologic functions such as kidney function decrease with age. For example, creatinine clearance, a measure of kidney function, is directly related to the age of the patient, which must be factored in when calculating test results.

Altitude

Red blood cells carry oxygen. Decreased oxygen levels at higher altitudes cause the body to produce more red blood cells to meet the body's oxygen requirements; the higher the altitude, the greater the increase. Thus red blood cell (RBC) counts and related determinations such as hemoglobin (Hgb) and hematocrit (Hct) have higher normal ranges at higher elevations.

Dehydration

Dehydration (decrease in total body fluid) that occurs for example, with persistent vomiting or diarrhea, causes **hemoconcentration**, a condition in which blood components that cannot easily leave the bloodstream become concentrated in the smaller plasma volume.

Blood components affected include RBCs, enzymes, iron (Fe), calcium (Ca), sodium (Na), and coagulation factors. Consequently, results on specimens from dehydrated patients may not accurately reflect the patient's status. In addition, it is often difficult to obtain blood specimens from dehydrated patients.

Diet

Blood composition is significantly altered by ingestion of food. For example:

- Glucose (blood sugar) levels increase dramatically with the ingestion of carbohydrates or sugar-laden substances but return to normal within 2 hours if the patient has normal glucose metabolism.
- Ingestion of lipids (such as fats found in foods such as butter and cheese and in some IV feeding preparations) increases blood lipid content, a condition called **lipemia**. High levels of lipids cause the serum or plasma to appear milky (cloudy white) or turbid, and the specimen is described as being **lipemic** (Fig. 9-1).

memory • jogger   To associate lipemic with fat, think "fat lip" or visualize a fat white cloud, because fat makes the specimen cloudy white.

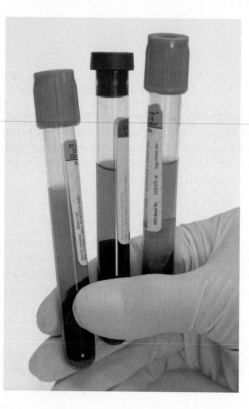

FIGURE 9-1

Left to right, Lipemic, icteric, and normal specimen.

Lipemia can be present for up to 12 hours, which is why accurate testing of triglycerides (a type of lipid) requires a 12-hour fast. In addition, some chemistry tests cannot be performed on lipemic specimens because the cloudiness interferes with the testing procedure.

key • point   When a test requires a fasting specimen but the serum or plasma sample submitted is lipemic, it is a clue that the patient most likely was not fasting.

- Some test methods that detect occult (hidden) blood in stool specimens also detect similar substances in meat and certain vegetables. Consequently, a special diet that eliminates these foods must be followed for several days before the specimen is collected.
- Fluid intake can also affect blood composition. Excessive fluid intake can decrease Hgb levels, and alter electrolyte balance. Consumption of caffeine beverages can affect cortisol levels. Chronic consumption or recent ingestion of large amounts of alcohol can cause hypoglycemia, and increased triglycerides.

key • point   Requiring a patient to fast or follow a special diet eliminates most dietary influences on testing.

Diurnal/Circadian Variations

The levels of many blood components normally exhibit **diurnal** (happening daily) or **circadian** (having a 24-hour cycle) variations or fluctuations. Factors that play a role in diurnal variations include posture, activity, eating, daylight and darkness, and being awake or asleep. For example, maximum renin and TSH levels normally occur in the predawn hours of the morning during sleep, while peak cortisol levels normally occur later in the morning, around 8:00 AM. Other blood components that exhibit diurnal variation with highest levels occurring in the morning include bilirubin, hemoglobin, insulin, iron, potassium, testosterone, and red blood cells. Blood levels of eosinophils, creatinine, glucose, triglyceride, and phosphate are normally lowest in the morning. Diurnal variations can be large. For example the levels of cortisol, TSH, and iron can differ by 50% or more between morning and late afternoon.

key • point   Tests influenced by diurnal variation are often ordered as timed tests, and it is important to collect them as close to the time ordered as possible.

Drug Therapy

Some drugs alter physiologic functions, causing changes in the concentrations of certain blood analytes. The effect may be desired or an unwanted side effect or sensitivity.

Consequently, it is not uncommon for physicians to monitor levels of specific blood analytes while a patient is receiving drug therapy. The following are just a few examples of drugs that can alter physiologic function and the analytes they affect:

- Chemotherapy drugs can cause a decrease in blood cells, especially WBCs and platelets.
- Many drugs are toxic to the liver, evidenced by increased levels of liver enzymes such as aspartate aminotransaminase (AST), also called serum glutamic-oxaloacetic transaminase (SGOT), and alkaline phosphatase (ALP) and lactate dehydrogenase (LDH), and decreased production of clotting factors.
- Opiates such as morphine increase levels of liver and pancreatic enzymes.
- Steroids and diuretics can cause pancreatitis and an increase in amylase and lipase values.
- Thiazide diuretics can elevate calcium and glucose levels and decrease sodium and potassium levels.

Drugs can also interfere in the actual test procedure, causing false increases or decreases in test results. A drug may compete with the test reagents for the substance being tested, causing a falsely low or false-negative result, or the drug may enhance the reaction, causing a falsely high or false-positive result.

fyi An acronym for substances that interfere in the testing process is CRUD, which stands for "compounds reacting unfortunately as the desired."

Although it is ultimately up to the physician to prevent or recognize and eliminate drug interferences, this can be a complicated issue that requires cooperation between the physician, pharmacy, and laboratory to make certain that test results are not affected by medications. Phlebotomists can play a role in this effort by noting on the requisition when they observe medication being administered just prior to blood collection.

key · point According to CAP guidelines, drugs that interfere with blood tests should be stopped or avoided 4 to 24 hours prior to obtaining the blood sample for testing. Drugs that interfere with urine tests should be avoided for 48 to 72 hours prior to the urine sample collection.

Exercise

Exercise affects a number of blood components, raising levels of some and lowering levels of others. Effects vary, depending on the patient's physical condition and the duration and intensity of the activity. Levels typically return to normal soon after the activity is stopped. The following are examples of how exercise affects blood components:

- Arterial pH and PCO_2 levels are reduced by exercise.
- Glucose, creatinine, insulin, lactic acid, and protein can be elevated by moderate muscular activity.
- Skeletal muscle enzyme levels are increased by exercise, with levels of creatine kinase (CK) and LDH remaining elevated for 24 hours or more.
- Vigorous exercise shortly before blood collection can increase cholesterol levels by 6%.

fyi   Athletes generally have higher resting levels of skeletal muscle enzymes, and exercise produces less of an increase.

Fever

Fever affects the levels of a number of hormones. Fever-induced hypoglycemia increases insulin levels followed by a rise in glucagon levels. Fever also increases cortisol and may disrupt its normal diurnal variation.

Gender

A patient's gender affects the concentration of a number of blood components. Most differences are apparent only after sexual maturity and are reflected in separate normal values for males and females. For example, RBC, Hgb, and Hct normal values are higher for males than for females.

Jaundice

Jaundice, also called **icterus**, is a condition characterized by increased **bilirubin** (a product of the breakdown of red blood cells) in the blood, leading to deposits of yellow bile pigment in the skin, mucous membranes, and sclera (whites of the eyes), giving the patient a yellow appearance. The term **icteric** means relating to or marked by jaundice and is used to describe serum, plasma, or urine specimens that have an abnormal deep yellow to yellow-brown color due to high bilirubin levels (see Fig. 9-1). The abnormal color can interfere in chemistry tests based on color reactions, including reagent strip analyses on urine.

key • point   Jaundice in a patient may indicate liver inflammation caused by hepatitis B or C virus.

Position

Body position before and during blood collection can influence specimen composition. Going from supine (lying down on the back) to an upright sitting or standing position causes blood fluids to filter into the tissues, decreasing plasma volume in an adult up to 10%. Only protein-free fluids can pass through the capillaries, consequently the blood concentration of components that are protein in nature or bound to protein, such as aldosterone, bilirubin, blood cells, calcium, cholesterol, iron, protein, and renin, increases. In most cases the concentration of freely diffusible blood components is not affected by postural changes. Nevertheless, a significant increase in potassium (K^+) levels occurs within 30 minutes of standing that has been attributed to the release of intracellular potassium from muscle. Other examples of the effects of posture changes include

- A change in position from lying to standing can cause up to a 15% variation in total and high-density lipoprotein (HDL) cholesterol results.

key • point The National Cholesterol Education Program recommends that lipid profiles be collected in a consistent manner after the patient has been either lying or sitting quietly for a minimum of 5 minutes.

- Plasma aldosterone and renin change more slowly but can double within an hour. Consequently, patients are required to be recumbent (lying down) for at least 30 minutes prior to aldosterone specimen collection, and plasma renin-activity levels require documentation of the patient's position during collection.
- The RBC count on a patient who has been standing for approximately 15 minutes will be higher than a basal state RBC count on the patient.

key • point Calling outpatients into the drawing area and having them sit in the drawing chair while paperwork related to the draw is readied can help minimize effects of postural changes on some analytes.

Pregnancy

Pregnancy causes physiologic changes in many body systems. Consequently, results of a number of laboratory tests must be compared to normal ranges established for pregnant populations. For example, body fluid increases, which are normal during pregnancy, have a diluting effect on the red blood cells, leading to lower red blood counts.

Smoking

A number of blood components are affected by smoking. The extent of effects depends upon the number of cigarettes smoked. Patients who smoke prior to specimen collection may have increased cholesterol, cortisol, glucose, and triglyceride levels and white blood counts. Chronic smoking often leads to decreased pulmonary function and increased red blood cell counts and hemoglobin levels. Smoking can also affect the body's immune response, typically lowering the concentrations of immunoglobulins IgA, IgG, and IgM, but increasing levels of IgE.

fyi Skin puncture specimens may be difficult to obtain from smokers because of impaired circulation in the fingertips.

Stress

Emotional stress such as anxiety, fear, or trauma can cause transient (short-lived) elevations in white blood cells (WBCs). For example, studies of crying infants demonstrated marked increases in WBC counts, which returned to normal within 1 hour after crying stopped. Consequently, CBC or WBC specimens on an infant are ideally obtained after the infant has been sleeping or resting quietly for at least 30 minutes. If they are collected while an infant is crying, it should be noted on the report.

fyi Studies in psychoneuroimmunology (PNI), a field that deals with the interactions between the brain, the endocrine system, and the immune system, have demonstrated that receptors on the cell membrane of WBCs can sense stress in a person and react by increasing cell numbers.

Stress also causes decreases in serum iron and increases in adrenal hormones such as cortisol. Other hormones that can be affected include aldosterone, and thyroid-stimulating hormone (TSH) and growth hormone (GH) in children.

Temperature and Humidity

Environmental factors such as temperature and humidity can affect test values by influencing the composition of body fluids. Acute heat exposure causes interstitial fluid to move into the blood vessels, increasing plasma volume and influencing its composition. Extensive sweating without fluid replacement, on the other hand, can cause hemoconcentration. Environmental factors associated with geographic location are accounted for when reference values are established.

fyi Temperature and humidity in the laboratory are closely monitored to maintain specimen integrity and to ensure proper functioning of equipment.

PROBLEM SITES

Burns, Scars, and Tattoos

Avoid burned, scarred, or tattooed areas. Veins are difficult to palpate or penetrate in these areas. Healed burn sites and other areas with extensive scarring may have impaired circulation and yield erroneous test results. Newly burned areas are painful and also susceptible to infection. Tattooed areas can have impaired circulation, may be more susceptible to infection, and contain dyes that can interfere in testing.

key • point If you have no choice but to draw in an area with a tattoo, try to insert the needle in a site that does not contain dye.

Damaged Veins

Some patient's veins feel hard and cordlike and lack resiliency because they are occluded or obstructed. These veins may be **sclerosed** (hardened) or **thrombosed** (clotted) from the effects of inflammation, disease, or chemotherapy drugs. Scarring caused by numerous venipunctures, as occurs in regular blood donors, persons with chronic illnesses, and illegal IV drug users, can also harden veins. Damaged veins are difficult to puncture; yield erroneous (invalid) test results because of impaired blood flow, and should be avoided.

key • point Choose another site, if possible, otherwise draw below (distal to) damaged veins.

Edema

Edema is swelling caused by the abnormal accumulation of fluid in the tissues. It sometimes results when fluid from an IV infiltrates the surrounding tissues. Specimens collected from edematous areas may yield inaccurate test results due to contamination with tissue fluid or altered blood composition caused by the swelling. In addition, veins are harder to locate, the tissue is often fragile and easily injured by tourniquet and antiseptic application, and healing may be prolonged in these areas. Another site should be chosen, if possible.

key • point Phlebotomists on early morning rounds in hospitals or nursing homes are often the first ones to notice edema from infiltrated IVs and should alert the appropriate personnel to the problem.

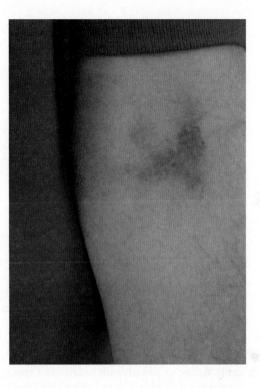

FIGURE 9-2

Remains of a hematoma that formed during venipuncture.

Hematoma

A **hematoma** (Fig. 9-2) is a swelling or mass of blood (often clotted) that can be caused by blood leaking from a blood vessel during or following venipuncture. A large bruise eventually spreads over the surrounding area. Venipuncture through an existing hematoma is painful and can result in collection of a specimen that is contaminated with hemolyzed blood from outside the vein and unsuitable for testing. Venipuncture in the area surrounding a hematoma may also be painful. In addition, obstruction of blood flow by the hematoma and the effects of the coagulation process may lead to inaccurate test results on the specimen.

c a u t i o n   Never perform venipuncture through a hematoma. If there is no alternative site, perform the venipuncture distal to the hematoma to ensure the collection of free-flowing blood.

Mastectomy

Blood should never be drawn from an arm on the same side as a **mastectomy** (breast removal) without first consulting the patient's physician. Lymph node removal, which is typically part of the procedure, causes **lymphostasis** (obstruction or stoppage of normal lymph flow). Impaired lymph flow makes the arm susceptible to swelling and infection. Applying a tourniquet to the arm can cause injury. Effects of lymphostasis can also change blood composition in that arm and lead to erroneous test results.

> **key • point** When a mastectomy has been performed on both sides, the patient's physician should be consulted to determine a suitable site. Generally, the side of the most recent mastectomy is the one avoided.

Obesity

Obese patients often present a challenge to the phlebotomist. Veins on obese patients may be deep and difficult to find. Proper tourniquet selection and application is the first step to a successful venipuncture. Conventional latex tourniquets may be too short to fit around the arm without rolling and twisting. A long length of Penrose drain tubing or a long Velcro closure strap often works better than a latex or vinyl strap. A blood pressure cuff can also be used.

Check the antecubital area first. Obese patients often have a double crease in the antecubital area with an easily palpable median cubital vein between the two creases. If no vein is easily visible or palpable on tourniquet application, ask the patient what sites have been successful for past blood draws. Most patients who are "difficult draws" know what sites work best. If the patient has never been drawn before or does not remember, another site to try is the cephalic vein. To locate the cephalic vein, rotate the patient's arm so that the hand is prone. In this position, the weight of excess tissue often pulls downward, making the cephalic vein easier to feel and penetrate with a needle.

VASCULAR ACCESS DEVICES (VADS) AND SITES

Arterial Line

An **arterial line** (A-line or Art-line) is a catheter that is placed in an artery. It is most commonly placed in a radial artery and is typically used to provide accurate and continuous measurement of a patient's blood pressure. It may also be used to collect blood gas and other blood specimens and for the administration of drugs such as dopamine. Only specially trained personnel should access arterial lines. Never apply a tourniquet or perform venipuncture on an arm with an arterial line.

Arteriovenous Shunt or Fistula

An **arteriovenous (AV) shunt**, **fistula**, or **graft** (Fig. 9-3) is the permanent, surgical fusion of an artery and a vein that is typically created to provide access for dialysis. It is commonly located on the back of the arm above the wrist. The connection of the artery and vein

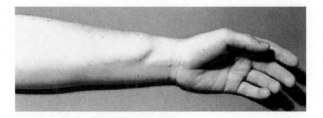

FIGURE 9-3
Arteriovenous (AV) shunt or fistula.

creates a loop close to the surface of the skin that can usually be easily seen and felt and is identified by a distinctive buzzing sensation called a "thrill" when palpated.

caution   Never apply a blood pressure cuff or tourniquet or perform venipuncture on an arm with a shunt.

Heparin or Saline Lock

A **heparin** or **saline lock** (Fig. 9-4) is a catheter or cannula connected to a stopcock or a cap with a diaphragm (thin rubberlike cover) that provides access for administering medication or drawing blood. It is often placed in a vein in the lower arm above the wrist and can be left in place for up to 48 hours. To keep it from clotting, the device is flushed and filled with heparin or saline, respectively. A saline lock is sometimes flushed with heparin also. Heparin readily adheres to surfaces and to remove all traces is difficult. Consequently, a 5-mL discard tube should be drawn first when blood specimens are collected from either type of device. Drawing coagulation specimens from either type is not recommended because traces of heparin or dilution with saline can negatively affect test results. Only specially trained personnel should draw blood from heparin and saline locks.

FIGURE 9-4
Saline lock with needleless entry stopcock.

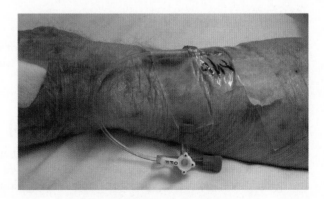

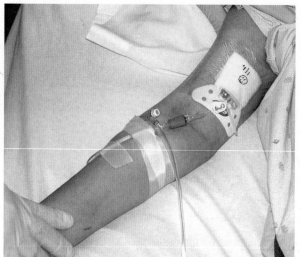

FIGURE 9-5
Patient's arm with an intravenous (IV) line.

Intravenous Sites

Intravenous (IV) means of, pertaining to, or within a vein. An intravenous line, referred to simply as an IV, is a catheter inserted in a vein to administer fluids. It is preferred that blood specimens not be drawn from an arm with an IV (Fig. 9-5) as they can be contaminated or diluted with the IV fluid, causing erroneous test results. This is especially true if the specimen is drawn above the IV. When a patient has an IV in one arm, blood specimens should be collected from the other arm. If a patient has IVs in both arms, or the other arm is also unavailable for some reason, it is preferred that the specimen be collected by capillary puncture. Many specimens (e.g., CBCs) can be easily collected this way. A specimen that cannot be collected by capillary puncture (e.g., a coagulation specimen) may be collected below the IV (never above) following the steps in Procedure 9-1.

Previously Active IV Sites

Previously active IV sites present a potential source of error in testing. Blood specimens should not be collected from a known previous IV site within 24 to 48 hours of the time the IV was discontinued. Follow facility protocol.

Central Vascular Access Devices (CVADs)

A **central vascular access device (CVAD)**, also called an **indwelling line**, consists of tubing inserted into a main vein or artery. CVADs are used primarily for administering fluids and medications, monitoring pressures, and drawing blood. Having a CVAD is practical for

PROCEDURE 9-1

Performing Venipuncture Below an IV

Purpose: To obtain a blood specimen by venipuncture below an IV

Equipment: Applicable ETS or syringe system supplies and equipment

Step	Explanation/Rationale
1. Ask the patient's nurse to turn off the IV for at least 2 minutes prior to collection	A phlebotomist is not qualified to make IV adjustments. Turning off the IV for 2 minutes allows IV fluids to dissipate from the area
2. Apply the tourniquet distal to the IV	Avoids disturbing the IV
3. Select a venipuncture site distal to the IV	Venous blood flows up the arm toward the heart. Drawing below an IV affords the best chance of obtaining blood that is free of IV fluid contamination
4. Perform the venipuncture in a different vein than the one with the IV if possible	IV fluids can be present below an IV because of backflow and may still be there after the IV is shut off, because of poor venous circulation
5. Ask the nurse to restart the IV after the specimen has been collected	IV flow rates must be precise, and starting or adjusting them is not part of a phlebotomist's scope of practice
6. Document that the specimen was collected below an IV, indicate the type of fluid in the IV, and identify which arm	This aids laboratory personnel and the patient's physician in the event that test results are questioned

patients who need IV access for an extended time and is especially beneficial for patients who do not have easily accessible veins.

caution Only specially trained personnel should access CVADs to draw blood. However, the phlebotomist may assist by transferring the specimen to the appropriate tubes.

Most CVADs are routinely flushed with heparin or saline to reduce risk of thrombosis. A small amount of blood must be drawn from the line and discarded before a blood specimen can be collected, to help ensure that it is not contaminated with the flush solution. The amount of blood discarded depends upon the dead space volume of the line. Two times the dead space volume is discarded for non-coagulation tests and six times (normally about 5

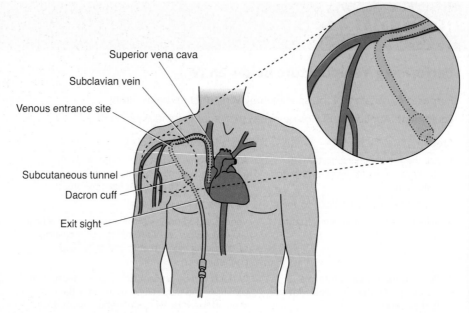

Superior vena cava

Subclavian vein

Venous entrance site

Subcutaneous tunnel

Dacron cuff

Exit sight

FIGURE 9-6

Central venous catheter (CVC) placement.

mL) is generally recommended for coagulation tests, although it is preferred that specimens for coagulation tests not be drawn from CVADs. Three main types of CVADs are described as follows:

- **Central venous catheter (CVC)** or **central venous line:** a line inserted into a large vein such as the subclavian and advanced into the superior vena cava, proximal to the right atrium. The exit end is surgically tunneled under the skin to a site several inches away in the chest. One or more short lengths of capped tubing protrude from the exit site, which is normally covered with a transparent dressing (see Fig. 9-6 for CVC placement). There are a number of different types of CVCs, including Broviac, Groshong, and Hickman (Fig. 9-7).
- **Implanted port** (Fig. 9-8): a small chamber attached to an indwelling line that is surgically implanted under the skin and most commonly located in the upper chest or arm. The device is located by palpating the skin, and accessed by inserting a special needle through the skin into the self-sealing septum (wall) of the chamber. The site is not normally covered with a bandage when not in use.
- **Peripherally inserted central catheter (PICC)** (Fig. 9-9): a line inserted into the peripheral venous system (veins of the extremities) and threaded into the central venous system (main veins leading to the heart). It does not require surgical insertion and is typically placed in an antecubital vein just above or below the antecubital fossa.

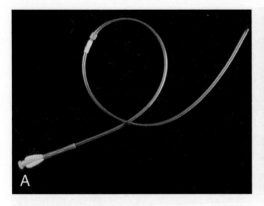
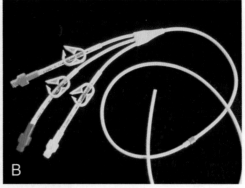

FIGURE 9-7

Central venous catheters. **A.** Groshong. **B.** Hickman. (Courtesy Bard Access Systems, Inc., Salt Lake City, UT.)

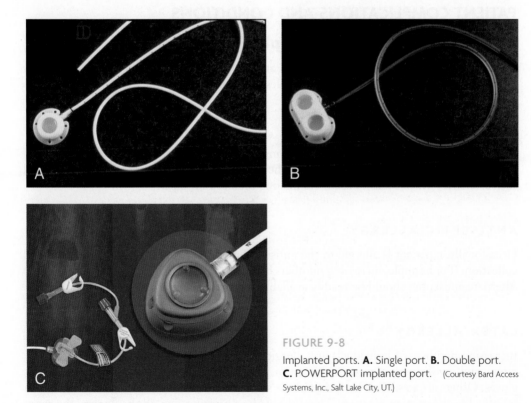

FIGURE 9-8

Implanted ports. **A.** Single port. **B.** Double port.
C. POWERPORT implanted port. (Courtesy Bard Access
Systems, Inc., Salt Lake City, UT.)

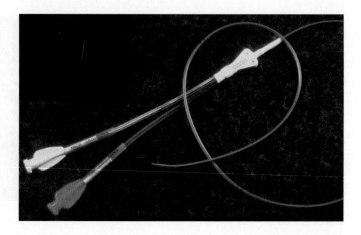

FIGURE 9-9

Groshong peripherally inserted central catheter. (Courtesy Bard Access Systems, Inc., Salt Lake City, UT.)

PATIENT COMPLICATIONS AND CONDITIONS

Allergies to Equipment and Supplies

Occasionally patients are encountered who are allergic to one or more of the supplies or equipment used in blood collection. Examples include the following.

ADHESIVE ALLERGY

Some patients are allergic to the glue used in adhesive bandages. Paper tape placed over a folded gauze square can be used instead, or the area can be wrapped with bandaging material such as Coban, which sticks to itself, eliminating the need for tape.

ANTISEPTIC ALLERGY

Occasionally, a patient is allergic to the antiseptic used in skin preparation prior to blood collection. (For example, increasing numbers of individuals are allergic to povidone-iodine.) Alternate antiseptics should be readily available for use in such cases.

LATEX ALLERGY

Increasing numbers of individuals are allergic to latex. Most latex allergies are seemingly minor and involve irritation or rashes from physical contact with latex products such as gloves. Others are so severe that being in the same room where latex materials are used can set off a life-threatening reaction. There should be a warning sign on the door to the room of any patient known to have a severe latex allergy, and it is vital that no items made of latex be brought into the room. This means the phlebotomist must wear nonlatex gloves, use a nonlatex tourniquet, and use nonlatex bandages when in the room, whether collecting blood from the patient or a roommate.

Excessive Bleeding

Normally, a patient will stop bleeding from the venipuncture site within a few minutes. Some patients, particularly those on aspirin or anticoagulant therapy, may take longer to stop bleeding. Pressure must be maintained over the site until the bleeding stops. If the bleeding continues after 5 minutes, the appropriate personnel should be notified.

c a u t i o n   Never apply a pressure bandage instead of maintaining pressure, and do not leave or dismiss a patient until bleeding has stopped or the appropriate personnel take charge of the situation.

Fainting

The medical term for fainting is **syncope (sin'ko-pea)**, described as a loss of consciousness and postural tone that results from insufficient blood flow to the brain. It can last for as little as a few seconds or as long as half an hour.

m e m o r y • j o g g e r   To remember that syncope means fainting, look for the word cope in syncope. If the body can't cope, the patient faints.

Any patient has the potential to faint during or immediately following venipuncture. Some patients become faint at just the thought or sight of their blood being drawn, especially if they are ill or have been fasting for an extended period. Other contributing factors include anemia, dehydration, emotional problems, fatigue, hypoglycemia, medications, nausea, and poor ventilation. Sudden faintness or loss of consciousness due to a nervous system response to abrupt pain, stress, or trauma is called **vasovagal** (relating to vagus nerve action on blood vessels) **syncope**.

A patient who feels faint at the time or has a history of fainting should be asked to lie down for the procedure. Inpatients who typically are already lying down, rarely faint during blood draws. Outpatients are more likely to faint, because they are usually sitting up during venipuncture.

Blood collection personnel should routinely ask patients how they are doing during a draw, watch for signs of fainting, and be prepared to protect the patient from falling. Signs to watch for include pallor (paleness), perspiration, and hyperventilation, or an indication from the patient that he or she is experiencing vertigo (a sensation of spinning), dizziness, light-headedness, or nausea. See Procedure 9-2 for steps to follow if a patient complains of feeling faint or exhibits symptoms of fainting during venipuncture.

c a u t i o n   The use of ammonia inhalants to revive patients can have unwanted side effects such as respiratory distress in asthmatic individuals and is not is recommended (see CLSI H3-A5, 11.8.1).

PROCEDURE 9-2

Steps to Follow if a Patient Starts to Faint During Venipuncture

Purpose: To properly handle a patient who feels faint or shows symptoms of fainting during a blood draw

Equipment: NA

Step	Explanation/Rationale
1. Release the tourniquet and remove and discard the needle as quickly as possible	Discontinuing the draw and discarding the needle protects the phlebotomist and the patient from injury should the patient faint
2. Apply pressure to the site while having the patient lower the head and breathe deeply	Pressure must be applied to prevent bleeding and bruising. Lowering the head and breathing deeply helps get oxygenated blood to the brain
3. Talk to the patient	Diverts patient's attention, helps keep the patient alert, and aids in assessing the patient's responsiveness
4. Physically support the patient	Prevents injury in case of collapse
5. Ask permission and explain what you are doing if it is necessary to loosen a tight collar or tie	Avoids misinterpretation of actions that are standard protocol to hasten recovery
6. Apply a cold compress or washcloth to the forehead and back of the neck	Part of the standard of care
7. Have someone stay with the patient until recovery is complete	Prevents patient from getting up too soon and possibly causing self-injury
8. Call first aid personnel if the patient does not respond	Emergency medicine is not in the phlebotomist's scope of practice
9. Document the incident according to facility protocol	Legal issues could arise, and further documentation is essential at that time

When a patient who has fainted regains consciousness, he or she must remain in the area for at least 15 minutes. The patient should be instructed *not* to operate a vehicle for at least 30 minutes. It is important for the phlebotomist to document the incident (following institution policy) in case of future litigation.

Nausea and Vomiting

It is not unusual to have a patient experience nausea before, during, or after a blood draw. A blood draw should not be attempted until the experience subsides.

key · point If the patient vomits during venipuncture the procedure must be terminated immediately.

The patient should be reassured and made as comfortable as possible. A feeling of nausea often precedes vomiting, so it is a good idea to give the patient an emesis basin or wastebasket to hold as a precaution. Ask the patient to breathe slowly and deeply. Apply a cold, damp washcloth or other cold compress to the patient's forehead. If the patient vomits, provide tissues or a washcloth to wipe the face and water to rinse the mouth unless the patient is NPO for surgery, other procedures, or otherwise not allowed to have water. Notify the patient's nurse, physician, or appropriate first aid personnel.

Pain

A small amount of pain is normally associated with routine venipuncture and capillary puncture. Putting patients at ease before blood collection helps them relax and can make the procedure less painful. Warning the patient prior to needle insertion helps avoid a startle reflex. A stinging sensation can be avoided by allowing the alcohol to dry completely prior to needle insertion.

Excessive, deep, blind, or lateral redirection of the needle is considered probing. It can be very painful to the patient; risks injury to arteries, nerves, and other tissues; and should never be attempted.

Marked or extreme pain, numbness of the arm, a burning or electric shock sensation, or pain that radiates up or down the arm during a venipuncture attempt indicates nerve involvement and requires immediate removal of the needle. If pain persists after needle removal, the patient's physician or other appropriate personnel should be consulted, and the incident documented. Application of an ice pack to the site after needle removal can help prevent or reduce inflammation associated with nerve involvement. Follow your healthcare facility's protocol.

> **c a u t i o n** If marked or extreme pain occurs, or the patient asks you to remove the needle for any reason, the venipuncture should be terminated immediately, even if there are no other signs of nerve injury.

Petechiae

Petechiae (Fig. 9-10) are tiny, nonraised red spots that appear on the patient's skin when a tourniquet is applied. The spots are minute drops of blood that escape the capillaries and come to the surface of the skin below the tourniquet, most commonly as a result of capillary wall defects or platelet abnormalities. They are not an indication that the phlebotomist has used incorrect procedure. However, they are an indication that the venipuncture site may bleed excessively.

Seizures/Convulsion

In the rare event that a patient has a seizure or goes into convulsions during blood specimen collection, it is important to discontinue the draw immediately. Hold pressure over the

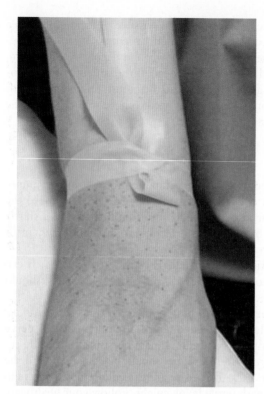

FIGURE 9-10

Petechiae. (Copyright Medical Training Solutions. Used with permission.)

site without overly restricting the patient's movement. Do not attempt to put anything into the patient's mouth. Try to prevent the patient from self-injury without completely restricting movement of the extremities. Notify the appropriate first aid personnel.

PROCEDURAL ERROR RISKS

Hematoma Formation

Hematoma formation is the most common complication of venipuncture. It is caused by blood leaking into the tissues during or following venipuncture and is identified by rapid swelling at or near the venipuncture site. (See Box 9-1 for situations that can trigger hematoma formation.) A hematoma is painful to the patient, often results in unsightly bruising, and can cause compression injuries to nerves and lead to lawsuits. Continuing to draw blood while a hematoma is forming risks injury to the patient and collection of a specimen contaminated with hematoma blood that has mixed with tissue fluids from outside the vein. Such a specimen has a high probability of being hemolyzed and rejected for testing. Even if it is not hemolyzed, it can still produce inaccurate test results. Presence of a hematoma makes the site unacceptable for subsequent venipunctures. (See Hematoma under Problem Sites, page 334).

BOX • 9-1 Situations That Can Trigger Hematoma Formation

- The vein is fragile or too small for the needle size.
- The needle penetrates all the way through the vein.
- The needle is only partly inserted into the vein.
- Excessive or blind probing is used to locate the vein.
- The needle is removed while the tourniquet is still on.
- Pressure is not adequately applied following venipuncture.

If a hematoma forms during blood collection, the phlebotomist should discontinue the draw immediately and hold pressure over the site for a minimum of 2 minutes. A small amount of blood under the skin is relatively harmless and generally resolves on its own. If the hematoma is large and causes swelling and discomfort, the patient should be offered a cold compress or ice pack to relieve pain and reduce swelling. Follow facility protocol.

fyi Acetaminophen or ibuprofen can help relieve discomfort from a hematoma. Ice applied in the first 24 hours helps manage the swelling and discomfort. After 24 hours, application of heat or warm moist compresses can help reabsorb accumulated blood.

Iatrogenic Anemia

Iatrogenic is an adjective used to describe an adverse condition brought on by the effects of treatment. Blood loss as a result of blood removed for testing is called iatrogenic blood loss. Removing blood on a regular basis or in large quantities can lead to iatrogenic anemia in some patients, especially infants.

fyi A primary reason for blood transfusion in neonatal ICU patients is to replace iatrogenic blood loss.

Blood loss to a point where life cannot be sustained is called **exsanguination**. Life is threatened if more than 10% of a patient's blood volume is removed at one time or over a short period of time. Coordination with physicians to minimize the number of times a patient is drawn, following quality assurance procedures to minimize redraws, and collecting minimum required specimen volumes, especially from infants, help reduce iatrogenic blood loss.

Inadvertent Arterial Puncture

Inadvertent arterial puncture is rare when proper venipuncture procedures are followed. It is most often associated with deep or blind probing, especially in the area of the basilic vein, which is in close proximity to the brachial artery. (This is one reason why the basilic vein is the last choice for venipuncture.) If an inadvertent arterial puncture goes undetected, leakage and accumulation of blood in the area can result in compression injury to a nearby nerve. Such injuries are often permanent and can lead to lawsuits. Arterial blood can usually be recognized by its bright red color, if the patient's pulmonary function is normal, or the fact that it spurts or pulses into the tube. If accidental arterial puncture is suspected, it is important for the phlebotomist to hold pressure over the site for a full 5 minutes after the needle is removed. Arterial puncture should not be used as a substitute for venipuncture, except in rare instances and with the approval of the patient's physician.

key • point Inadvertently collected arterial blood can usually be submitted for testing, rather than redrawing the patient. However, the specimen must be identified as arterial, since some test values are different for arterial specimens. Consult laboratory protocol.

Infection

Although a rare occurrence, infection at the site following venipuncture does happen. The risk of infection can be minimized by use of proper aseptic technique:

- Do not open adhesive tape or bandages ahead of time or temporarily tape them to lab coat cuffs or other contaminated items.
- Do not preload needles onto tube holders to have a supply for many draws ready ahead of time. The sterility of the needle is breached once the seal is broken.
- Do not touch the site with your finger, gauze, or any other nonsterile object after it has been cleaned, before or during needle insertion.
- Try to minimize the time between removing the needle cap and performing the venipuncture.
- Remind the patient to keep the bandage on for at least 15 minutes after specimen collection.

Nerve Injury

Poor site or improper vein selection, inserting the needle too deeply or quickly, movement by the patient as the needle is inserted, excessive or lateral redirection of the needle, or blind probing while attempting venipuncture can lead to injury of a main nerve (such as the median cutaneous), the risk of permanent damage, and the possibility of a lawsuit. Follow national guidelines for site selection, vein selection, and venipuncture technique to minimize the risk of problems. If initial needle insertion does not result in successful vein entry, and slight forward or backward redirection of the needle does not result in blood flow, the needle should be removed, and venipuncture attempted at an alternate site, preferably on the opposite arm.

> **caution** Extreme pain, a burning or electric shock sensation, numbness of the arm, and pain that radiates up or down the arm, are all signs of nerve involvement, and any one of them requires immediate removal of the needle. Application of an ice pack to the site after needle removal can help prevent or reduce inflammation associated with nerve involvement.

Reflux of Anticoagulant

In rare instances, it is possible for blood to **reflux** (backflow) into the patient's vein from the collection tube during the venipuncture procedure. Some patients have had adverse reactions to tube additives, particularly EDTA, attributed to reflux. Reflux can occur when the contents of the collection tube are in contact with the needle while the specimen is being drawn. To prevent reflux the patient's arm must be kept in a downward position so that the collection tube remains below the venipuncture site and fills from the bottom up. This prevents the needle from contacting blood in the tube. Back-and-forth movement of blood in the tube should also be avoided until the tube is removed from the evacuated tube holder. An outpatient can be asked to lean forward and extend the arm downward over the arm of the drawing chair to achieve proper positioning. Raising the head of the bed, extending the patient's arm over the side of the bed, or supporting the arm with a rolled towel can be used to help achieve proper positioning of a bedridden patient.

Vein Damage

Properly performed, an occasional venipuncture will not impair the patency of a patient's vein. Numerous venipunctures in the same area over an extended period of time, however, will eventually cause a buildup of scar tissue and increase the difficulty of performing subsequent venipunctures. Blind probing and improper technique when redirecting the needle can also damage veins and impair patency.

SPECIMEN QUALITY CONCERNS

The quality of a blood specimen can be compromised by improper collection techniques. A poor-quality specimen will generally yield poor-quality results that can affect the patient's care. Because it is not always apparent to the phlebotomist or testing personnel when the quality of a specimen has been compromised, it is very important for the phlebotomist to be aware of the following pitfalls of collection.

Hemoconcentration from Venous Stasis

Tourniquet application causes localized **venous stasis**, or stagnation of the normal venous blood flow. (A similar term for this is **venostasis**, the trapping of blood in an extremity by compression of veins.) In response, some of the plasma and filterable components of the blood pass through the capillary walls into the tissues. This results in hemoconcentration, a decrease in the fluid content of the blood with a subsequent increase in nonfilterable large molecule or protein-based blood components such as red blood cells. Other abnormally increased analytes include albumin, ammonia, calcium, cholesterol, coagulation factors, enzymes, iron, potassium, and total protein. Changes that occur within 1 minute of tourniquet application are slight; however, prolonged tourniquet application can lead to marked changes.

key • point   Cholesterol levels can increase up to 5% after 2 minutes of tourniquet application, and up to 15% after 5 minutes.

Massaging or squeezing the site, probing for veins, long-term IV therapy, drawing blood from sclerosed or occluded veins, and vigorous hand pumping (making and releasing a fist), can also result in the collection of specimens affected by hemoconcentration.

fyi   Vigorous fist pumping can significantly increase blood potassium levels.

Test results on hemoconcentrated specimens may not accurately reflect the patient's true status, and it is important that steps be taken to avoid them. A list of ways to prevent hemoconcentration during venipuncture is presented in Box 9-2.

BOX • 9-2   Ways to Help Prevent Hemoconcentration During Venipuncture

- Ask the patient to release the fist upon blood flow.
- Choose an appropriate patent vein.
- Do not allow the patient to pump the fist.
- Do not excessively massage the area when locating a vein.
- Do not probe or redirect the needle multiple times in search of a vein.
- Release the tourniquet within 1 minute.

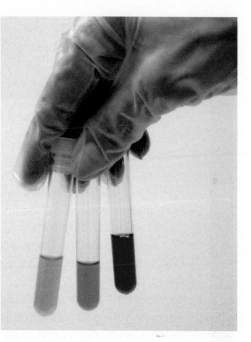

FIGURE 9-11

Left to right, Normal serum specimen, specimen with slight hemolysis, and grossly hemolyzed specimen.

Hemolysis

Hemolysis results when RBCs are damaged or destroyed and the hemoglobin they contain escapes into the fluid portion of the specimen. The red color of the hemoglobin makes the serum or plasma appear pink (slight hemolysis), dark pink to light red (moderate hemolysis), to red (gross hemolysis), and the specimen is described as being **"hemolyzed"** (Fig. 9-11). Hemolyzed specimens can be the result of patient conditions such as hemolytic anemia, liver disease, or a transfusion reaction, but they are more commonly the result of procedural errors in specimen collection or handling that damages the RBCs. Hemolysis can erroneously elevate levels of analytes such as enzymes, iron, magnesium, and potassium (K^+) and decrease red blood cell counts. Consequently, a specimen that is hemolyzed as a result of procedural error will most likely need to be redrawn. Box 9-3 lists procedural errors that can cause hemolysis.

Partially Filled Tubes

ETS tubes should be filled until the normal amount of vacuum is exhausted. Failing to do so results in a partially filled tube (Fig. 9-12) referred to as a short draw. Short draw serum tubes such as red tops and SSTs are generally acceptable for testing as long as the specimen is not hemolyzed and there is sufficient specimen to perform the test. Underfilled anticoagulant tubes and most other additive tubes, however, may not contain the proper blood-to-additive ratio for which the tube was designed.

BOX • 9-3   Procedural Errors That Can Cause Specimen Hemolysis

- Drawing blood from a vein that has a hematoma
- Failure to wipe away the first drop of blood (that may contain alcohol residue) during capillary puncture
- Forcing the blood from a syringe into an evacuated tube
- Frothing of the blood caused by improper fit of the needle on a syringe
- Mixing additive tubes too vigorously such as shaking them or inverting them too quickly or forcefully
- Partially filling a normal draw sodium fluoride tube
- Pulling back the plunger on a syringe too quickly
- Rough handling during transport, or horizontal transportation that allows back-and-forth movement of tube contents
- Squeezing the site during capillary specimen collection
- Using a needle with a too-small diameter for venipuncture
- Using a too-large tube with a small-diameter butterfly needle

---

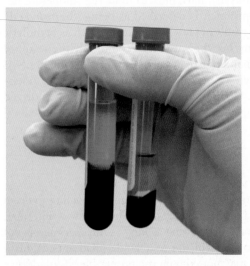

FIGURE 9-12

Two examples of under-filled light-blue-top tubes.

c a u t i o n   Never pour two partially filled additive tubes together to fill one tube, as this will also affect the blood-to-additive ratio.

Although in some cases underfilled additive tubes may be accepted for testing, the specimens can be compromised. For example:

- Excess EDTA in underfilled lavender-top tubes can shrink red blood cells and cause erroneously low blood cell counts and hematocrits.
- Excess heparin in plasma from underfilled green-top tubes may interfere with testing of some chemistry analytes.
- Excess sodium fluoride in underfilled gray-top tubes can result in hemolysis of the specimen.
- Underfilled coagulation tubes do not have the correct blood-to-additive ratio and will produce erroneous results.

Inadvertent (unintentional) short draws are usually the result of difficult draw situations in which blood flow stops or vacuum is lost during needle manipulation. Phlebotomists sometimes underfill tubes on purpose when it is inadvisable to obtain larger quantities of blood, such as when drawing from infants, children, or severely anemic individuals.

c a u t i o n   Some phlebotomists underfill tubes to save time. This practice is never recommended.

Partial vacuum tubes the same size as standard fill tubes but designed to contain a smaller volume of blood are available and should be used in situations where it is difficult or inadvisable to obtain larger amounts. These tubes are sometimes referred to as "short draw" tubes (Fig. 9-13), but they are designed to contain the proper blood-to-additive ratio even though they contain less blood. A line on the tube is typically used to indicate the fill level.

FIGURE 9-13

"Short draw" tube designed for partial filling. Line on tube indicates proper fill level.

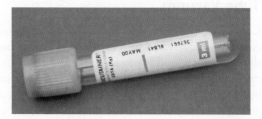

Specimen Contamination

Specimen contamination is typically inadvertent and generally the result of improper technique or carelessness such as

- Allowing alcohol residue, fingerprints, glove powder, baby powder, or urine from wet diapers to contaminate newborn screening samples, leading to specimen rejection
- Getting glove powder on blood films (slides) or in capillary specimens, resulting in misinterpretation of results. Calcium-containing powders can affect calcium results
- Unwittingly dripping perspiration into capillary specimens during collection or any specimen during processing or testing. The salt in sweat, for example, can affect sodium and chloride levels
- Using the correct antiseptic but not following proper procedure. For example, improperly cleaning blood culture bottle tops or the collection site, touching the site after it has been prepped (cleaned), or inserting the needle before the antiseptic on the arm or bottle tops is dry. (Traces of the antiseptic in the culture media can inhibit growth of bacteria and cause false-negative results.) Performing capillary puncture before the alcohol is dry causing hemolysis of the specimen and leading to inaccurate results or rejection of the specimen by the lab
- Using the wrong antiseptic to clean the site prior to specimen collection. For example, using alcohol to clean the site can contaminate an ethanol (blood alcohol) specimen. Using povidone- iodine (e.g., Betadine) to clean a skin puncture site can contaminate the specimen and cause erroneously high levels of uric acid, phosphate, and potassium

TROUBLESHOOTING FAILED VENIPUNCTURE

Failure to initially draw blood can be caused by a number of procedural errors. Being aware of these errors and knowing how to correct them may determine whether you obtain blood on the first try or have to repeat the procedure. If you fail to obtain blood, remain calm so that you can clearly analyze the situation and check the following:

Tube Position

Tube position is important. Check the tube to see that it is properly seated and the needle in the tube holder has penetrated the tube stopper. Reseat the tube to make certain the needle sleeve is not pushing the tube off the needle.

Tube Vacuum

Loss of tube vacuum can occur during venipuncture procedures if the needle bevel is not completely under the skin or the bevel backs out of the skin slightly. When this happens a short hissing sound is often heard, and there may be a spurt of blood into the tube before the blood flow stops. Tubes can also lose vacuum during shipping and handling, when they bump one another in trays, if they are dropped, or if they are pushed too far onto the needle prior to venipuncture. If you suspect that a tube has lost its vacuum, try a new one.

key • point A tube with vacuum problems at the start of a draw may be a sign that it is cracked or has been dropped. Cracked tubes present a safety hazard because they may leak or break with further handling. Never use a tube that has been dropped. Discard it instead.

Needle Position

Improper needle position is a common cause of failure to obtain blood. A seasoned phlebotomist uses visual cues to help determine if the needle is correctly positioned in the vein (Fig. 9-14A). Try first to visually determine if any of the following common

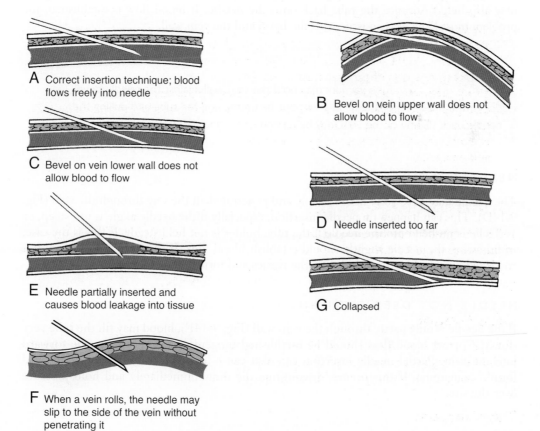

A Correct insertion technique; blood flows freely into needle

B Bevel on vein upper wall does not allow blood to flow

C Bevel on vein lower wall does not allow blood to flow

D Needle inserted too far

E Needle partially inserted and causes blood leakage into tissue

G Collapsed

F When a vein rolls, the needle may slip to the side of the vein without penetrating it

FIGURE 9-14

Proper and improper needle positioning. **A.** Correct needle insertion technique; blood flows freely into tube. **B.** Bevel on vein upper wall prevents blood flow. **C.** Bevel on vein lower wall prevents blood flow. **D.** Needle inserted too far penetrates through the vein. **E.** Partially inserted needle causes blood leakage into tissue. **F.** Needle slipped beside the vein, not into it; caused when a vein rolls to the side. **G.** Collapsed vein prevents blood flow.

problems with needle position or insertion have occurred. Some are harder to discern than others. Eliminate the ones that you can and try the remedy for the others to see if one works.

BEVEL AGAINST THE VEIN WALL

Blood flow can be impaired if the needle bevel is up against the upper or lower wall of the vein (Fig. 9-14B and C). This can happen if the needle angle is wrong. For example, an angle that is too shallow can cause the needle to contact the upper wall; an angle that is too steep can cause the needle to embed in the lower wall. This can also happen if the needle is inserted near a bend in the vein or at a point where the vein goes deeper into the skin. All of these situations are very hard to detect. Remove the tube from the holder needle to release vacuum pull on the vein, and pull the needle back slightly. (Rotating the bevel slightly may also help.) Advance the tube back onto the needle. If blood flow is established, the problem most likely was an issue with the bevel and the vein wall.

c a u t i o n Tube vacuum may hold the vein wall against the needle bevel. *Do not* rotate the bevel of the needle without first removing the tube and pulling the needle back slightly or the vein may be injured.

NEEDLE TOO DEEP

The needle may have gone in too deeply and penetrated all the way through the vein (Fig. 9-14D). This can happen on needle insertion, especially if the needle angle is too steep, or as a tube is pushed onto the needle if the tube holder is not held steady. If this is the case, withdrawing the needle slightly should establish blood flow. If the needle position is not corrected quickly, blood will leak into the tissues and form a hematoma.

NEEDLE NOT DEEP ENOUGH

If the needle is only partly through the vein wall (Fig. 9-14E), blood may fill the tube very slowly. Correct blood flow should be established by gently pushing the needle forward into the vein. Partial needle insertion can also cause blood to leak into the tissue and form a hematoma. If this occurs, discontinue the draw immediately and hold pressure over the site.

c a u t i o n Continuing the draw while a hematoma is forming increases the risk of injury to the patient and collection of blood from outside the vein that is contaminated with tissue fluids and very likely to be hemolyzed.

NEEDLE BESIDE THE VEIN

Veins are fairly tough and if a vein is not anchored well with the thumb, it may roll (move away) slightly and the needle may slip to the side of the vein instead of into it (Fig. 9-14F). Often the needle ends up beside the vein and slightly under it as well. (This is often the case with the basilic vein, which is not well anchored in the tissue to begin with.) If this happens, slip the tube off the needle to preserve the vacuum, withdraw the needle slightly until just the bevel is under the skin, anchor the vein securely, and redirect the needle into the vein. If redirection is unsuccessful, discontinue the draw and choose a new site. Do not search or probe for the vein or move the needle in a lateral (sideways) direction to find it.

fyi   When phlebotomists "miss" veins, they often tell patients that they have "veins that roll." This leads patients to mistakenly believe that there is a problem with their veins, when more than likely the problem is the phlebotomist's technique.

UNDETERMINED NEEDLE POSITION

If you cannot determine the position of the needle and the above solutions do not help, you may have to use your finger to relocate the vein. Remove the tube from the holder needle and withdraw the needle until the bevel is just under the skin. Clean your gloved finger with alcohol and palpate the arm above the point of needle insertion to try to determine needle position and vein location. Be careful not to feel too close to the needle, as this is painful to the patient. Once you have relocated the vein, pull the skin taut, and redirect the needle into it. If you cannot relocate the vein (or if access to it would require lateral redirection of the needle), discontinue the draw and select a new site.

c a u t i o n   *Do not* blindly probe the arm in an attempt to locate a vein. Probing is painful to the patient and can damage nerves or lead to inadvertent puncture of an artery.

Collapsed Vein

Sometimes the vacuum draw of a tube or the pressure created by pulling on a syringe plunger can be too much for a vein, causing it to collapse temporarily (Fig. 9-14G) and blood flow to cease. A vein may also collapse if the tourniquet is tied too tightly or too close to the venipuncture site. In this case, blood cannot be replaced as quickly as it is withdrawn and the vein collapses. In addition, veins sometimes collapse when the tourniquet is removed during the blood draw. This is often the case in elderly patients whose veins are fragile and collapse more easily.

fyi   Stoppage of blood flow upon tourniquet removal does not necessarily mean that the vein has collapsed. It may be that the needle is no longer positioned properly and a slight adjustment is needed to reestablish blood flow.

A clue that a normally visible vein has collapsed is that it disappears as soon as the vacuum tube is engaged or when the tourniquet is removed. To reintroduce tourniquet pressure, grasp the ends of the loose tourniquet with one hand and twist them together. That may be enough to reestablish blood flow. If the tourniquet cannot be retightened, use your finger to apply pressure to the vein several inches above the needle. Remove the tube from the needle and wait a few seconds for the blood flow to reestablish before reengaging it. Try using a smaller-volume tube or pull more slowly on the plunger if using a syringe. If the blood flow does not reestablish, remove the needle and attempt a second venipuncture at another site.

STUDY & REVIEW QUESTIONS

1. **Peak levels of this analyte typically occur at about 0800.**
   a. Bilirubin
   b. Cortisol
   c. Eosinophil
   d. Glucose

2. **Which of these tests are most affected if the patient is not fasting?**
   a. CBC and protime
   b. Glucose and triglycerides
   c. RA and cardiac enzymes
   d. Blood culture and thyroid profile

3. **Veins that feel hard and cordlike when palpated may be**
   a. Collapsed
   b. Fistulas
   c. Thrombosed
   d. Venules

4. **Tiny red spots that appear on a patient's arm when the tourniquet is applied are a sign that the**
   a. Patient is allergic to latex
   b. Patient is anemic
   c. Site may bleed excessively
   d. Tourniquet is too tight

5. **When the arm of the patient is swollen with excess fluids, the condition is called**
   a. Edema
   b. Hemoconcentration
   c. Icterus
   d. Syncope

6. **A patient has several short lengths of IV style tubing protruding from his chest. This is most likely a/an**
   a. A-line
   b. CVC
   c. Implanted port
   d. PICC

7. **Which of the following is most likely to cause reflux during venipuncture?**
   a. Allowing the tube to fill from the stopper end first
   b. Lateral redirection of the needle
   c. Releasing the tourniquet as soon as blood flows freely into the tube
   d. Using the wrong order of draw

8. **A patient complains of extreme pain when you insert the needle during a venipuncture attempt. The pain does not subside, but the patient does not feel any numbness or burning sensation. You know the needle is in the vein because the blood is flowing into the tube. You only have two tubes to fill, and the first one is almost full. What should you do?**
   a. Ask the patient if he or she wants you to continue the draw
   b. Discontinue the draw and attempt collection at another site
   c. Distract the patient with small talk and continue the draw
   d. Tell the patient to hang in there as you only have one tube left

9. **Which of the following situations can result in hemoconcentration?**
   a. Leaving the tourniquet on longer than a minute
   b. Mixing the specimen too vigorously
   c. Partially filling a normal draw tube
   d. Using a needle that is too small for size of the tube

10. **You are in the process of collecting a specimen by venipuncture. You hear a hissing sound, there is a spurt of blood into the tube, and blood flow stops. What has most likely happened?**
   a. Reflux has occurred
   b. The needle has gone through the back of the vein
   c. The tube has lost its vacuum
   d. The vein has collapsed

CASE · STUDY · 9-1

Physiological Variables, Problem Sites, and Patient Complications

Charles is a phlebotomist who works in a physician's office laboratory. One morning shortly after the drawing station opens he is asked to collect blood specimens for a CBC and a glucose test from a very heavyset woman who appears quite ill. The patient tells Charles that she vomited all night and was unable to eat or drink anything. She also mentions that she has had a mastectomy on the left side and the last time she had blood collected she was stuck numerous times before the phlebotomist was able to successfully collect the specimen.

QUESTIONS:
1. What physiologic variables may be associated with the collection of this specimen and how should they be dealt with?
2. What complications might Charles expect and how should he prepare for them?
3. How should Charles go about selecting the blood collection site?
4. What options does Charles have if he is unable to select a proper venipuncture site?

CASE · STUDY · 9-2

Troubleshooting Failed Venipuncture

A phlebotomist named Sara is in the process of collecting a protime and CBC from a patient. The needle is in the patient's vein. As Sara pushes the first tube onto the needle in the tube holder there is a spurt of blood into the tube and she hears a hissing sound. Then the blood stops flowing. She repositions the needle but is not able to establish blood flow.

QUESTIONS:
1. Why did blood spurt into the tube and then stop?
2. What clues are there to determine what the problem is?
3. What can Sara do to correct the problem?

Bibliography and Suggested Readings

Bishop, M. L., Duben-Engelkirk, J. L., & Fody, E. P. (2005). Clinical chemistry: principles, procedures, correlations (5th ed). Philadelphia: Lippincott Williams & Wilkins.

Burtis, C. A., Ashwood, E.R. (2001). Tietz fundamentals of clinical chemistry (5th ed). Philadelphia: W. B. Saunders.

Cavalieri, T. A, Chopra, A., & Bryman P. N. When outside the norm is normal: interpreting lab data in the aged. Geriatrics 1992;47(5):66–70

College of American Pathologists. (2005). So you're going to collect a blood specimen (11th ed). Northfield, IL.

Dale, J. C. Preanalytical variables in laboratory testing. Laboratory Medicine, September 1998.

Ernst, D. J. (2005). Applied phlebotomy. Baltimore: Lippincott Williams & Wilkins.

Henry, J. B. (2001). Clinical diagnostic and management of laboratory methods (20th ed). Philadelphia: W. B. Saunders.

Lippi, G., Salvagno, G. L., Montagnana, M., & Guidi, G. C. Short-term venous stasis influences routine coagulation testing. Blood Coagulation & Fibrinolysis 2005;16(6):453–458.

Magee, L. S. Preanalytical variables in the chemistry laboratory. Becton Dickinson Lab Notes 2005;15(1).

Malcolm L., Brigden, M. L., & Heathcote, J. C. Problems in interpreting laboratory tests, what do unexpected results mean? Postgraduate Medicine 2000;107(7). Accessed 11-04-05.

Managing Preanalytical Variability in Hematology. Becton Dickinson Lab Notes 2004;14 (1).

Mayo Foundation for Medical Education and Research. Postural and venous stasis-induced changes in total calcium. Mayo Clinic Proceedings 2005;80:1100–1101. Letters to the editor.

National Committee for Clinical Laboratory Standards. H3-A5. (December 2003). Procedures for the collection of diagnostic blood specimens by venipuncture (4th ed). Wayne, PA: CLSI/NCCLS.

National Committee for Clinical Laboratory Standards, H4-A5 (2004). Procedures and devices for the collection of diagnostic capillary blood specimens; approved standard (5th ed). Wayne, PA: CLSI/NCCLS.

Rock R. C. Interpreting laboratory tests: a basic approach. Geriatrics 1984;39(1):49–54

CAPILLARY PUNCTURE EQUIPMENT AND PROCEDURES

key•terms

arterialized	feather	newborn/neonatal screening
blood film/smear	interstitial fluid	osteochondritis
calcaneus	intracellular fluid	osteomyelitis
CBGs	lancet	PKU
cyanotic	microcollection containers	plantar surface
differential	microhematocrit tubes	whorls

objectives

Upon successful completion of this chapter, the reader should be able to:

1. Define the key terms and abbreviations listed at the beginning of this chapter.
2. List and describe the various types of equipment needed for capillary specimen collection.
3. Describe the composition of capillary specimens, identify which tests have different reference values when collected by capillary puncture methods, and name tests that cannot be performed on capillary specimens.
4. Identify indications for performing capillary puncture on adults, children, and infants.
5. List the order of draw for collecting capillary specimens.
6. Describe proper procedure for selecting the puncture site and collecting capillary specimens from adults, infants, and children.
7. Describe how both routine and thick blood smears are made and reasons for making them at the collection site.
8. Explain the clinical significance of capillary blood gas, neonatal bilirubin, and newborn screening tests and describe how specimens for these tests are collected.

Drops of blood for testing can be obtained by puncturing or making an incision in the capillary bed in the dermal layer of the skin with a lancet, other sharp device, or laser. Terms typically used to describe this technique include capillary, dermal, or skin puncture, regardless of the actual type of device or method used to penetrate the skin, and the specimens obtained are respectively referred to as capillary, dermal, or skin puncture specimens. (To best reflect the nature and source of the specimen, and for simplification and consistency, the terms capillary specimen and capillary puncture are used in this chapter.) With the advent of laboratory instrumentation capable of testing small quantities, many specimens for laboratory tests can now be collected in this manner. Capillary specimen collection is especially useful in pediatric patients in whom removal of larger quantities of blood can have serious consequences. Collection sites include the fingers of adults and children over the age of two and the heels of infants. Although steps may differ slightly, procedures in this chapter were written to conform to CLSI Standard H4-A5, *Procedures and Devices for the Collection of Diagnostic Capillary Blood Specimens.*

CAPILLARY PUNCTURE EQUIPMENT

In addition to blood collection supplies and equipment described in Chapter 7, the following special equipment may be required for skin puncture procedures.

Lancet/Incision Device

A **lancet** is a sterile, disposable, sharp-pointed or bladed instrument that either punctures or makes an incision in the skin to obtain capillary blood specimens for testing. Lancets are available in a range of lengths and depths to accommodate various specimen collection requirements. Selection depends upon the age of the patient, collection site, volume of specimen required, and the puncture depth needed to collect an adequate specimen without injuring bone. Lancets are specifically designed for either finger puncture (Fig. 10-1), or heel puncture (Fig. 10-2), and must have OSHA-required safety features, such as permanently retractable blades, to reduce the chance of accidental sharps injuries.

LASER LANCET

A revolutionary device, the Lasette *plus* (Fig. 10-1C) (Cell Robotics, Albuquerque, NM), perforates the skin with a laser instead of a sharp instrument. The laser vaporizes water in the skin to produce a small hole in the capillary bed. Because no sharp instrument is involved, there is no risk of accidental sharps injury, and no need for sharps disposal. A special single-use disposable insert prevents cross-contamination between patients. The Lasette is cleared by the FDA for use on the fingers of adults and children 5 years of age and older. Use on children younger than 5 years of age is subject to a physician's discretion.

Collection Devices

MICROCOLLECTION CONTAINERS

Microcollection containers (Fig. 10-3), also called microtubes, are special small plastic tubes used to collect the tiny amounts of blood obtained from capillary punctures. They are

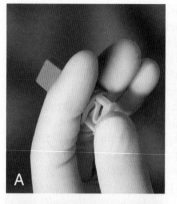

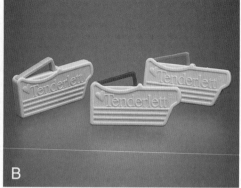

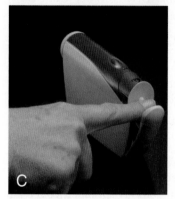

FIGURE 10-1

Several types of finger puncture lancets. **A.** Vacutainer brand Genie Lancets   (Courtesy Becton Dickinson, Franklin Lakes, NJ.) **B.** Tenderlett Toddler, Junior, and Adult lancet devices.   (Courtesy ITC, Edison, NJ.) **C.** Lasette Plus laser lancet.   (Courtesy Cell Robotics, Albuquerque, NM.)

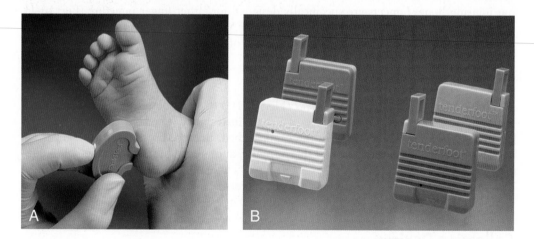

FIGURE 10-2

Several types of heel puncture lancets. **A.** BD QuikHeel infant lancet, also available in a preemie version. (Courtesy Becton Dickinson, Franklin Lakes, NJ.) **B.** Tenderfoot toddler *(pink)*, newborn *(pink/blue)*, preemie *(white)*, and micro-preemie heel incision devices *(blue)*.   (Courtesy ITC, Edison, NJ.)

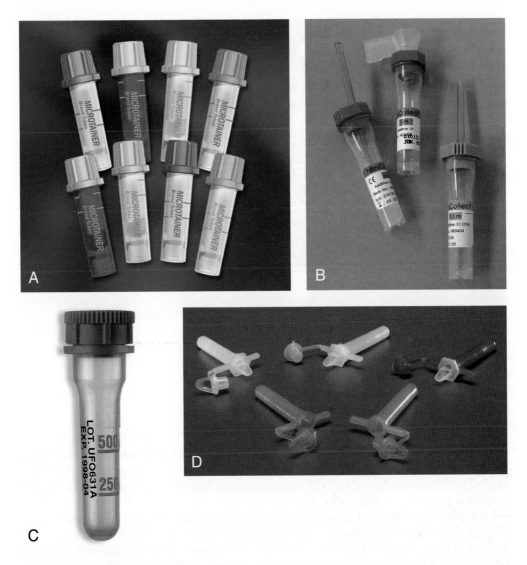

FIGURE 10-3

Examples of microcollection containers. **A.** Microtainers (Courtesy Becton Dickinson, Franklin Lakes, NJ.) **B.** MiniCollect Capillary Blood Collection Tubes. (Courtesy Greiner Bio-One, Kremsmuenster, Austria.) **C.** Capiject EDTA Capillary Blood Collection Tube. (Terumo, Somerset, NJ.) **D.** Samplette capillary blood collection collectors (Courtesy Tyco Healthcare, Kendall, Mansfield, MA.)

often referred to as "bullets" because of their size and shape. Some come fitted with narrow plastic capillary tubes (see Fig. 10-3B) to facilitate specimen collection. Most have color-coded bodies or stoppers that correspond to color-coding of ETS blood collection tubes and markings for minimum and maximum fill levels that are typically measured in microliters (μL) such as 250 μL and 500 μL, respectively (see Fig. 10-3C). Some manufacturers print lot numbers and expiration dates on each tube.

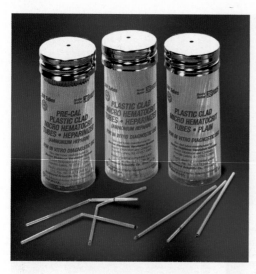

FIGURE 10-4

Microhematocrit tubes   (Courtesy Becton Dickinson, Franklin Lakes, NJ.)

> c a u t i o n   Sometimes venous blood obtained by syringe during difficult draw situations, is put into microcollection containers. When this is done, the specimen must be labeled as venous blood. Otherwise it will be assumed to be a capillary specimen, which may have different normal values.

MICROHEMATOCRIT TUBES AND SEALANTS

Microhematocrit tubes (Fig. 10-4) are disposable, narrow-bore plastic or plastic-clad glass capillary tubes that fill by capillary action and typically hold 50 to 75 μL of blood. They are primarily used for manual hematocrit (Hct) also called packed cell volume (PVC) determinations. The tubes come coated with ammonium heparin, for collecting Hct tubes directly from a capillary puncture, or plain, to be used when an Hct tube is filled with blood from a lavender-top tube. Heparin tubes typically have a red band on one end; nonadditive tubes have a blue band. Smaller microhematocrit tubes designed for use with special microcentrifuges such as those available from StatSpin, Inc. (Norwood, MA) require as little as 9 μL of blood and are often used in infant and child anemia screening programs and pediatric clinics. Plastic or clay sealants that come in small trays are used to seal one end of microhematocrit tubes. Traditionally, the dry end of the tube was inserted into the clay to plug it. Because of safety concerns, it is now recommended that sealing methods be used that do not require manually pushing the tube into the sealant or products be used that measure Hct without centrifugation.

CAPILLARY BLOOD GAS EQUIPMENT

The following special equipment (Fig. 10-5) is used to collect **capillary blood gas (CBG)** specimens:

- *CBG collection tubes:* CBG collection tubes are long thin narrow-bore capillary tubes. They are normally plastic for safety and are available in a number of different sizes to

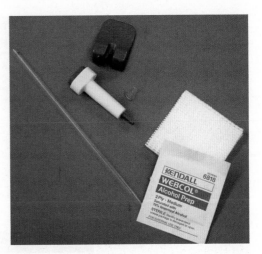

FIGURE 10-5

Capillary blood gas collection equipment.

accommodate volume requirements of various testing instruments. The most common CBG tubes are 100 mm in length with a capacity of 100 μL. A color-coded band identifies the type of anticoagulant that coats the inside of the tube; it is normally green, indicating sodium heparin.

- *Stirrers:* Stirrers are small metal filings (often referred to as "fleas") or small metal bars that are inserted into the tube after collection of a CBG specimen to aid in mixing the anticoagulant.
- *Magnet:* Both ends of a CBG tube are sealed immediately after specimen collection to prevent exposure to air, and a magnet is used to mix the specimen. The magnet typically has an opening in the center or side so that it can be slipped over the capillary tube and moved back and forth along the tube length, pulling the metal stirrer with it, and mixing the anticoagulant into the blood specimen.
- *Plastic caps:* Plastic end caps or closures are used to seal CBG tubes and maintain anaerobic conditions in the specimen. CBG tubes typically come with their own caps.

MICROSCOPE SLIDES

Microscope slides are used to make blood films for hematology determinations. (See Chapter 7, General Blood Collection Equipment and Supplies.)

Warming Devices

Warming the site increases blood flow as much as seven times. This is especially important when performing heelsticks on newborns. Heel-warming devices (Fig. 10-6) are commercially available. To avoid burning the patient, the devices provide a uniform temperature that does not exceed 42°C. A towel or diaper dampened with warm tap water can also be used to wrap a hand or foot prior to skin puncture. However, care must be taken not to get the water so hot that it scalds the patient.

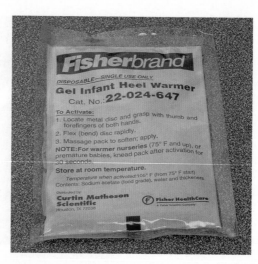

FIGURE 10-6
Infant heel warmer.

CAPILLARY PUNCTURE PRINCIPLES

Composition of Capillary Specimens

Capillary specimens are a mixture of arterial, venous, and capillary blood, along with **interstitial fluid** (fluid in the tissue spaces between the cells) and **intracellular fluid** (fluid within the cells) from the surrounding tissues. Because arterial blood enters the capillaries under pressure, capillary blood contains a higher proportion of arterial blood than venous blood and therefore more closely resembles arterial blood in composition. This is especially true if the area has been warmed, since warming increases arterial flow into the area.

Reference Values

Because the composition of capillary blood differs from that of venous blood, reference (normal) values may also differ. For example, the concentration of glucose is normally higher in capillary blood specimens, while total protein (TP), calcium (Ca^{2+}), and potassium (K^+), concentrations are lower.

key · point Although potassium values are normally lower in properly collected skin puncture specimens, levels may be falsely elevated if there is tissue fluid contamination or hemolysis of the specimen.

Indications for Capillary Puncture

A properly collected capillary specimen can be a practical alternative to venipuncture when small amounts of blood are acceptable for testing. Capillary puncture can be an appropriate choice for adults and older children under the following circumstances:

- There are no accessible veins
- Available veins are fragile or must be saved for other procedures such as chemotherapy

- The patient has thrombotic or clot-forming tendencies
- To obtain blood for POCT procedures such as glucose monitoring

Capillary puncture is the preferred method of obtaining blood from infants and very young children for the following reasons:

- Infants have a small blood volume; removing quantities of blood typical of venipuncture or arterial puncture can lead to anemia.
- Large quantities removed rapidly can cause cardiac arrest. Life is threatened if more than 10% of a patient's blood volume is removed at once or over a short period.
- Obtaining blood from infants and children by venipuncture is difficult and may damage veins and surrounding tissues.
- An infant or child can be injured by the restraining method used while performing a venipuncture.
- Capillary blood is the preferred specimen for some tests, such as newborn screening tests.

c a u t i o n   Capillary puncture is generally *not* appropriate for patients who are dehydrated or have poor circulation to the extremities from other causes such as shock, as specimens may be hard to obtain and may not be representative of blood elsewhere in the body.

Tests That Cannot Be Collected by Capillary Puncture

Although today's technology allows many tests to be performed on very small quantities of blood, and a wide selection of devices are available to make collection of skin puncture specimens relatively safe and easy, some tests cannot be performed on skin puncture specimens. These include most erythrocyte sedimentation rate methods, coagulation studies that require collection of a plasma specimen, blood cultures, and tests that require large volumes of serum or plasma.

Order of Draw

The order of draw for collecting multiple specimens by capillary puncture is not the same as for venipuncture. Puncturing the skin releases tissue thromboplastin, which activates the coagulation process in the blood drops. Specimens must be collected quickly to minimize the effects of platelet clumping and microclot formation and ensure that an adequate amount of specimen is collected before the site stops bleeding. Hematology specimens are collected first because they are most affected by the clotting process. Serum specimens are collected last because they are supposed to clot. The CLSI order of draw for capillary specimens is

- EDTA specimens
- Other additive specimens
- Serum specimens

CAPILLARY PUNCTURE STEPS

Capillary punctures have the same general steps regardless of whether they are fingersticks or heelsticks. The first four steps are the same as Chapter 5 venipuncture steps 1 through 4.

Step 1: Review and accession test request

Step 2: Approach, identify, and prepare patient

Step 3: Verify diet restrictions and latex sensitivity

Step 4: Sanitize hands and put on gloves

Step 5: Position Patient

Position is important to patient comfort and the success of specimen collection. For finger punctures, the patient's arm must be supported on a firm surface with the hand extended and palm up. A young child is typically held in the lap by a parent or guardian parent who restrains the child with one arm and holds the child's arm steady with the other. For heel punctures, an infant should be supine (lying face up) with the foot lower than the torso so the force of gravity can assist blood flow.

Step 6: Select the Puncture/Incision Site

General site selection criteria include one that is warm, pink or normal color, and free of scars, cuts, bruises, or rashes. It should not be **cyanotic** (bluish in color from lack of oxygen), edematous (swollen), or infected. Swollen or previously punctured sites should be avoided, as accumulated tissue fluid can contaminate the specimen and negatively affect test results. Specific locations for capillary puncture include fingers of adults and heels of infants.

key · point CLSI has deleted the great (big) toe as a recommended capillary collection site.

ADULTS AND OLDER CHILDREN

The CLSI recommended site for capillary puncture on adults and children over 1 year old is the palmar surface of the distal or end segment of the middle or ring finger of the nondominant hand. The puncture site should be in the central, fleshy portion of the finger, slightly to the side of center and perpendicular to the grooves in the **whorls** (spiral pattern) of the fingerprint (see Fig. 10-7). Finger puncture precautions are summarized and explained as follows:

- *Do not* collect blood from fingers on the same side as a mastectomy without consultation with the patient's physician.
- *Do not* puncture fingers of infants and children under the age of 1 year. The amount of tissue between skin surface and bone is so small that bone injury is very likely. Infection and gangrene have been identified as complications of finger punctures in newborns.

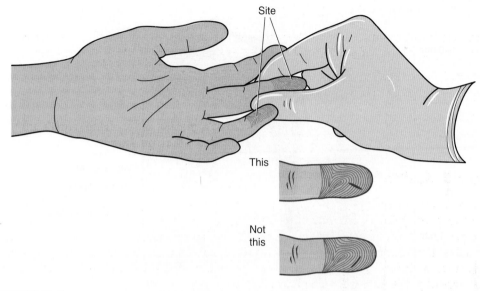

FIGURE 10-7
Recommended site and direction of finger puncture.

- *Do not* puncture the side or very tip of the finger. The distance between the skin surface and the bone is half as much at the side and tip as it is in the central portion of the end of the finger.
- *Do not* puncture the index finger. The index finger is more sensitive and can be calloused and harder to poke. Also, the patient will use that finger more and notice the pain longer.
- *Do not* puncture the fifth or little finger. The tissue between skin surface and bone is the thinnest in this finger, and bone injury is likely.
- *Do not* puncture the thumb. It has a pulse, indicating an artery in the puncture area, and the skin is generally thick and calloused, making it hard to obtain a good specimen.
- *Do not* puncture parallel to the grooves or lines of the fingerprint. A parallel puncture will allow blood to run down the finger rather than form a rounded drop, and make collection difficult.

INFANTS

The heel is the recommended site for collection of capillary puncture specimens on infants less than 1 year old. However, it is important to perform the puncture in an area of the heel where there is little risk of puncturing the bone. Puncture of the bone can cause painful **osteomyelitis** (os'te-o-mi'el-i'tis), inflammation of the bone marrow and adjacent bone, or **osteochondritis** (os'te-o-kon-dri'tis), inflammation of the bone and cartilage, as a result of

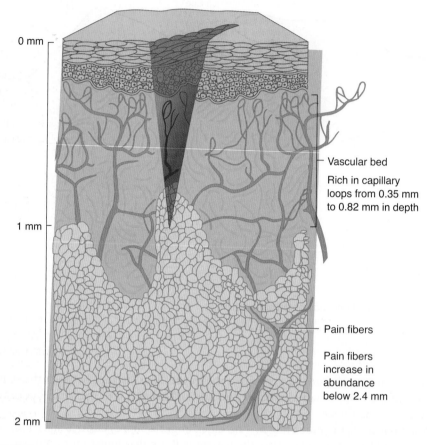

FIGURE 10-8

Cross section of full-term infant's heel showing lancet penetration depth needed to access the capillary bed.

infection. Additional punctures through a previous puncture site that is inflamed can spread an infection.

Studies have shown that the **calcaneus** (kal-ka'ne-us) or heel bone of small or premature infants may be as little as 2.0 mm below the skin surface on the plantar or bottom surface of the heel and half that distance at the **posterior curvature** (back) of the heel. Punctures deeper than this may cause bone damage. The vascular or capillary bed (see Fig. 10-8) in the skin of a newborn is located at the dermal–subcutaneous junction between 0.35 and 1.6 mm beneath the skin surface, so punctures 2.0 mm deep or less will provide adequate blood flow without risking bone injury. Pain fibers increase in abundance below the capillary bed, so deeper punctures are also more painful.

According to CLSI, to avoid puncturing bone the only safe areas for heel puncture are on the plantar surface of the heel, medial to an imaginary line extending from the middle of the great toe to the heel or lateral to an imaginary line extending from between the fourth

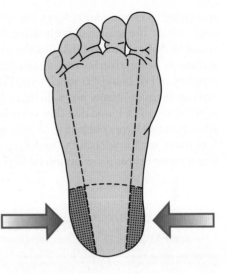

FIGURE 10-9

Infant heel. *Shaded areas indicated by arrows* represent recommended safe areas for heel puncture.

and fifth toes to the heel (see Fig. 10-9). Punctures in other areas risk bone, nerve, tendon, and cartilage injury.

> m e m o r y • j o g g e r   One way to remember that the safe areas for heel puncture are the medial or lateral plantar surfaces of the heel is to think of the phrase "Make little people happy." Using the first letter of each word, "M" stands for medial, "L" stands for lateral, "P" stands for plantar, and "H" stands for heel.

CLSI infant capillary puncture precautions are summarized as follows:

- *Do not* puncture earlobes.
- *Do not* puncture deeper than 2.0 mm. Deeper punctures risk injuring the bone, even in the safest puncture areas.
- *Do not* puncture through previous puncture sites. This can be painful and can spread previously undetected infection.
- *Do not* puncture the area between the imaginary boundaries. The calcaneus may be as little as 2.00 mm deep in this area.
- *Do not* puncture the posterior curvature of the heel, as the bone can be as little as 1 mm deep in this area.
- *Do not* puncture in the area of the arch and other areas of the foot other than the heel, as arteries, nerves, tendons, and cartilage may be injured.
- *Do not* puncture severely bruised areas. It is painful, and impaired circulation or byproducts of the healing process can negatively affect the specimen.

Step 7: Warm the Site if Applicable

Warming increases blood flow up to sevenfold and, except for PO_2 levels, does not significantly alter results of routinely tested analytes. Increased blood flow makes specimens easier and faster to obtain and reduces the tendency to compress or squeeze the site, which can contaminate the specimen with tissue fluid and hemolyze red blood cells. Because the increase is due to arterial flow into the area, a specimen obtained from a warmed site is described as being **arterialized**. Consequently, warming the site is essential when collecting capillary pH or blood gas specimens. Warming is typically recommended for heelstick procedures because infants normally have high red blood counts and other factors that result in relatively thick blood that flows slowly. Warming may also be required before fingersticks when patients have cold hands. Warming can be accomplished by wrapping the site for 3 to 5 minutes with a washcloth, towel, or diaper that has been moistened with comfortably warm water or using a commercial heel warming device.

> c a u t i o n The temperature of the material used to warm the site must not exceed 42°C (108°F), as higher temperatures can burn the skin, especially the delicate skin of an infant.

Step 8: Clean and Air-Dry Site

The collection site must be cleaned with an antiseptic prior to puncture, so that skin flora (microorganisms on the skin) do not infiltrate the puncture wound and cause infection. The CLSI- recommended antiseptic for cleaning a capillary puncture site is 70% isopropanol.

> c a u t i o n *Do not* use povidone-iodine to clean skin puncture sites because it greatly interferes with a number of tests, most notably uric acid, phosphorus, and potassium.

After cleaning, allow the site to air-dry to ensure maximum antiseptic action and minimize the chance of alcohol contamination of the specimen. Residual alcohol, in addition to causing a stinging sensation, causes rapid hemolysis of red blood cells. It has also been shown to interfere with glucose testing.

Step 9: Prepare Equipment

Gloves are put on at this point if not put on in step 4. Select collection devices according to the tests that have been ordered and place them within easy reach, along with several layers of gauze or gauze-type pads. Select a new, sterile lancet/incision device according to the site selected, age of the patient, and amount of blood to be collected. Prepare equipment in view of the patient or guardian to provide assurance that it is new and being handled aseptically. Verify lancet sterility by checking to see that packaging is intact before opening. Open the package or protective cover in an aseptic manner and do not allow the device opening to rest or brush against any nonsterile surface. If the lancet/incision device has a protective shield or locking feature that prevents accidental activation, remove or release it per manufacturer's instructions. Hold the device between the thumb and index fingers or as described by the manufacturer.

Step 10: Puncture the Site and Discard Lancet

FINGER PUNCTURE

Grasp the patient's finger between your nondominant thumb and index finger. Hold it securely in case of sudden movement. Place the lancet device flat against the skin in the central, fleshy pad of the finger, slightly to the side of center and perpendicular to the fingerprint whorls as described in step 6.

key • point With very young children it is usually best to grasp all four of their fingers between your fingers and thumb. If you grasp only one finger, the child may twist it trying to pull away. When holding all the fingers, it is easiest to puncture the middle finger, as it is normally the longest and sticks out farthest.

HEEL PUNCTURE

Grasp the foot gently but firmly with your nondominant hand. Encircle the heel by wrapping your index finger around the arch and your thumb around the bottom. Wrap the other fingers around the top of the foot. Place the lancet flat against the skin on the medial or lateral plantar surface of the heel.

BOTH FINGER PUNCTURE AND HEEL PUNCTURE

Use enough pressure to keep the device in place without deeply compressing the skin. Warn the patient (or patient's parent or guardian) of impending puncture, and activate the release mechanism to trigger the puncture. Remove the device from the skin immediately following puncture and discard it in a sharps container.

Step 11: Wipe Away the First Blood Drop

Position the site downward and apply gentle pressure toward the site to encourage blood flow. Wipe away the first drop of blood with a dry gauze pad. The first drop is normally contaminated with excess tissue fluid, and may contain alcohol residue that can keep the blood from forming a well-rounded drop and also hemolyze the specimen.

key • point Some POCT instruments may allow use of the first drop so follow manufacturer instructions.

Step 12: Fill and Mix Tubes/Containers in Order of Draw

Continue to position the site downward to enhance blood flow and apply gentle intermittent pressure to tissue surrounding a heel puncture site or proximal to a finger puncture site.

> c a u t i o n Do not use strong repetitive pressure or "milk" the site, as hemolysis and tissue fluid contamination of the specimen can result.

Collect subsequent blood drops using devices appropriate for the ordered tests. Collect slides, platelet counts, and other hematology specimens first to avoid the effects of platelet aggregation (clumping) and clotting. Collect other anticoagulant containers next, and serum specimens last according to the CLSI order of draw for capillary specimens explained above.

To fill a collection tube or device, touch it to the drop of blood formed on the surface of the skin.

- If making a blood film, touch the appropriate area of the slide to the blood drop.
- A microhematocrit or narrow-bore capillary tube will fill automatically by "capillary" action if held in a vertical position above, or a horizontal position beside, the blood drop while touching one end to the blood drop. While maintaining contact with the blood drop, the opposite end of the tube may need to be lowered slightly and brought back into position now and then as it fills. Do not remove the tube from the drop or continually hold or tip the tube below the site. This can result in air spaces in the specimen that cause inaccurate test results. When the tube is full, plug the opposite or dry end with clay or other suitable sealant.
- To fill a microcollection container or microtube, hold it upright just below the blood drop. Touch the tip of the tube's "scoop" to the drop of blood and allow the blood to run down the inside wall of the tube. The scoop should touch only the blood and not the surface of the skin. This allows blood to be collected before it runs down the surface of the finger or heel.

> c a u t i o n Do not use a scooping motion against the surface of the skin and attempt to collect blood as it flows down the finger. Scraping the scoop against the skin activates platelets, causing them to clump, and can also hemolyze the specimen.

You may need to tap microcollection tubes gently now and then to encourage the blood to settle to the bottom. When filled to an appropriate level, seal containers with the covers provided. Mix additive tubes by gently inverting them 8 to 10 times or per manufacturer's instructions.

Step 13: Place Gauze and Apply Pressure

After collecting specimens, apply pressure to the site with a clean gauze pad until bleeding stops. Keep the site elevated while applying pressure.

Step 14: Label Specimen and Observe Special Handling Instructions

Label the specimens with the appropriate information (see Chapter 8). Labels must be directly affixed to microcollection containers. Microhematocrit tubes can be placed in a non-additive tube or an appropriately sized aliquot tube and identifying information written on the label; or follow laboratory protocol. Follow any special handling required such as cooling in crushed ice (e.g., ammonia), transportation at body temperature (e.g., cold agglutinin), or light protection (e.g., bilirubin).

Step 15: Check the Site and Apply Bandage

The site must be examined to verify that bleeding has stopped. If bleeding persists beyond 5 minutes, notify the patient's nurse or physician. If bleeding has stopped and the patient is an older child or adult, apply a bandage and advise the patient to keep it in place for at least 15 minutes.

> c a u t i o n   *Do not* apply bandages to infants and children under 2 years old as they pose a choking hazard. In addition, bandage adhesive can stick to the paper-thin skin of newborns and tear it when the bandage is removed.

Step 16: Dispose of Used and Contaminated Materials

Equipment packaging and bandage wrappers are normally discarded in the regular trash. Some facilities require contaminated items such as blood-soaked gauze to be discarded in biohazard containers. Follow facility protocol.

Step 17: Thank Patient, Remove Gloves, and Sanitize Hands

Thanking the patient is courteous and professional. Gloves must be removed in an aseptic manner and hands washed or decontaminated with hand sanitizer as an infection control precaution.

Step 18: Transport Specimen to the Lab

Prompt delivery to the lab protects specimen integrity and is typically achieved by personal delivery, transportation via a pneumatic tube system, or a courier service.

FINGERSTICK PROCEDURES

Most capillary punctures are fingersticks. Fingerstick procedures are illustrated in Procedure 10-1.

PROCEDURE 10-1

Fingerstick Procedure

Purpose: To obtain a blood specimen for patient diagnosis or monitoring from a finger puncture

Equipment: Gloves; warming device (optional), antiseptic prep pad; safety finger puncture lancet, microcollection tubes or other appropriate collection devices; gauze pads; sharps container; permanent ink pen; bandage

Step	Explanation/Rationale
1–3. See Chapter 8 Venipuncture Steps 1 through 3	See Chapter 8 Procedure 8-2: steps 1 through 3
4. Sanitize hands and put on gloves	Proper hand hygiene plays a major role in infection control by protecting the phlebotomist, the patient, and others from contamination. Gloves are put on at this point
5. Position patient	The patient's arm must be supported on a firm surface with the hand extended and the palm up. A young child may have to be held on the lap and restrained by a parent or guardian
6. Select the puncture/incision site	Select a site in the central, fleshy portion and slightly to the side of center of a middle or ring finger that is warm, pink or normal color, and free of scars, cuts, bruises, infection, rashes, swelling, or previous punctures
7. Warm the site if applicable	Warming makes blood collection easier and faster, and reduces the tendency to squeeze the site. It is not normally part of a routine fingerstick unless the hand is cold, in which case, wrap it in a comfortably warm washcloth or towel for 3 to 5 minutes or use a commercial warming device
8. Clean and air-dry site	CLSI recommends 70% isopropanol for cleaning capillary puncture sites. Cleaning removes or inhibits skin flora that could infiltrate the puncture and cause infection. Letting the site dry naturally permits maximum antiseptic action, prevents contamination caused by wiping, and avoids stinging on puncture and specimen hemolysis from residual alcohol

PROCEDURE 10-1 *(Continued)*

Step	Explanation/Rationale
9. Prepare equipment	Select a fingerstick lancet according to the age of the patient and amount of blood to be collected. Verify lancet sterility by checking to see that packaging is intact before opening; open and handle aseptically to maintain sterility. Select collection devices according to the ordered tests. Place items within easy reach along with several layers of gauze or gauze-type pads. Remove or release any lancet locking mechanism and hold the lancet between the thumb and index finger or per manufacturer instructions
10. Puncture the site and discard lancet/incision device 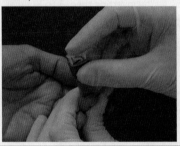	Grasp the patient's finger between your nondomi nant thumb and index finger, holding it securely in case of sudden movement. Place the lancet flat against the skin in the central, fleshy pad of the fin ger, slightly to the side of center to avoid bone injury and perpendicular to the fingerprint whorls so the blood will form easily collected drops and not run down the fingerprint. Warn the patient or parent/guardian, trigger the puncture, and discard the lancet in sharps container
11. Wipe away the first blood drop 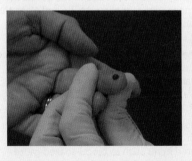 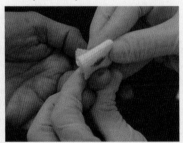	Apply gentle pressure until a blood drop forms, and use a clean gauze pad to wipe it away. This prevents contamination of the specimen with excess tissue fluid and rids the site of alcohol residue that could prevent formation of well-rounded drops and also hemolyze the specimen

(Continued)

Step	Explanation/Rationale
12. Fill and mix tubes/containers in order of draw	Collect subsequent blood drops using devices appropriate for the ordered tests and in the CLSI order of draw to minimize effects of clotting on specimens. Hold a microhematocrit tube above or beside the site and touch one end to the blood drop. You may need to lower the opposite end of the tube slightly as it fills but do not remove it from the drop as this creates air spaces in the specimen that compromise results. When the tube is full, plug the opposite or dry end with clay or other suitable sealant. Hold a microcollection tube below the blood drop. Touch the scoop to the blood drop and allow it to run down the inside wall of the tube. The tube may need a gentle tap occasionally to settle blood to the bottom. Seal tubes when full and mix additive tubes by gently inverting them 8 to 10 times.

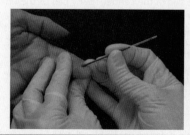 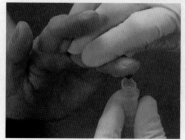

Step	Explanation/Rationale
13. Place gauze and apply pressure	Apply pressure with a clean gauze pad and elevate the site until bleeding stops
14. Label specimen and observe special handling instructions	Specimens must be labeled with the appropriate information (see Chapter 8). Affix labels directly to microcollection containers. Place microhematocrit tubes in a nonadditive or aliquot tube and place the label on this container. Follow any special handling required
15. Check the site and apply bandage	Examine the site to verify that bleeding has stopped, apply a bandage if the patient is an older child or adult, and advise patient to keep it in place for at least 15 minutes. If bleeding persists beyond 5 minutes, notify the patient's nurse or physician
16. Dispose of used and contaminated materials	Discard equipment packaging and bandage wrappers in the trash. Follow facility protocol for discarding contaminated items such as blood-soaked gauze
17. Thank patient, remove gloves, and sanitize hands	Thanking the patient is courteous and professional. Remove gloves aseptically and wash or decontaminate hands with sanitizer as an infection control precaution
18. Transport specimen to the lab	Prompt delivery to the lab is necessary to protect specimen integrity

HEELSTICK PROCEDURES

Heel punctures are performed on infants under 1 year of age. Heelstick procedure is illustrated in Procedure 10-2.

PROCEDURE 10-2

Heelstick Procedure

Purpose: To obtain a blood specimen for patient diagnosis or monitoring from a heel puncture

Equipment: Gloves; warming device, antiseptic prep pad; safety heel puncture lancet, microcollection tubes or other appropriate collection devices; gauze pads; sharps container; permanent ink pen

Step	Explanation/Rationale
1–3. See Chapter 8 venipuncture steps 1 through 3	See Chapter 8 Procedure 8-2: steps 1 through 3
4. Sanitize hands and put on gloves	Proper hand hygiene plays a major role in infection control by protecting the phlebotomist, the patient, and others from contamination. Gloves should be put on at this point
5. Position patient	For heel puncture an infant should be lying face up with the foot lower than the torso so gravity can assist blood flow
6. Select the puncture/incision site	Select a site on the medial or lateral plantar surface of the heel that is warm, normal color, and free of cuts, bruises, infection, rashes, swelling, or previous punctures
7. Warm the site if applicable	Warming makes blood collection easier and faster and reduces the tendency to squeeze the site. Warm the heel by wrapping it in a comfortably warm washcloth, towel, or diaper for 3 to 5 minutes or use a commercial heel-warming device
8. Clean and air-dry site	CLSI recommends 70% isopropanol for cleaning capillary puncture sites. Cleaning removes or inhibits skin flora that could infiltrate the puncture and cause infection. Letting the site dry naturally permits maximum antiseptic action, prevents contamination caused by wiping, and avoids stinging on puncture and specimen hemolysis from residual alcohol

(Continued)

PROCEDURE 10-2   *(Continued)*

Step	Explanation/Rationale
9. Prepare equipment	Select a heel puncture device. Verify packaging is intact to assure sterility. Open and handle aseptically to maintain sterility. Select blood collection devices according to the ordered tests. Place items within easy reach along with several layers of sterile gauze. Release any locking mechanism, and hold the lancet between the thumb and index finger

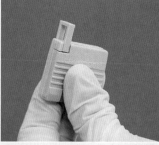

Step	Explanation/Rationale
10. Puncture site and discard lancet/incision device	Grasp the foot gently, but firmly with your nondominant hand. Encircle the heel with your index finger around the arch, thumb around the bottom, and other fingers around the top of the foot. Place the lancet flat against the skin on the medial or lateral plantar surface of the heel, using enough pressure to keep it in place without deeply compressing the skin. Trigger the puncture, and discard the lancet in a sharps container

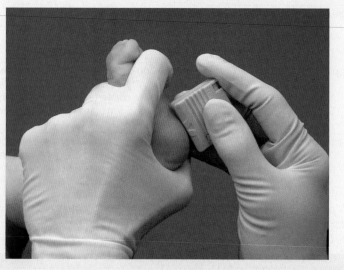

PROCEDURE 10-2   *(Continued)*

Step	Explanation/Rationale
11. Wipe away the first blood drop	Position the foot downward and apply gentle pressure to the site to encourage blood flow. Wipe away the first blood drop with a gauze pad to prevent contamination of the specimen with excess tissue fluid and rid the site of alcohol residue that could prevent formation of well-rounded drops and also hemolyze the specimen
12. Fill and mix tubes/containers in order of draw	Collect subsequent blood drops using appropriate devices for the ordered tests and fill them in the same manner described in fingerstick procedure step 12. Follow CLSI order of draw for capillary specimens to minimize effects of clotting
13. Place gauze and apply pressure	Apply pressure with a clean gauze pad and elevate the foot until bleeding stops
14. Label specimen and observe special handling instructions	Specimens must be labeled with the appropriate ID information (see Chapter 8). Affix labels directly to microcollection containers. Place microhematocrit tubes in a nonadditive or aliquot tube and place the label on this container. Follow any special handling required
15. Check the site	Examine the site to verify that bleeding has stopped. If bleeding persists beyond 5 minutes, notify the patient's nurse or physician. Do not apply a bandage to an infant as it can become a choking hazard and can also tear the skin when removed
16. Dispose of used and contaminated materials	Discard equipment packaging and bandage wrappers in the trash. Follow facility protocol for discarding contaminated items such as blood-soaked gauze
17. Thank parent or guardian, remove gloves, and sanitize hands	Thanking the parent or guardian is courteous and professional. Remove gloves aseptically and wash or decontaminate hands with sanitizer as an infection control precaution
18. Transport specimen to the lab	Prompt delivery to the lab is necessary to protect specimen integrity

SPECIAL CAPILLARY PUNCTURE PROCEDURES

Capillary Blood Gases

Capillary puncture blood is less desirable for blood gas analysis because of its partial arterial composition to begin with and because it is temporarily exposed to air during collection, which can alter test results. Consequently, **capillary blood gas specimens** (CBGs) are rarely collected on adults. However, because arterial punctures can be hazardous to infants and young children, blood gas analysis on these patients is sometimes performed on capillary specimens.

CBG specimens are collected from the same sites as routine capillary puncture specimens. Warming the site for 5 to 10 minutes prior to collection is necessary to increase blood flow and arterialize the specimen. Proper collection technique is essential to minimize exposure of the specimen to air. Collection of a capillary blood gas specimen by heel puncture is illustrated in Procedure 10-3.

PROCEDURE 10-3

Collection of a Capillary Blood Gas (CBG) Specimen by Heel Puncture

Purpose: To obtain a specimen for blood gas analysis by capillary puncture

Equipment: Gloves, warming device, antiseptic prep pad, safety lancet, special capillary tube with caps, metal filings (fleas) or stirrer bar, magnet, sterile gauze pads; sharps container; permanent ink pen

Step	Explanation/Rationale
1–6. Same as routine heelstick procedures	See capillary puncture steps 1 through 6
7. Warm the site	Warming the site is required to arterialize the specimen. It also makes blood collection easier and faster and reduces the tendency to squeeze the site. Warm the heel by wrapping it in a comfortably warm washcloth, towel, or diaper for 3 to 5 minutes or use a commercial heel-warming device
8. Clean and air-dry site	CLSI recommends cleaning a heel puncture site with 70% isopropanol to remove or inhibit skin flora that could infiltrate the puncture and cause infection. Letting the site dry naturally permits maximum antiseptic action, prevents contamination caused by wiping, and avoids stinging on puncture and specimen hemolysis from residual alcohol
9. Prepare equipment	Place a metal stirrer bar or fleas in the capillary tube to help mix the specimen during collection. Place tube caps and magnet within easy reach along with several layers of sterile gauze. Select, open, prepare, and hold a sterile puncture device as described in Heelstick Procedure 10-2 step 9
10. Puncture site and discard lancet	Grasp the heel and puncture the site as described in Heelstick Procedure 10-2 step 10. Immediately discard the puncture device

PROCEDURE 10-3   *(Continued)*

Step	Explanation/Rationale
11. Wipe away the first drop of blood	Wiping the first drop removes excess tissue fluid and alcohol residue that could affect test results
12. Fill the capillary tube with blood	Collect the specimen quickly to minimize exposure of the blood drops to air and carefully to prevent introduction of air spaces in the tube. The tube must be completely full with no air spaces or results will be inaccurate
13. Immediately cap both ends of the tube	The tube must be sealed as soon as possible to prevent exposure to air and protect blood gas composition
14. Mix the specimen with the magnet	Run the magnet back and forth the full length of the tube several times. The magnet pulls the metal stirrer or fleas with it, mixing the blood with the heparin and preventing clotting
15. Label the tube	Specimens must be labeled with the appropriate ID information
16. Place tube in ice slurry	Place the tube horizontally in ice slurry. Cooling slows WBC metabolism and prevents changes in pH and blood gas values
17. Check the puncture site	Examine the site to verify that bleeding has stopped. If bleeding persists beyond 5 minutes, notify the patient's nurse or physician. Do not apply a bandage to an infant as it can become a choking hazard and can also tear the skin when removed
18. Dispose of used and contaminated materials	Discard equipment packaging and bandage wrappers in the trash. Follow facility protocol for discarding contaminated items such as blood-soaked gauze
19. Thank parent or guardian, remove gloves, and sanitize hands	Thanking the parent or guardian is courteous and professional. Remove gloves aseptically and wash or decontaminate hands with sanitizer as an infection control precaution
20. Transport specimen to the lab	Prompt delivery to the lab is necessary to protect specimen integrity

Neonatal Bilirubin Collection

Neonates (newborns) are commonly tested to detect and monitor increased bilirubin levels caused by overproduction or impaired excretion of bilirubin. Overproduction of bilirubin occurs from accelerated red blood cell hemolysis associated with hemolytic disease of the newborn (HDN). Impaired bilirubin excretion often results from temporary abnormal liver function commonly associated with premature infants. High levels of bilirubin result in jaundice (yellow skin color).

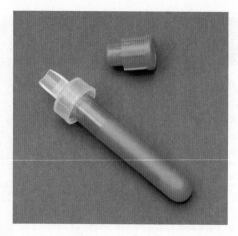

FIGURE 10-10

Amber-colored microcollection container used to protect a bilirubin specimen from effects of ultraviolet light.

Bilirubin can cross the blood–brain barrier in infants, accumulating to toxic levels that can cause permanent brain damage or even death. A transfusion may be needed if levels increase at a rate equal to or greater than 5.0 mg/dL per hour or when levels exceed 18.0 mg/dL. Bilirubin breaks down in the presence of light. Consequently, jaundiced infants are often placed under special ultraviolet (UV) lights to lower bilirubin levels.

caution   The UV light must be turned off when collecting a bilirubin specimen to prevent it from breaking down bilirubin in the specimen as it is collected.

Proper collection of bilirubin specimens is crucial to the accuracy of results. Specimens are normally collected by heel puncture. They must be collected quickly to minimize exposure to light and must be protected from light during transportation and handling. Specimens are often collected in amber-colored microcollection containers (Fig. 10-10) to reduce light exposure. Specimens must be collected carefully to avoid hemolysis, which could falsely decrease bilirubin results. Because determination of the rate of increase in bilirubin levels depends on accurate timing, specimens should be collected as close as possible to the time requested.

Newborn/Neonatal Screening

Newborn/neonatal screening is the routine testing of newborns for the presence of certain genetic (inherited), metabolic (chemical changes within living cells), hormonal, and functional disorders that can cause severe mental handicaps or other serious abnormalities if not detected and treated early. Some states also screen for infectious agents such as toxoplasma and HIV. Screening for **phenylketonuria (PKU)**, **galactosemia**, and **hypothyroidism** is required by law in all 50 states and U.S. territories. The number and type of other newborn screening tests varies by state. The March of Dimes recommends that all newborns be screened for 29 specific disorders, including hearing loss, for which there is effective treatment (see Table 10-1).

TABLE 10-1   March of Dimes Recommended Newborn Screening Tests by Category

Disorder Category	Description	Consequence if Untreated	Screening Tests
Organic acid metabolism disorders	Inherited disorders resulting from inactivity of an enzyme involved in the breakdown, of amino acids and other body substances such as lipids, sugars, and steroids	Toxic acids build up in the body and can lead to coma and death within the first month of life	IVA (isovaleric acidemia) GA I (glutaric acidemia) HMG (3-OH,3-CH₃-glutaric aciduria) MCD (multiple carboxylase deficiency) MUT (methylmalonic acidemia from mutase deficiency) Cbl A, B (methylmalonic acidemia) 3MCC (3-methylcrotonyl-CoA carboxylase deficiency) PROP (propionic acidemia) BKT (beta-ketothiolase deficiency)
Fatty acid oxidation disorders	Disorders involving inherited defects in enzymes that are needed to convert fat into energy	The body is unable to produce alternate fuel when it runs out of glucose as can happen with illness or skipping meals. Glucose deprivation negatively affects the brain and other organs, and can lead to coma and death	MCAD (medium-chain acyl-CoA dehydrogenase deficiency) VLCAD (very long-chain acyl-CoA dehydrogenase deficiency) LCHAD (long-chain L-3-OH-acyl-CoA dehydrogenase deficiency) TFP (trifunctional protein deficiency) CUD (carnitine uptake defect)
Amino acid metabolism disorders	A diverse group of disorders. Some involve lack of an enzyme needed to breakdown an amino acid. Others involve deficiencies of enzymes that aid in the elimination of nitrogen from amino acid molecules	Toxic levels of amino acids or ammonia can build up in the body, causing a variety of symptoms and even death. Severity of symptoms varies by disorder	PKU (phenylketonuria) MSUD (maple syrup urine disease) HCY (homocystinuria) CIT (citrullinemia) ASA (argininosuccinic acidemia) TYR I (tyrosinemia type I)
Hemoglo-binopathies	Inherited disorders of the red blood cells that result in varying degrees of anemia and other health problems	Anemias that vary in severity by disorder and by individual	Hb SS (sickle cell anemia) Hb S/Th (hemoglobin S/beta thalassemia) Hb S/C (hemoglobin S/C disease)

Disorder Category	Description	Consequence if Untreated	Screening Tests
Others	Mixed group of inherited and noninherited disorders	Severity varies from mild to life threatening, depending on the disorder	CH (congenital hypothyroidism) BIOT (biotinidase deficiency) CAH (congenital adrenal hyperplasia due to 21-hydroxylase deficiency) GALT (classical galactosemia) HEAR (hearing loss) CF (cystic fibrosis)

TABLE 10-1 *(Continued)*

Most newborn screening tests are ideally performed when an infant is between 24 and 72 hours old. Because of early hospital release some infants are tested before they are 24 hours old. Early testing for some tests such as PKU may not give accurate results, so some states require repeat testing approximately 2 weeks later. On-line information on newborn screening can be found at the National Newborn Screening and Genetic Resource Center at www.genes-r-us.uthscsa.edu/.

c a u t i o n   If an infant requires a blood transfusion, newborn screening samples should be collected before it is started, as dilution of the sample with donor cells invalidates test results.

PHENYLKETONURIA

Phenylketonuria (PKU) is a genetic disorder characterized by a defect in the enzyme that breaks down the amino acid phenylalanine, converting it into the amino acid tyrosine. Without intervention, phenylalanine, which is in almost all food, accumulates in the blood and is only slowly metabolized by an alternate pathway that results in increased phenylketones in the urine. PKU cannot be cured but it can normally be treated with a diet low in phenylalanine. If left untreated or not treated early on, phenylalanine can rise to toxic levels and lead to brain damage and mental retardation. PKU testing typically requires the collection of two specimens, one shortly after an infant is born and another after the infant is 10 to 15 days old. The incidence of PKU in the United States is approximately 1 in 10,000 to 25,000 births.

HYPOTHYROIDISM

Hypothyroidism is a disorder that is characterized by insufficient levels of thyroid hormones. If left untreated, the deficiency hinders growth and brain development. Some forms of neonatal hypothyroidism are not inherited but temporarily acquired when the mother has the condition. Newborn screening tests detect both inherited and noninherited forms.

In the United States and Canada, the newborn screening test for hypothyroidism measures total thyroxine (T_4). Positive results are confirmed by measuring thyroid-stimulating hormone (TSH) levels. The disorder is treated by supplying the missing thyroid hormone orally. The incidence of hypothyroidism is 1 in 4000 births.

GALACTOSEMIA

Galactosemia is an inherited disorder characterized by lack of the enzyme needed to convert the milk sugar galactose into glucose needed by the body for energy. Within a week of birth, an infant with galactosemia will fail to thrive due to anorexia, diarrhea, and vomiting unless galactose and lactose (lactose breaks down to galactose and glucose) are removed from the diet. Untreated, the infant may starve to death. Untreated infants that survive typically fail to grow, are mentally handicapped, and have cataracts. Treatment involves removing all milk and dairy products from the infant's diet. Several less severe forms of galactosemia that may not need treatment can also be detected by newborn screening. The incidence of galactosemia is 1 in 60,000 to 80,000 births.

BLOOD SPOT COLLECTION

All newborn screening tests except hearing tests are typically performed on a few drops of blood obtained by heel puncture. The blood drops are collected by absorption onto circles printed on a special type of filter paper that is typically part of the test requisition (Fig. 10-11). The blood-filled circles are referred to as blood spots.

fyi New laboratory techniques can screen for as many as 30 different disorders in the blood spots on one requisition.

To fill the circles, heel puncture is performed, and the first blood drop is wiped away in the normal manner. The filter paper is brought close to the heel, and a large drop of free flowing blood is applied to the center of the first circle on the printed side of the paper. The paper must not be allowed to touch the surface of the heel. This can result in smearing, blotting and stoppage of blood flow, and incomplete penetration of blood through the paper. The original position of the paper must be maintained and blood must continue flowing until it completely fills the circle on both sides of the paper. The same process is continued until all circles are filled. Unfilled or incompletely filled circles can result in inability to perform all required tests. Circles must be filled from one side of the paper only and by one large drop that spreads throughout the circle. Application of multiple drops or filling circles from both sides of the paper causes layering of blood and possible misinterpretation of results.

caution Do not contaminate the filter paper circles by touching them with or without gloves or allowing any other object or substance to touch them before, during, or after specimen collection. Substances that have been identified as contaminants in newborn screening specimens include alcohol, formula, lotion, powder, and urine.

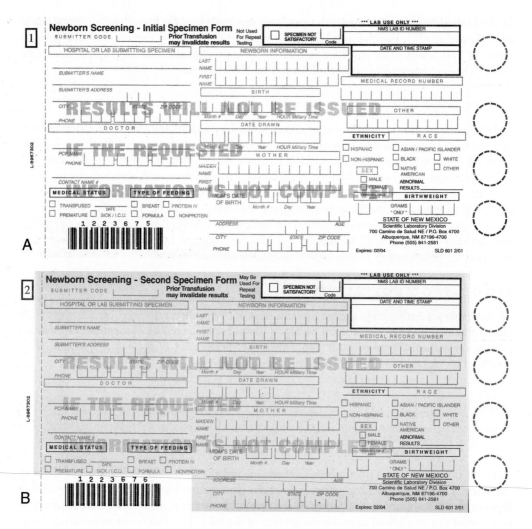

FIGURE 10-11

Newborn screening specimen form. (Courtesy Daniel Gray, State of New Mexico Scientific Laboratory, Albuquerque, NM.)

After collection, the specimen must be allowed to air-dry in an elevated horizontal position away from heat or sunlight. Specimens should not be hung to dry or stacked together before or after the drying process. Hanging may cause the blood to migrate and concentrate toward the low end of the filter paper and lead to erroneous test results on the sample. Stacking can result in cross-contamination between specimens, which also causes erroneous results. When dry, the requisition containing the sample is normally placed in a special envelope and sent to a state public health laboratory or other approved laboratory for testing. Results are sent to the infant's physician or other healthcare provider. The procedure for collecting blood spots for newborn screening is shown in Procedure 10-4.

PROCEDURE 10-4

Newborn Screening Blood Spot Collection

Purpose: To obtain a newborn screening blood sample by heel puncture

Equipment: Gloves, warming device, antiseptic prep pad, safety lancet, newborn screening filter paper, sterile gauze pads; sharps container; permanent ink pen

Step	Explanation/Rationale
1–4. Follow Chapter 8 venipuncture steps 1 through 4	See Chapter 8 Procedure 8-2: steps 1 through 4
5. Position patient	See Heelstick Procedure 10-2: step 5
6. Select the puncture/incision site	See Heelstick Procedure 10-2: step 6
7. Warm the site if applicable	See Heelstick Procedure 10-2: step 7
8. Clean and air-dry site	See Heelstick Procedure 10-2: step 8
9. Prepare equipment	See Heelstick Procedure 10-2: step 9
10. Puncture site and discard lancet	See Heelstick Procedure 10-2: step 10
11. Wipe away the first blood drop	See Heelstick Procedure 10-2: step 11
12. Bring the filter paper close to the heel	Ensures that drops fill the circles properly. The paper must not actually touch the heel or smearing, incomplete penetration of the paper, blotting, and stoppage of blood flow can result
13. Generate a large, free-flowing drop of blood	It takes a large, free-flowing blood drop to fill a circle. Small drops can result in incomplete filling and the tendency to layer successive drops in a circle to fill it
14. Touch the blood drop to the center of the filter paper circle	The drop must touch the center of the circle for blood to uniformly spread out to the perimeter
15. Fill the circle with blood	Blood drop position is maintained until blood soaks through the circle, completely filling both sides of the paper. Do not fill spots from the reverse side to finish filling the circles as this causes layering and erroneous results
16. Fill remaining blood spot circles	Fill all circles the same way. Unfilled or incompletely filled circles can result in inability to perform all required tests
17. Place gauze and apply pressure	Apply pressure with a clean gauze pad and elevate the site until bleeding stops
18. Label specimen	Specimens must be appropriately identified
19. Check the site	Check the site to verify that bleeding has stopped, but do not apply a bandage as it can become a choking hazard and can also tear the skin when removed

(Continued)

PROCEDURE 10-4 *(Continued)*

Step	Explanation/Rationale
20. Dispose of used materials	Equipment packaging and bandage wrappers can be discarded in the trash. Follow facility protocol for discarding contaminated items such as blood-soaked gauze
21. Allow the specimen to air-dry	The specimen must be allowed to air-dry in an elevated horizontal position away from heat or sunlight. It should not be hung to dry or stacked with other specimens before or after the drying process. Hanging causes blood to migrate to the low end of the filter paper and leads to erroneous test results
22. Dispatch specimen to testing facility	When dry, the sample-containing requisition is normally placed in a special envelope and sent to the appropriate laboratory for testing

Routine Blood Film/Smear Preparation

A **blood film** or **smear** (a drop of blood spread thin on a microscope slide) is required to perform a manual **differential** (Diff), a test in which the number, type, and characteristics of blood cells are determined by examining a stained blood smear under a microscope. A manual differential may be performed as part of a complete blood count or to confirm abnormal results of a machine-generated differential or platelet count. Two blood smears are normally prepared and submitted for testing. Although a common practice in the past, today blood smears are rarely made at the bedside. They are typically made in the hematology department from blood collected in an EDTA tube, either by hand or using an automated machine that makes a uniform smear from a single drop of blood.

key·point Blood smears prepared from EDTA specimens should be made within 1 hour of collection to eliminate cell distortion caused by the anticoagulant.

A few special tests require evaluation of a blood smear made from a fresh drop of blood from a fingertip. An example is a leukocyte alkaline phosphatase (LAP) stain or score, which usually requires four fresh peripheral blood (blood from an extremity) smears. Skin puncture collection of peripheral smears is typically preferred. In addition, some hematologists prefer blood smears made from blood that has not been in contact with EDTA.

When collected with other skin puncture specimens, blood smears should be collected first to avoid effects of platelet clumping. Blood smear preparation from a capillary puncture is illustrated in Procedure 10-5.

Preparing a Blood Smear From a Capillary Puncture.

Purpose: To prepare two routine blood films (smears) for hematology or other studies using blood obtained by capillary puncture

Equipment: Gloves, alcohol prep pad, lancet/incision device, 2 plain or frosted glass slides free of cracks or chipped edges, gauze pads, bandage, and a pencil

Step	Explanation/Rationale
1. Perform capillary puncture	Blood to make the slide can be obtained by normal finger or heel puncture, following capillary puncture steps 1 through 9 until this point
2. Wipe away first blood drop	Wiping the first drop removes excess tissue fluid and alcohol residue that could distort cell morphology
3. Touch a slide the next blood drop 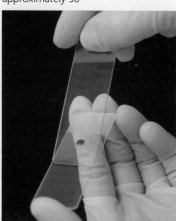	The drop should be 1 to 2 mm in diameter and centered on the slide adjacent to the frosted end or 1/2 to 1 inch from one end of a plain slide
4. Hold the blood drop slide between the thumb and forefinger of the nondominant hand. With the other hand, rest the second slide in front of the drop at an angle of approximately 30°	The second slide is called the pusher or spreader slide and is held at one end, between the thumb and index finger in either a vertical or horizontal position. If blood is of normal thickness, a 30° angle will create a smear that covers approximately 3/4 of the remaining area of slide

(Continued)

PROCEDURE 10-5 *(Continued)*

Step	Explanation/Rationale
5. Pull the spreader slide back to the edge of the blood drop. Stop it as soon as it touches the drop, and allow the blood to spread along its width 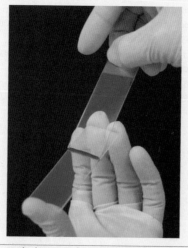	The blood must spread the width of the pusher slide or a bullet-shaped film will result
6. Push the spreader slide away from the drop in one smooth motion, carrying it the entire length and off the end of the blood drop slide 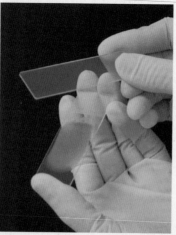	Let the weight of the spreader slide carry the blood and create the film or smear. *Do not* push down on the spreader slide as this creates lines and ridges and an unacceptable blood film

PROCEDURE 10-5 *(Continued)*

Step	Explanation/Rationale
7. Place the drop of blood for the second smear on the spreader slide. Use the slide with the first smear as the spreader slide for the second smear and make it in the same manner as the first one	This way, two smears can be made using only two slides
8. Place gauze over the wound and ask the patient to apply pressure	A conscious, mentally alert patient can apply pressure. Otherwise the phlebotomist must apply pressure
9. Label frosted blood slides by writing the patient information in pencil on the frosted area. If using a preprinted label, attach it over the writing or in the empty space at the blood drop end if it is a plain slide	*Do not* use ink as it may dissolve during the staining process
10. Allow the blood films to dry naturally and place them in a secondary container for transport	*Never* blow on a slide to dry it as red blood cell distortion may result. Be aware that unfixed slides are capable of transmitting disease and handle accordingly
11. Thank patient, remove gloves, and sanitize hands	Thanking the patients, parents and guardians is courteous and professional. Remove gloves aseptically and wash hands or use a hand sanitizer as an infection control precaution
12. Transport specimen to the lab	Prompt delivery to the lab is necessary to protect specimen integrity

To manually prepare a smear from an EDTA specimen the tube of blood must first be mixed for a minimum of 2 minutes to ensure a uniform specimen. A plain capillary tube or pipet is then used to dispense a drop of blood from the specimen tube onto the slide. A device called DIFF-SAFE (Fig. 10-12A–C) (Alpha Scientific, Malvern, PA) allows a slide to be made from an EDTA tube without removing the tube stopper. The device is inserted through the rubber stopper of the specimen tube and then pressed against the slide to deliver a uniform drop of blood.

c a u t i o n   Blood smears are considered biohazardous or infectious until they are stained or fixed.

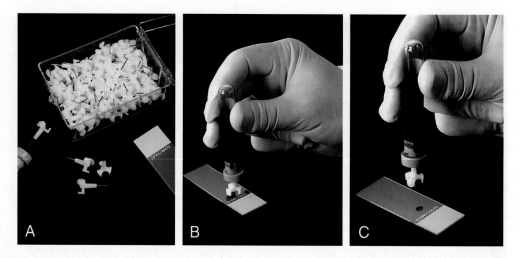

FIGURE 10-12

A. DIFF-SAFE blood drop delivery device. **B.** Applying a blood drop to a slide using a DIFF-SAFE device.
C. Blood drop on slide.   (Courtesy Alpha Scientific, Malvern, PA.)

Making a good blood smear is a skill that takes practice to perfect. Improperly made blood smears may not contain a normal, even distribution of blood cells and can produce erroneous results. An acceptable smear covers about 1/2 to 3/4 of the surface of the slide and has no holes, lines, or jagged edges. It should show a smooth transition from thick to thin when held up to the light. The thinnest area of a properly made smear, often referred to as the **feather**, is one cell thick and is the most important area because that is where a differential is performed.

Smears that are uneven, too long (i.e., cover the entire length of the slide), too short, too thick, or too thin are not acceptable. The length and thickness of the smear can usually be controlled by adjusting the size of the drop or the angle of the spreader slide. Dirt, fingerprints, or powder on the slide, or fat globules and lipids in the specimen can result in holes in the smear. A chipped pusher slide, a blood drop that has started to dry out, or uneven pressure as the smear is made can cause the smear to have ragged edges. Table 10-2 lists common problems associated with routine blood smear preparation.

Thick Blood Smear Preparation

Thick blood smears are most often requested to detect the presence of malaria, a disorder caused by four species of parasitic sporozoan (types of protozoa) organisms called plasmodia. These organisms are transmitted to humans by the bite of infected female anopheles mosquitoes. Symptoms of malaria include serial bouts of fever and chills at regular intervals, related to the multiplication of certain forms of the organism within the red blood cells and the consequent rupture of those cells. The progressive destruction of red blood cells in certain types of malaria causes severe anemia.

TABLE 10-2   Common Problems Associated with Routine Blood Smear Preparation

Problem	Probable Cause
Absence of feather	Spreader slide lifted before the smear was completed
Holes in the smear	Dirty slide
	Fat globules in the blood
	Blood contaminated with glove powder
Ridges or uneven thickness	Too much pressure applied to spreader slide
Smear is too thick	Blood drop too large
	Spreader slide angle too steep
	Patient has high red blood cell count
Smear is too short	Blood drop too small
	Spreader slide angle too steep
	Spreader slide pushed too quickly
	Patient has high red blood cell count
Smear is too long	Blood drop too large
	Spreader slide angle too shallow
	Spreader slide pushed too slowly
	Patient has a low hemoglobin
Smear too thin	Blood drop too small
	Spreader slide angle too shallow
	Patient has a low hemoglobin
Streaks or tails in feathered edge	Blood drop started to dry out
	Edge of spreader slide dirty or chipped
	Spreader slide pushed through blood drop
	Uneven pressure applied to spreader slide

Malaria is diagnosed by the presence of the organism in a peripheral blood smear. Diagnosis often requires the evaluation of both regular and thick blood smears. Presence of the organism is observed most frequently in a thick smear; however identification of the species requires evaluation of a regular blood smear. Malaria smears may be ordered stat or at timed intervals and are most commonly collected just prior to the onset of fever and chills.

To prepare a thick smear, a very large drop of blood is placed in the center of a glass slide and spread with the corner of another slide or cover slip until it is the size of a dime. The smear is allowed to dry for a minimum of 2 hours before staining with fresh diluted Giemsa stain, a water-based stain that lyses the red blood cells and makes the organism easier to see.

STUDY & REVIEW QUESTIONS

1. **Which of the following tests requires an arterialized specimen?**
   a. Bilirubin
   b. CBGs
   c. Electrolytes
   d. Glucose

2. **Skin puncture supplies include all of the following except**
   a. Gauze pad
   b. Lancet
   c. Microcollection device
   d. Povidone-iodine pad

3. **Skin puncture blood contains**
   a. Arterial blood
   b. Interstitial fluids
   c. Venous blood
   d. All of the above

4. **The concentration of this substance is higher in capillary blood than in venous blood**
   a. Blood urea nitrogen
   b. Carotene
   c. Glucose
   d. Total protein

5. **Skin puncture is typically performed on adults when**
   a. Patients have thrombotic tendencies
   b. There are no accessible veins
   c. Veins need to be saved for other procedures
   d. All of the above

6. **If collected by capillary puncture, which test specimen is collected first?**
   a. CBC
   b. Electrolytes
   c. Glucose
   d. Phosphorus

7. **Which of the following conditions disqualifies a site for capillary puncture?**
   a. Cyanotic
   b. Edematous
   c. Swollen
   d. All of the above

8. **The least hazardous area of an infant's foot for capillary puncture is the**
   a. Arch
   b. Central area of the heel
   c. Medial or lateral plantar surface of the heel
   d. Posterior curvature of the heel

9. **According to CLSI, a heel puncture lancet should not puncture deeper than**
   a. 1.5 mm
   b. 2.0 mm
   c. 2.5 mm
   d. 3.0 mm

10. **Which of the following is a proper skin puncture procedure?**
    a. Clean the site thoroughly with povidone-iodine
    b. Milk the site to keep the blood flowing freely
    c. Puncture parallel to the grooves of the fingerprint
    d. Wipe away the first drop of blood

11. **When making a routine blood smear, the "pusher slide" is normally used at an angle of**
    a. 15°   c. 45°
    b. 30°   d. 60°

12. **The blood specimen for this test is placed in circles on special filter paper**
    a. Bilirubin   c. PKU
    b. CBGs   d. Malaria

CASE · STUDY · 10-1

Capillary Puncture Procedure

A phlebotomist is sent to collect a CBC specimen on a 5-year-old pediatric patient. The patient has an IV in the left forearm. The right arm has no palpable veins so the phlebotomist decides to perform skin puncture on the middle finger of the right hand. This is the phlebotomist's first job, and although he is quite good at routine venipuncture, he has not performed very many skin punctures. The child is uncooperative and the mother tries to help steady the child's hand during the procedure. The phlebotomist is able to puncture the site, but the child pulls the hand away. Blood runs down the finger. The phlebotomist grabs the child's finger and tries to fill the collection device with the blood as it runs down the finger. The child continues to try to wriggle the finger free. The phlebotomist finally fills the container to the minimum level. When the specimen is tested, the platelet count is abnormally low. A slide is made and platelet clumping is observed. A new specimen is requested. Hemolysis is later observed in the specimen.

QUESTIONS
1. How might the circumstances of collection have contributed to the platelet clumping in the specimen?
2. What most likely caused the hemolysis?
3. What factors may have contributed to the specimen collection difficulties?

Bibliography and Suggested Readings

Bishop, M. L., Duben-Engelkirk, J. L., & Fody, E. P. (2001). Clinical chemistry: principles, procedures, correlations (4th ed). Philadelphia: Lippincott Williams & Wilkins.

Fischbach, F. (2003). A manual of laboratory & diagnostic tests (7th ed). Philadelphia: Lippincott Williams & Wilkins.

Harmening, D. (2002). Clinical hematology and fundamentals of hemostasis (4th ed). Philadelphia: FA Davis.

Joint Commission on the Accreditation of Healthcare Organizations, 2002-2003. (2002). Comprehensive accreditation manual for pathology and clinical laboratory sciences. Joint Commission Resources. Oakbrook Terrace, IL: JCAHO.

Lotspeich-Steininger, C. A., Stiene-Martin, E. A., & Koepke, J. A. (1998). Clinical hematology: principles, procedure, correlations (2nd ed). Philadelphia: Lippincott-Raven.

National Committee for Clinical Laboratory Standards LA4-A4. (2003). Blood collection on filter paper for newborn screening programs; approved standard (4th ed). Wayne, PA: CLSI/NCCLS.

National Committee for Clinical Laboratory Standards, H-18A3. (2004). Procedures for the handling and processing of blood specimens: approved guideline. Wayne, PA: CLSI/NCCLS.

National Committee for Clinical Laboratory Standards, H4-A5. (2004). Procedures and devices for the collection of diagnostic capillary blood specimens; approved standard-(5th ed). Wayne, PA. CLSI/NCCLS.

IV

Special Procedures

SPECIAL COLLECTIONS AND POINT-OF-CARE TESTING

key·terms

ACT	ETOH	lookback
aerobic	FAN	lysis
agglutination	FUO	Na$^+$
anaerobic	GTT	NIDA
ARD	HCG	peak level
autologous donation	HMT	POCT
bacteremia	hyper/hypoglycemia	PP
BT	hyper/hypokalemia	septicemia
chain of custody	hyper/hyponatremia	TDM
Cl$^-$	iCa^{2+}	TnI
compatibility	INR	TnT
drug screening	K$^+$	trough level

objectives

Upon successful completion of this chapter, the reader should be able to:

1. Define the key terms and abbreviations at the beginning of this chapter.

2. Explain the principle behind each special collection procedure, identify the steps involved, and list any special supplies or equipment required.

3. Describe patient identification and specimen labeling procedures required for blood bank tests, and identify the types of specimens typically required.

4. Describe sterile technique in blood culture collection, explain why it is important, and list the reasons why a physician might order blood cultures.

5. List examples of coagulation specimens and describe how to properly collect and handle them.

6. Describe chain of custody procedures and identify the tests that may require them.

7. Explain the importance of timing, identify the role of drug half-life providing names of drugs as examples; and describe peak, trough, and therapeutic levels in therapeutic drug monitoring.

8. Define point-of-care testing (POCT), explain the principle behind the POCT examples listed in this chapter, and identify any special equipment required.

SPECIAL PROCEDURES

Most laboratory tests require blood specimens collected using routine venipuncture or capillary puncture procedures. Some tests, however, require special or additional collection procedures or are performed on other body substances such as feces or urine. Collecting specimens for these tests may require special preparation, equipment, handling, or timing. The following are some of the most commonly encountered special test procedures.

Blood Bank Specimens

Blood bank specimens yield information that determines which blood products can be transfused safely into a patient. Faithful attention to protocol when collecting blood bank specimens is crucial to safe transfusions. Follow facility specific procedures.

SPECIMEN REQUIREMENTS

Blood bank tests require collection of one or more plain (no serum separator gel) red stopper tubes or a lavender or pink top EDTA tube.

IDENTIFICATION AND LABELING REQUIREMENTS

Blood bank specimens require strict patient identification and specimen labeling procedures. Mislabeled or incompletely, inaccurately, or unlabeled specimens will not be accepted for testing. An error in specimen identification or labeling requires re-collection and causes a delay in patient treatment. An undetected error can result in administration of an incompatible blood product and the possibility of a fatal transfusion reaction. Typical labeling requirements for blood bank specimens are shown in Box 11-1.

BOX • 11-1   Labeling Requirements for Blood Bank Specimens

- Patient's full name (including middle initial)
- Patient's hospital identification number (or social security number for outpatients)
- Patient's date of birth
- Date and time of collection
- Phlebotomist's initials
- Room number and bed number (optional)

SPECIAL IDENTIFICATION SYSTEMS

A variety of special blood bank identification systems are available. One system uses a special ID bracelet such as the Typenex Blood Recipient Identification Band (Fenwal Biotech Division, a division of Travenol Laboratories, Chicago, IL) 1 or the Securline Blood Bank (Precision Dynamics Corporation, San Fernando, CA) that is attached to the patient's wrist.

With this system, the patient's identity is confirmed and the information written on a self-carbon adhesive label on the special bracelet, which contains a unique ID number. The adhesive label is peeled from the bracelet, leaving a carbon copy of the information, including the unique ID number, on the bracelet. The adhesive label is placed on the patient's specimen (Fig. 11-1). Additional ID number labels from the bracelet are sent to the lab with the specimen to be used in the crossmatch process or eventually attached to the unit of blood or other blood products used for transfusion. Figure 11-2 shows a blood bank ID bracelet and a patient's specimen with additional numbered labels attached to it. Prior to transfusion, the nurse must match the numbers on the patient's blood bank ID bracelet with the numbers on the unit of blood. Some facilities require the unique number and patient's name to be brought to the blood bank as an additional identification check when picking up the blood products.

Electronic blood bank ID systems are also available. One example is the MedPoint Transfusion System (Bridge Medical Inc., Solana Beach, CA). It is a portable bedside bar code scanning system that provides electronic verification and tracing of the blood transfusion process. The hardware includes a portable data terminal and a printer (Fig. 11-3). At the time of specimen collection, the phlebotomist scans his or her ID badge and then the patient's bar-coded wristband. A matching specimen label with the bar-coded identifier is printed at the bedside, ensuring positive patient identification. The bar-coded data are used throughout the transfusion process and appear on the unit of blood prepared for transfusion. The patient's wristband and the unit of blood are scanned and a match is electronically verified before transfusion of the unit is begun.

FIGURE 11-1

A phlebotomist compares labeled blood bank tube with blood bank ID bracelet.

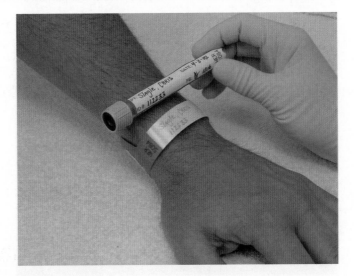

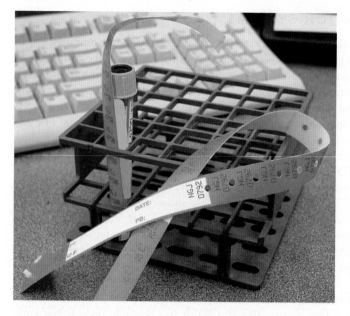

FIGURE 11-2

Securline Blood Bank recipient identification band and blood sample with additional numbers from a similar band attached to a blood sample.   (Precision Dynamics Corporation, San Francisco, CA.)

Type and Screen and Crossmatch

One of the most common tests performed by the blood bank is a blood type and screen. This test determines a patient's blood type (ABO) and Rh factor (positive or negative). When required, a crossmatch is performed using the patient's type and screen results to help select a donor unit of blood. During a crossmatch, the patient's plasma or serum and the donor red cells are mixed together to determine **compatibility** (suitability to be mixed). A transfusion of incompatible blood can be fatal because of **agglutination** (clumping) and **lysis** (rupturing) of the red blood cells within the patient's circulatory system.

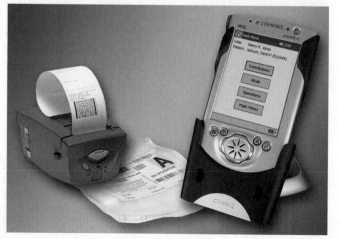

FIGURE 11-3

Bridge Medical MedPoint transfusion system.   (Bridge Medical Inc., Solana Beach, CA.)

Blood Donor Collection

Blood donor collection involves collecting blood to be used for transfusion purposes rather than for diagnostic testing. Blood is collected from volunteers in amounts referred to as units. Donor collection requires special training and exceptional venipuncture skills. Facilities that provide blood donor services are called blood banks. Blood banks follow guidelines set by the American Association of Blood Banks (AABB) for purposes of quality assurance and standardization. United States Food and Drug Administration (FDA) regulation is required, since blood and blood products are considered pharmaceuticals.

key•point All potential blood donors must be interviewed to determine eligibility to donate blood as well as to obtain information for the records that must be kept for all blood donors.

DONOR ELIGIBILITY

To donate blood, a person must be within the ages of 17 and 66 years and weigh at least 110 lb. Minors must have written permission from their parents. Adults over the age of 66 years may be allowed to donate at the discretion of the blood bank physician. A brief physical examination, as well as a complete medical history, is needed to determine the patient's health status. This information is collected each time a person donates, no matter how many times a person has donated before. All donor information is strictly confidential. In addition, the donor must give written permission for the blood bank to use his or her blood. Donor unit collection principles are listed in Box 11-2.

BOX • 11-2 Donor Unit Collection Principles

- Donor units are normally collected from a large antecubital vein.
- The vein is selected in a manner similar to routine venipuncture and cleaned in a manner similar to blood culture collection (see page 406).
- The collection unit is a sterile, closed system consisting of a bag to contain the blood connected by a length of tubing to a sterile 16- to18-gauge needle.
- The bag fills by gravity and must be placed lower than the patient's arm.
- The collection bag contains an anticoagulant and preservative solution and is placed on a mixing unit while the blood is being drawn.
- The unit is normally filled by weight but typically contains around 450 mL of blood when full. Only one needle puncture can be used to fill a unit. If the unit only partially fills and the procedure must be repeated, an entire new unit must be used.

LOOKBACK PROGRAM

A unit of blood can be separated into several components: red blood cells, plasma, and platelets. All components of the unit must be traceable to the donor for federally required **lookback** programs. A lookback program requires notification to all blood recipients when a donor for a blood product they have received has turned positive for a transmissible disease.

AUTOLOGOUS DONATION

Autologous donation is the process by which a person donates blood for his or her own use. This is done for elective surgeries when it is anticipated that a transfusion will be needed. Using one's own blood eliminates many risks associated with transfusion, such as disease transmission and blood or plasma incompatibilities. Although blood is normally collected several weeks prior to the scheduled surgery, the minimum time between donation and surgery can be as little as 72 hours. To be eligible to make an autologous donation, a person must have a written order from a physician.

CELL SALVAGING

During some surgical procedures, the patient's blood is salvaged, washed, and reinfused. Prior to reinfusion it is recommended that the salvaged blood be tested for residual free hemoglobin. A high free hemoglobin level indicates that too many red cells were destroyed during the salvage process and renal dysfunction could result if the blood were reinfused. Free hemoglobin can be detected using point-of-care instruments such as the HemoCue Plasma/Low Hemoglobin analyzer (Fig.11-4).

Blood Cultures

A physician may order blood cultures when a patient experiences **fever of unknown origin (FUO)** or there is reason to suspect **bacteremia** (bacteria in the blood) or **septicemia** (microorganisms or their toxins in the blood). Blood cultures help determine the presence and extent of infection, as well as indicate the type of organism responsible and the antibiotic to which it is most susceptible. They are also useful in assessing the effectiveness of antibiotic therapy once treatment is initiated.

key·point   Blood cultures are typically ordered immediately before or after anticipated fever spikes when bacteria are most likely to be present. Therefore timely collection is essential.

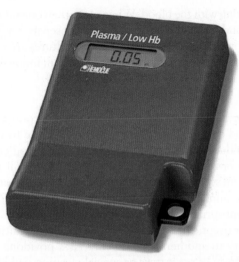

FIGURE 11-4

HemoCue Plasma/Low Hb.   (HemoCue, Inc., Mission
Viejo, CA.)

SPECIMEN REQUIREMENTS

Blood culture specimens are most commonly collected in special bottles (Fig. 11-5) containing nutrient broth (referred to as media) that encourages the growth of microorganisms. They are typically collected in sets of two: one **aerobic** (with air), and one **anaerobic** (without air). The anaerobic bottle is filled first when a syringe is used to collect the blood. When a butterfly is used it is preferable to fill the aerobic bottle first because air in the tubing will be drawn into

FIGURE 11-5

BACTEC blood culture bottles. Anaerobic/F,
Aerobic/F, and Myco/F-lytic.   (Becton Dickinson,
Franklin Lakes, NJ.)

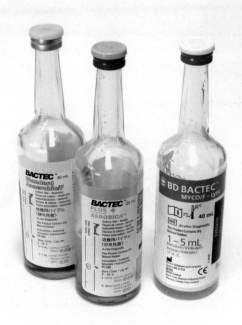

it along with the blood. When more than one set is ordered for collection at the same time, the second set should be obtained from a separately prepared site on the opposite arm. However, in some cases, "second-site" blood cultures are more useful when drawn 30 minutes apart. If timing is not specified on the requisition, follow laboratory protocol.

SKIN ANTISEPSIS

Skin antisepsis, the destruction of microorganisms on the skin, is a critical part of the blood culture collection procedure. Failure to carefully disinfect the venipuncture site can introduce skin surface bacteria into the blood culture bottles and interfere with interpretation of results. The laboratory must report all microorganisms detected, so it is up to the patient's physician to determine whether the organism is clinically significant or merely a contaminant. If a contaminating organism is misinterpreted as pathogenic, it could result in inappropriate treatment.

Antiseptic or sterile technique for blood culture collection varies slightly from one laboratory to another. Traditionally 10% povidone or 1–2% tincture of iodine compounds in the form of swabsticks or special cleaning pad kits such as benzalkonium chloride (Fig. 11-6) have been used to clean the collection site. When using a povidone-iodine swabstick (Fig. 11-7), the swab should be placed at the site of the needle insertion and moved outward in concentric circles without going over any area more than once, as shown in (Fig. 11-8). The area covered should be 3 to 4 inches in diameter. Because of the incidence of iodine sensitivities, some healthcare facilities are using chlorhexidine gluconate/isopropyl alcohol antiseptic preparations in blood culture preparation kits that have a one-step application and are effective with a 30-second scrub.

> 🔑 **key · point**   According to CLSI: Chlorhexidine gluconate is the recommended blood culture site disinfectant for infants 2 months and older and patients with iodine sensitivity.

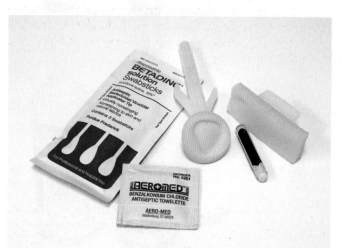

FIGURE 11-6

Four types of blood culture cleaning supplies. *Left to right,* Betadine swabsticks   (The Purdue Frederick Co., Norwalk, CT.); *center,* Benzalkonium Chloride   (Aero-Med, Glastonbury, CT), Chloroprep (Medi-Flex Hospital Products, Inc., Overland Park, KS), Frepp/Sepp II   (MediFlex Inc., Overland Park, KS).

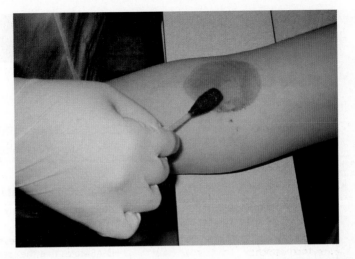

FIGURE 11-7

Cleaning a blood culture site using a povidone-iodine swabstick.

COLLECTION PROCEDURE

Blood culture specimen collection procedure is shown in Procedure 11-1.

MEDIA INOCULATION METHODS

Media inoculation can occur several different ways, directly into the bottle during specimen collection or after collection as when blood has been collected in a syringe.

Direct Inoculation   To collect the specimen directly into the blood culture media use a butterfly and specially designed holder (Fig.11-9). Connect the special holder to the Luer connector of the butterfly collection set. Fill the aerobic vial first because the butterfly tubing has air in it. Avoid backflow by keeping the culture bottle or tube lower than the collection site and preventing the culture media from contacting the stopper or needle during blood collection. Mix each container after removing it from the needle holder. After filling both containers and collecting any other tests, remove the needle from the patient's arm, activate the safety device, and hold pressure over the site.

FIGURE 11-8

Pattern of concentric circles used when cleaning a blood culture site.

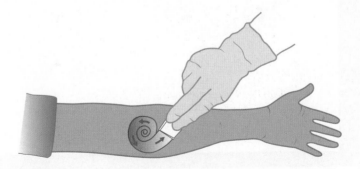

PROCEDURE 11-1

Blood Culture Specimen Collection

Purpose: Collect a blood culture specimen

Equipment: Gloves, suitable skin antiseptic; blood culture bottles; butterfly and blood culture tube holder or needle, syringe, and transfer device; alcohol pads; bandage; permanent ink pen

Step	Explanation/Rationale
1. Follow normal identification protocol; explain collection procedure	Patient must be properly identified and consent to the procedure
2. Identify venipuncture site and release tourniquet 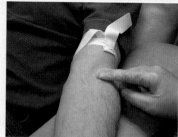	Proper disinfection takes time, and CLSI Standard H3-A5 states that the tourniquet should not be left on longer than 1 minute
3. Aseptically select and assemble equipment 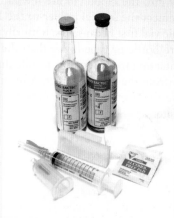	Aseptic technique when handling equipment aids in accurate diagnosis by reducing the risk of false positive results due to contamination

Step	Explanation/Rationale
4. Perform friction scrub 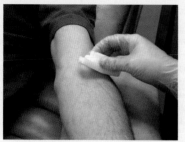	Bacteria exist on the skin surface and can be temporarily removed by vigorous scrubbing with an effective antiseptic solution for the amount of time designated by the procedure method, generally 30–60 seconds

△ **c a u t i o n** Do not scrub the skin of neonates too aggressively as this may be abrasive and cause the skin to tear

Step	Explanation/Rationale
5. Allow the site to dry	Antisepsis does not occur instantly. The 30-second wait allows time for the antiseptic to be effective against skin surface bacteria
6. Cleanse the culture bottle stoppers while the site is drying 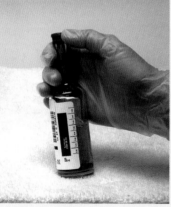 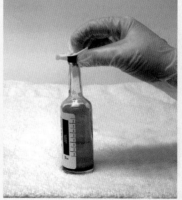	Tops of the culture bottles must be free of contaminants when inoculated. Some manufacturers recommend prepping the septum with iodine to provide visual confirmation that it was cleaned prior to inoculation. Others suggest placing a clean alcohol prep pad on top of each bottle after cleaning. Typically, culture bottles with plastic caps can be cleaned with 70% isopropyl alcohol after removing the cap and be covered with an alcohol pad until ready to inoculate

(Continued)

PROCEDURE 11-1   *(Continued)*

Step	Explanation/Rationale
7. Mark the minimum and maximum fill on the culture bottles	Blood culture bottles have vacuum, but it is not always measured as in evacuated tubes. Most culture bottles do have fill lines on the sides that can be marked. Marking the bottles ensures that enough, but not too much, blood enters the bottle. Typically, adult blood cultures require 10 to 20 mL per set, while pediatric blood cultures require 1–2 mL per set. Consult manufacturer's instructions as volume requirements may vary depending on the system used
8. Reapply the tourniquet and perform the venipuncture without touching or repalpating the site	The tourniquet must be reapplied to aid in venipuncture and care must be taken so that the site is not recontaminated in the process. Ensuring antiseptic technique and sterility of the site is critical to accurate diagnosis. However, if the patient has "difficult" veins and a need to relocate them is anticipated, the gloved palpating finger must be cleaned in the same manner as the site, including the 30-second contact time. Repalpating should only be done above or below the site of needle entry
9. Inoculate the media as required	Media inoculation can occur directly into the bottle during specimen collection or after collection when a syringe is used. With either method, if an iodine preparation was used to clean the bottle tops it must be dry or removed to prevent contamination of the specimen

Step	Explanation/Rationale
10. Clean the patient's skin, if applicable	If an iodine preparation was used to clean the arm it should be removed with alcohol or suitable cleanser. Iodine left on the skin can be irritating and even toxic to those with iodine sensitivity. Iodine contamination of a blood sample can also cause erroneous results for other tests
11. Label the specimen containers with required identification information, including the site of collection (e.g., right arm)	Noting the collection site is necessary in case there is a localized infection. Some facilities require that labeling information include the amount of blood added to each bottle
12. Dispose of used and contaminated materials	Materials such as needle caps and wrappers are normally discarded in the regular trash. Some facilities require that contaminated items such as blood-soaked gauze be discarded in biohazard containers
13. Thank patient, remove gloves, and sanitize hands	Thanking the patient is courteous and professional. Gloves must be removed in an aseptic manner and hands washed or decontaminated with hand sanitizer as an infection control precaution
14. Transport specimens to the lab	Prompt delivery to the lab protects specimen integrity and is typically achieved by personal delivery, transportation via a pneumatic tube system, or a courier service

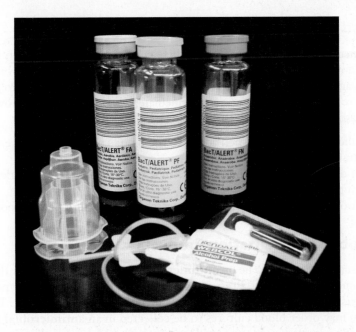

FIGURE 11-9

BacT/Alert blood culture supplies including a specially designed holder for a butterfly needle.   (bioMerieux, Durham, NC)

key · point Blood culture specimens are always collected first in the order of draw to prevent contamination from other tubes.

Syringe Inoculation When the syringe method is used, the blood must be transferred to the bottles after the draw is completed. New OSHA regulations require use of a safety transfer device for this procedure. To transfer blood from the syringe to the culture bottles, activate the needle safety device as soon as the needle is removed from the vein. Remove the needle and attach a safety transfer device to the syringe. Push the culture bottle into the device until the needle inside it penetrates the bottle stopper. Allow the blood to be drawn from the syringe by the vacuum in the container. The plunger may need to be held back to keep from expelling too much blood into the bottle. Never push the plunger to expel the blood into the vial. This can hemolyze the specimen and cause aerosol formation when the needle is removed.

If a transfer safety device is not available and a needle must be used, use extreme caution upon blood transfer. The practice of changing needles prior to this transfer is no longer recommended. Several recent studies have shown that changing needles has little effect on reducing contamination rates and may actually increase risk of needlestick injury to the phlebotomist. Never hold the culture bottle in your hand during the inoculation process. Place it on a solid surface or in a rack. When delivering blood to the bottles, direct the flow along the side of the container. As with the transfer device, do not push on the syringe plunger.

INTERMEDIATE COLLECTION TUBE

Blood is sometimes collected in an intermediate collection tube rather than blood culture bottles. A yellow top sodium polyanethol sulfonate (SPS) tube is acceptable for this purpose. Other anticoagulants such as citrate, heparin, EDTA, and oxalate may be toxic to bacteria and are not recommended. Use of an intermediate tube is discouraged, however, for the following reasons:

- SPS in the collection tube when added to the blood culture bottle increases the final concentration of SPS.
- Transfer of blood from the intermediate tube to the blood culture bottles presents another opportunity for contamination.
- Transfer of blood to the culture bottles presents an exposure risk to laboratory staff.

Antimicrobial Neutralization Products

It is not unusual for patients to be on **antimicrobial** (antibiotic) **therapy** at the time blood culture specimens are collected. Presence of the antimicrobial agent in the patient's blood can inhibit the growth of the microorganisms in the blood culture bottle. In such cases, the physician may order blood cultures to be collected in an **antimicrobial removal device (ARD)** (Becton Dickinson) or **fastidious antimicrobial neutralization (FAN)** (bioMerieux) bottles. An ARD contains a resin that removes antimicrobials from the blood.

FAN bottles contain activated charcoal that neutralizes the antibiotic. The blood can then be processed by conventional technique without the risk of inhibiting the growth of microorganisms. ARDs and FANs should be delivered to the lab for processing as soon as possible.

Coagulation Specimens

There are a number of important things to remember when collecting specimens for coagulation tests.

- At one time it was customary to draw a *"clear"* or discard tube prior to collection of a blue top. A few milliliters of blood were collected into a plain red top tube to clear the needle of thromboplastin contamination picked up as it penetrated the skin. The clearing tube was discarded if it was not needed for other tests. New studies have shown that a "clear" tube is not necessary when collecting for a PT or PTT. A clear tube is required for all other coagulation tests (e.g., factor VIII) because CLSI still recommends that they be the second or third tube drawn.
- Sodium citrate tubes for coagulation studies must be filled until the vacuum is exhausted to obtain a *9:1 ratio of blood to anticoagulant.* Even when the tubes are properly filled, this ratio is altered if the patient's hemoglobin level is abnormally high or low. In such cases, laboratory personnel may request specimen collection in a special tube that has had the anticoagulant volume adjusted Do not use blue top tubes that are designed for fibrin degradation (FDP) or fibrin split products (FSP) tests for other coagulation tests. FDP/FSP tubes have a different additive and a different fill volume.

> c a u t i o n   All anticoagulant tubes must be gently inverted from 3-8 times immediately after collection to avoid microclots that can invalidate test results.

- Never pour two partially filled tubes together to create a full tube, as the anticoagulant-to-blood ratio will be greatly increased.
- Cooling on ice during transport may be required for some test specimens to protect the coagulation factors. Some coagulation factors such as factors V and VIII are not stable. If the tests cannot be performed in a timely manner, the specimen needs to be centrifuged and the plasma frozen.
- If a coagulation specimen must be drawn from an indwelling catheter, CLSI recommends drawing and discarding 5 mL of blood or 6 times the dead space volume of the catheter before collecting the specimen. If heparin has been introduced into the line, it should be flushed with 5 mL of saline before drawing the discard blood and collecting the specimen.

D-Xylose Absorption

The D-xylose absorption test is a noninvasive way to help diagnose malabsorption, or failure of the small intestine to absorb nutrients. D-Xylose is a simple sugar called a pentose that is

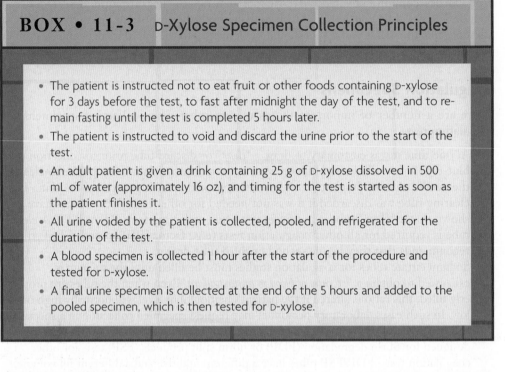

BOX • 11-3 D-Xylose Specimen Collection Principles

- The patient is instructed not to eat fruit or other foods containing D-xylose for 3 days before the test, to fast after midnight the day of the test, and to remain fasting until the test is completed 5 hours later.
- The patient is instructed to void and discard the urine prior to the start of the test.
- An adult patient is given a drink containing 25 g of D-xylose dissolved in 500 mL of water (approximately 16 oz), and timing for the test is started as soon as the patient finishes it.
- All urine voided by the patient is collected, pooled, and refrigerated for the duration of the test.
- A blood specimen is collected 1 hour after the start of the procedure and tested for D-xylose.
- A final urine specimen is collected at the end of the 5 hours and added to the pooled specimen, which is then tested for D-xylose.

present in certain fruit. It is not normally present in blood or urine unless foods containing it are eaten. D-xylose test procedure principles are listed in Box 11-3.

If absorption is normal, D-xylose will be absorbed into the bloodstream from the small intestine, pass through the liver, and be excreted by the kidneys, thus appearing in the blood and urine. If absorption is abnormal, low blood and urine values will be obtained. Falsely low blood and urine values may result from other problems such as bacterial overgrowth of the small intestine, renal disease, or delayed gastric emptying time.

2-Hour Postprandial Glucose

Postprandial (PP) means after a meal. Glucose levels in blood specimens obtained 2 hours after a meal are rarely elevated in normal persons but may be significantly increased in diabetic patients. Therefore, a glucose test on a specimen collected 2 hours after a meal (**2-hour PP**) is an excellent screening test for diabetes and other metabolism problems. A 2-hour PP test is also used to monitor insulin therapy. Correct timing of specimen collection is very important. Glucose levels in specimens collected too early or late may be falsely elevated or decreased, respectively, leading to misinterpretation of results. Two-hour PP procedure principles are shown in Box 11-4.

Glucose Tolerance Test

A **glucose tolerance test (GTT)** is used to diagnose carbohydrate metabolism problems. The major carbohydrate in the blood is glucose, the body's source of energy. The GTT, also

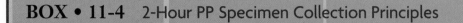

BOX • 11-4   2-Hour PP Specimen Collection Principles

- The patient is placed on a high-carbohydrate diet for 2 to 3 days prior to the test.
- The patient fasts prior to the test. This means no eating, smoking, or drinking other than water for at least 10 hours before the test.
- A fasting glucose specimen may be collected before the start of the test.
- The patient is instructed to eat a special breakfast (typically one containing the equivalent of 100 grams of glucose) or given a measured dose of glucose beverage on the day of the test.
- A blood glucose specimen is collected 2 hours after the patient finishes eating.

called the oral glucose test (OGTT), evaluates the body's ability to metabolize glucose. The two major types of disorders involving glucose metabolism are those in which the blood glucose level is increased (**hyperglycemia**), as in diabetes mellitus, and those in which the blood glucose levels are decreased (**hypoglycemia**). Insulin, produced by the pancreas, is primarily responsible for regulating blood glucose levels. The GTT evaluates insulin response to a measured dose of glucose (Fig. 11-10) by recording glucose levels on specimens collected at specific time intervals. Insulin levels are sometimes measured also. GTT length is typically 1 hour for gestational diabetes, and 3 hours for other glucose metabolism evaluations. The test rarely exceeds 6 hours. Results are plotted on a graph, creating a so-called GTT curve (Fig. 11-11).

There are a number of variations of the GTT procedure, involving different doses of glucose and timing of collections. The method used to collect the blood, however, should be consistent for all specimens. That is, if the first specimen is collected by venipuncture, all succeeding specimens should be venipuncture specimens. If skin puncture is used to collect the first specimen, all succeeding specimens should also be skin puncture specimens.

GTT PREPARATION AND PROCEDURE

Preparation for a GTT is very important. The patient must eat balanced meals containing approximately 150 grams (g) of carbohydrate for 3 days before the test, and must fast for at least 12 hours, but not more than 16 hours prior to the test. The patient is allowed to drink water during the fast and during the test to avoid dehydration and because urine specimens may be collected as part of the procedure. No other food or beverages are allowed. The patient is also not allowed to smoke or chew gum, as these activities stimulate the digestive process and may cause erroneous test results. The patient should receive both verbal and written instructions to ensure compliance. The GTT procedure is shown in Procedure 11-2.

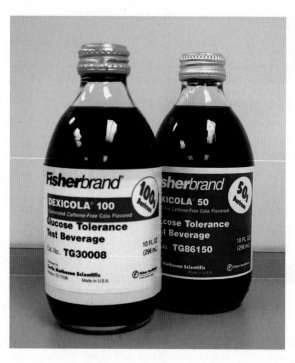

FIGURE 11-10

Commercial Glucose Tolerance Test Beverage, 50 gram & 100 gram doses.

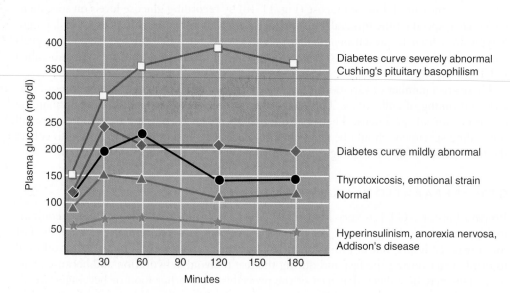

FIGURE 11-11

Glucose tolerance test (GTT) curves.

PROCEDURE 11-2

GTT Procedure

Purpose: Perform a glucose tolerance test

Equipment: Gloves, alcohol prep pads, ETS holder, tubes, and needle, glucose beverage, urine containers (if applicable) bandage, permanent ink pen

Step	Explanation/Rationale
1. Follow normal identification protocol, explain collection procedure, and advise patient that water *is* allowed, but drinking other beverages, eating food, smoking, or chewing gum is *not* allowed throughout the test period	Patient must be properly identified and must understand and consent to the procedure. Eating, drinking beverages other than water, smoking, and chewing gum all affect test results
2. Draw fasting specimen and check for glucose	If the fasting glucose result is abnormal, the patient's physician must be consulted before continuing the test. The test is not normally performed if the patient's blood glucose is over 200 mg/dL
3. Ask the patient to collect a fasting urine specimen if urine testing has been requested	The GTT can be requested with or without urine testing
4. Give the patient the determined dose of glucose beverage	A typical adult patient dose is 75 g. Children and small adults are given approximately 1 g of glucose per kilogram of weight. The dose for detecting gestational diabetes is normally between 50 and 75 g
5. Remind the patient to finish the beverage within 5 minutes	Results may be inaccurate if the patient takes longer to drink the beverage, as the glucose may start to be metabolized by the body, affecting test results
6. Note the time that the patient finishes the beverage, start the timing for the test and calculate the collection times for the rest of the specimens based on this time	GTT specimens are typically collected 30 minutes, 1 hour, 2 hours, 3 hours, and so forth, after the patient finishes the glucose beverage
7. Give a copy of the collection times to the patient	Patients (especially outpatients) must be aware of the collection times so that they are available for the draw
8. Collect blood and urine specimens (if applicable) as close to the computed times as possible	Timing of specimen collection is critical for computation of the GTT curve and correct interpretation of results
9. Label all specimens with the exact time collected and the time interval of the test (1/2 hour, 1 hour etc.) in addition to patient identification information	Each specimen must be correctly identified for accurate computation of the GTT curve and interpretation of results. Actual time of collection must be recorded

(Continued)

PROCEDURE 11-2 *(Continued)*

Step	Explanation/Rationale
10. Deliver or send specimens to the lab as soon as possible	Glucose specimens must be separated from the cells or tested within 2 hours of collection for accurate results. Specimens collected in sodium fluoride are stable for 24 hours and are sometimes held and tested all together. Follow facility protocol

caution If the patient vomits during the procedure, his or her physician must be consulted to determine if the test should be continued.

In normal patients, blood glucose levels peak within 30 minutes to 1 hour following glucose ingestion. The peak in glucose levels triggers the release of insulin, which brings glucose levels back down to fasting levels within about 2 hours, and no glucose spills over into the urine.

Diabetics have inadequate or absent insulin response, consequently glucose levels peak at higher levels and are slower to return to fasting levels. If blood is not drawn on time, it is important for the phlebotomist to note the discrepancy so that the physician can take this into consideration.

Lactose Tolerance Test

A lactose tolerance test (Box 11-5) is used to determine if a patient lacks the enzyme (mucosal lactase) that is necessary to convert the milk sugar lactose into glucose and galactose. A person lacking the enzyme suffers from gastrointestinal distress and diarrhea following ingestion of milk and other lactose-containing foods. Symptoms are relieved by eliminating milk from the diet.

A lactose tolerance test is typically performed in the same manner as a 2-hour GTT; however, an equal amount of lactose is substituted for the glucose. Blood samples are drawn at the same times as for a GTT. If the patient has mucosal lactase, the resulting glucose curve will be similar to a GTT curve, and the result is considered negative. If the patient is lactose intolerant (lacking the enzyme lactase), the glucose curve will be flat, rising no more than 10 mg/dL from the fasting level. Some individuals normally have a flat GTT curve (resulting in a false-positive result), and it is suggested that they have a 2-hour GTT performed the day before the lactose tolerance so results can be evaluated adequately. False-positive results have also been demonstrated in patients with small bowel resections and with disorders such as slow gastric emptying, Crohn's disease, and cystic fibrosis. A lactose tolerance test can also be performed on breath samples (see Chapter 13).

> **BOX • 11-5**   Lactose Tolerance Test Principles
>
> - It is suggested that a 2-hour GTT be performed the day before the lactose tolerance test.
> - A 2-hour lactose tolerance test is performed in the same manner as the GTT; however, an equal amount of lactose is substituted for the glucose.
> - Blood samples for glucose testing are drawn at the same times used in the previous GTT test.
> - If the patient has mucosal lactase, the resulting glucose curve will be similar to the GTT curve.
> - If the patient lacks the enzyme (is lactose intolerant), glucose levels will rise no more than 20 mg/dL from the fasting level, resulting in a "flat" curve.
> - False-positive results have been demonstrated in patients with small bowel resections, and disorders such as slow gastric emptying, Crohn's disease, and cystic fibrosis.

Paternity/Parentage Testing

Paternity testing is performed to determine the probability that a specific individual fathered a particular child. Generally, paternity test results exclude the possibility of paternity, rather than prove paternity. Testing may be requested by physicians, lawyers, child support enforcement bureaus, or individuals. Paternity testing requires chain-of-custody protocol and specific identification procedures that may include fingerprinting. A photo identification document such as a passport is usually required. The mother, child, and alleged father are all tested. Blood samples are preferred for testing; however, buccal (cheek) swabs are increasingly being used.

Blood sample testing usually includes ABO and Rh typing. If the putative (assumed) or alleged parent is not excluded by basic red cell antigen testing, further testing is performed until the individual is excluded or the likelihood of parentage is established. Further testing includes identifying extended red cell antigens, red cell enzymes and serum proteins, white cell enzymes, and HLA (human leukocyte antigen), or white cell antigens.

DNA profiles can also be performed on buccal samples, which are collected by rubbing a swab against the inside of the cheek to collect loose cells. DNA extracted from the cells is "mapped" to create a DNA profile. DNA profiles of the individuals involved are compared to determine an alleged father's probability of paternity.

Paternity testing can also be performed before the infant is born on specimens obtained by amniocentesis or by chorionic villus sampling. (Chorionic villi are projections of vascular tissue that have the same genetic makeup as the fertilized egg and become the fetal portion of the placenta.)

TABLE 11-1   Examples of Categories of Drugs That Typically Require Therapeutic Monitoring

Drug Category	Examples	Use
Antibiotics	Aminoglycosides (gentamicin, tobramycin, amikacin), chloramphenicol, vancomycin	Treat infections caused by bacteria that are resistant to other antibiotics
Anticancer drugs	Methotrexate	Psoriasis, rheumatoid arthritis (RA), non-Hodgkin's lymphoma, osteosarcoma
Antiepileptics	Carbamazepine (Tegretol), ethosuximide, *gabapentin, *lamotrigine, phenobarbital, phenytoin, valproic acid	Epilepsy, seizure prevention, mood stabilization
Bronchodilators	Theophylline, caffeine	Asthma, chronic obstructive pulmonary disorder (COPD), neonatal apnea
Cardiac drugs	Digitoxin, digoxin, procainamide, quinidine	Congestive heart failure (CHF), angina, arrhythmia
Immuno-suppressants	Azathioprine, cyclosporine, sirolimus, tacrolimus	Autoimmune disorders, prevent organ transplant rejection
Protease inhibitors	Atazanavir, indinavir, lopinavir, nelfinavir, ritonavir	HIV/AIDS
Psychiatric drugs	Antidepressants (such as imipramine, amitriptyline, nortriptyline, doxepin, desipramine), lithium, valproic acid	Bipolar disorder (manic depression), depression

* May not always require monitoring.

Therapeutic Drug Monitoring (TDM)

The drug dosage necessary to produce a desired effect varies widely among patients. **Therapeutic drug monitoring (TDM)**, the testing of drug levels at specific intervals, is used in the management of patients being treated with certain drugs, to help establish a drug dosage, maintain the dosage at a therapeutic (beneficial) level, and avoid drug toxicity. Drugs that are monitored typically have a narrow therapeutic range, which means the amount required to be effective is fairly close to the amount that can cause side effects or toxicity. Table 11-1 lists examples of categories of drugs that require monitoring.

When a patient takes a drug dose, the amount in the bloodstream rises initially. It eventually peaks, and then falls, typically reaching its lowest or trough level just before the next dose is due. For a drug to be beneficial, the **peak (maximum) level** must not exceed toxic levels, and the **trough (minimum) level** must remain within the therapeutic range. Consequently, timing of specimen collection in regard to dosage administration is critical for safe and beneficial treatment and must be consistent. A team effort is essential and requires coordination with pharmacy, nursing, and the lab. The phlebotomist, a key player in this team effort, must understand the importance of peak and trough levels and collect the specimens in a timely manner.

- Peak levels screen for drug toxicity and specimens are collected when the highest serum concentration of the drug is anticipated. Peak times are influenced by many factors but typically occur approximately 30 minutes after intravenous (IV) administration, 60 minutes after intramuscular (IM) administration, and 1 to 2 hours after oral intake. Careful coordination of sample collection with dosing is critical.

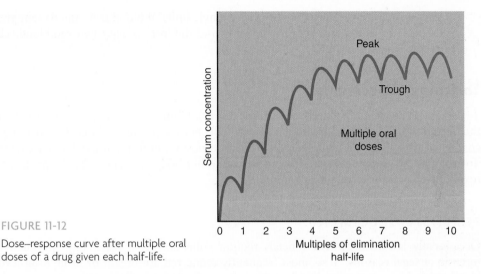

FIGURE 11-12

Dose–response curve after multiple oral doses of a drug given each half-life.

- Trough levels are monitored to ensure that levels of the drug stay within the therapeutic range. Trough level specimens are easiest to collect, because they are collected when the lowest serum concentration of the drug is expected, usually immediately prior to administration of the next scheduled dose.

Collection timing is most critical for aminoglycoside drugs, such as amikacin, gentamicin, and tobramycin, which have short half-lives. A half-life is the time required for the body to metabolize half the amount of the drug. (Figure 11-12 depicts dose–response curve based on doses of drug given each half-life) The timing is less critical for drugs that have longer half-lives, such as phenobarbital and digoxin.

The FDA has approved some manufacturer's gel tubes for all analytes, including TDM; however, other manufacturer's gel tubes may affect TDM results. Refer to manufacture package inserts and test methodologies used in the laboratory for specific requirements.

Therapeutic Phlebotomy

Therapeutic phlebotomy involves the withdrawal of large volumes of blood, usually measured by the unit (as in blood donation), or approximately 500 mL. It is performed by phlebotomists who have been specially trained in the procedure or in donor phlebotomy, as the procedure is similar to collecting blood from donors. It is used as a treatment for certain medical conditions such as polycythemia and hemochromatosis.

- *Polycythemia* is a disease involving overproduction of red blood cells by the body, which is detrimental to the patient's health and the most common reason for performing therapeutic phlebotomy. The patient's red blood cell levels are monitored regularly, usually by the hematocrit test. Periodic removal of blood when the hematocrit exceeds a certain level is used to help keep the patient's red blood cell levels within the normal range.
- *Hemochromatosis* is a disease characterized by excess iron deposits in the tissues. It can be caused by a defect in iron metabolism or result from multiple blood transfusions

or excess iron intake. Periodic removal of single units of blood from the patient gradually depletes iron stores because the body uses the iron to make new red blood cells to replace those removed.

Toxicology Specimens

Toxicology is the scientific study of toxins (poisons). Clinical toxicology is concerned with the detection of toxins and treatment for the effects they produce. Forensic toxicology is concerned with the legal consequences of toxin exposure, both intentional and accidental. Toxicology tests examine blood, hair, urine, and other body substances for the presence of toxins, often present in very small amounts.

FORENSIC SPECIMENS

Occasionally law enforcement officials request collection of a toxicology specimen for forensic or legal reasons. Tests most frequently requested are breath or urine drug levels, blood alcohol concentration (BAC), and specimens for DNA analysis. When forensic specimens are collected, a special protocol, referred to as **chain of custody**, must be strictly followed. Chain of custody requires detailed documentation that tracks the specimen from the time it is collected until the results are reported. The specimen must be accounted for at all times. If documentation is incomplete, legal action may be compromised.

A special chain-of-custody form (Fig. 11-13) is used to identify the specimen and the person or persons who obtained and processed the specimen. Information on the form also includes the time, date, and place the specimen was obtained, along with the signature of the person from whom the specimen was obtained. Patient identification and specimen collection takes place in the presence of a witness, frequently a law enforcement officer, in which case, protocol and packaging are completed by the officer before the specimen is sent to a crime laboratory for analysis. A phlebotomist involved in drawing a blood alcohol specimen for legal reasons can be summoned to appear in court.

BLOOD ALCOHOL (ETHANOL) SPECIMENS

Normally a physician orders a blood alcohol (**ethanol [ETOH]**) test on a patient for medical reasons related to treatment or other clinical purposes. Blood alcohol determinations for industrial purposes are becoming more common and may be required in connection with on-the-job injury, employee insurance programs, and employee drug screening. Sometimes a law enforcement agency requests a blood alcohol test on an individual. Both industrial and legal samples require that chain-of-custody protocol be strictly followed. Refer to the specific state law for legal regulations and requirements.

Skin Preparation   The antiseptic used to clean the venipuncture site must not contain alcohol or other volatile organic substances or results will be compromised. Therefore, 70% isopropyl alcohol used for routine venipuncture site preparation or other alcohols such as methanol and ethyl alcohol cannot be used for blood alcohol specimen collection. Tincture of iodine contains alcohol and likewise should not be used to clean the site. The most

SONORA
Laboratory Sciences

3401 E. Harbour Dr., Phoenix, Arizona 85034
602 431-5000
800 SONORA-1
800 766-6721

ORDERING PHYSICIAN/COMPANY OR FACILITY

2013AC
SOEHS-T'BIRD SAMARITAN MEDICAL
                    CENTER   2013A

5555 W THUNDERBIRD RD

GLENDALE, AZ   85306
602 588-5555   *RT14

CHAIN OF CUSTODY REQUISITION FORM

Failure to complete form properly could invalidate chain of custody.

DONOR INSTRUCTIONS   (To be completed by donor)

******************** IDENTIFICATION IS REQUIRED AT TIME OF COLLECTION ********************

DONOR AFFIDAVIT

I certify that the specimen identified by the ID number on this form was provided by me on this date and is not adulterated. In my presence, the specimen was sealed with an evidence seal taken from this form. The ID Number on the seal and on this form are identical. I have initialed the seal. By my signature I consent to the release of laboratory test results to the doctor, facility, individual or company shown on this form.

Donor Signature   Donor Name **(Print Clearly)**   Date

Birthdate   Social Security Number   Daytime Phone

You have the right to list any drugs, prescription or non prescription, that you may have taken in the last two weeks or other relevant medical information. Please do so, if desired, in the space provided: _____

COLLECTOR INSTRUCTIONS   (To be completed by collector)

1. Check donor identification **(preferably a picture I.D.)**
2. RECORD SPECIMEN TEMP:_____ (90° - 100°)
3. Specimen lid is tight, sealed properly with evidence seal, <u>and</u> initialed by donor.
4. I.D. number on specimen and form must match.
5. Place specimen in tamper-proof bag and seal in the presence of the donor.
6. Form is completed and signed by donor.
7. Collector signs this form, indicates date, time and collection site.

I certify that the specimen identified by this form was collected according to specified procedures, was properly identified and prepared for transport to the laboratory.

Check One Box
☐ Pre-Employment
☐ Post-accident
☐ Random
☐ Reasonable Cause
☐ Periodic
☐ Other_____

Collector Signature   Printed Name   Date   Collection Time

Collection Site   Address   Phone

COMMENTS:_____

LABORATORY USE ONLY

SPECIMEN RECEIVED BY:

SIGNATURE   PRINTED NAME   DATE

SPECIMEN SEAL CONDITION: ☐ INTACT   ☐ NOT INTACT

COMMENTS: _____

TESTS

[X] 2406 (FORENSIC COM-
          PREHENSIVE)

SOCIAL SECURITY NUMBER
____ ____ ____

DEPT:_____

PHONE:_____

COLLECTION TIME/DATE
_____/_____

************ SPECIMEN I.D. NUMBER 293012 ****************************

293012   293012   EVIDENCE SEAL   SPECIMEN I.D. NUMBER   EVIDENCE SEAL
                                            293012
293012   293012   Donor Initials

293012   293012   EVIDENCE SEAL   ___/___/___   EVIDENCE SEAL
                                            Date

ORIGINAL TO LABORATORY

FIGURE 11-13

Chain of custody requisition form.   (Courtesy Sonora Laboratory Sciences, Phoenix, AZ.)

frequently used antiseptics for ETOH specimen collection are povidone-iodine and aqueous benzalkonium chloride (BZK). If an alternative antiseptic is not available, regular soap and water can be used.

Specimen Requirements   A glass **gray top**, **sodium fluoride tube**, with or without an anticoagulant (depending upon the need for serum, plasma, or whole blood in the test procedure), is typically required for specimen collection. Because alcohol is volatile (easily vaporized or evaporated), the tube should be filled until the vacuum is exhausted, and the stopper should not be removed until absolutely necessary.

> **key · point**   Glass tubes are preferred for blood alcohol specimens because of the porous nature of plastic tubes.

DRUG SCREENING

Many healthcare organizations, sports associations, and major companies require preemployment **drug screening**. Random screening (without prior notice) may be performed on employees or athletes. Tests may detect a specific drug or screen for up to 30 different drugs, depending upon the circumstance. Testing is typically performed on urine rather than blood because it is easy to obtain and a wide variety of drugs or their metabolites (products of metabolism) can be detected in urine for a longer period of time (see Table 11-2 for a list of drugs commonly detectable by drug screening, along with the length of time after use that the drug is detectable in the body). Figure 11-14 shows the Triage Urine Drug Abuse Screen device (Biosite, Culver City, CA) that simultaneously tests for eight major classes of drugs of abuse.

There are legal implications to drug screening and chain-of-custody protocol is required whether it is performed for legal reasons or not. The following are urine drug screen patient preparation and collection requirements defined by the **National Institute on Drug Abuse (NIDA)**.

Patient Preparation Requirements

- Explain the test purpose and procedure.
- Advise the patient of legal rights.
- Obtain a witnessed signed consent form.

Specimen Collection Requirements

- A special area must be maintained for urine collection.
- A proctor is required to be present at the time of collection to verify that the specimen came from the correct person.
- A split sample may be required for confirmation or parallel testing.
- The specimen must be labeled appropriately to establish a chain of custody.

TABLE 11-2 Drugs Commonly Detectable at Drug Screening

Drug or Drug Families	Common Names	Detectable (time)	Comment
Alcohol		2–12 hours	
Amphetamines	Methamphetamine, speed, crystal, crank, ice	1–3 days 2–7 days	Single/light use Frequent/chronic use
Barbiturates	Downers, Seconal, Fiorinal, Tuinal, Phenobarbital	2 days to 4 weeks	Varies considerably with drugs in this class
Benzodiazepines	Valium, Librium, Xanax, Dalmane, Serax	1 week to >30 days	Varies considerably with drugs in this class
Cocaine (as metabolite)	Crack	1–3 days 3–14 days	Single/light use Frequent use/free base
Cannabinoids	Marijuana, grass hash	1–7 days >30 days	Single/light use Frequent/chronic use
Methadone	Dolophine	1–4 days	Single/light use
Opiates	Heroin, morphine, codeine, Dilaudid hydrocodone	2–4 days >7 days	Single/light use Frequent/chronic use
Phencyclidine	PCP, angel dust	2–7 days >30 days	Single/light use Frequent/chronic use
Propoxyphene	Darvon, Darvocet	1–2 days >7 days	Single/light use Frequent/chronic use

Courtesy Tox Talk, Sonora Laboratory Sciences, Phoenix, AZ (1996).

FIGURE 11-14

Triage urine drug of abuse (DOA) screen.

(Biosite, San Diego, CA.)

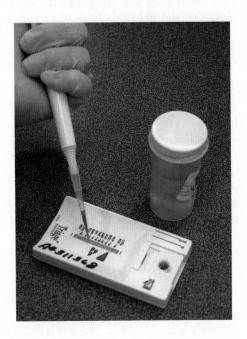

• To avoid tampering, a specimen must be sealed and placed in a clocked container during transport from the collection site to the testing site. Documentation must be carefully maintained from courier to receiver.

Trace Elements

Trace elements or metals include aluminum, arsenic, copper, lead, iron, and zinc. These elements are measured in such small amounts that traces of them in the glass, plastic, or stopper material of evacuated tubes may leach into the specimen, causing falsely elevated test values. For this reason, specimens for these tests must be collected in special trace-element-free tubes. These tubes are made of materials that have been specially manufactured to be as free of trace elements as possible. An insert with each carton of tubes gives a detailed analysis of residual amounts of metals contained in the tubes. These tubes are typically royal blue and contain EDTA, heparin, or no additive. The type of additive is indicated on the label, e.g., red for no additive, lavender for EDTA, and green for heparin.

POINT-OF-CARE TESTING

Point-of-care testing (POCT), also known as alternate site testing (AST) or ancillary, bedside, or near-patient testing, brings laboratory testing to the location of the patient. It has been made possible by advances in laboratory instrumentation that have led to the development of small, portable, and often hand-held testing devices. Its benefits include convenience to the patient and a short turnaround time (TAT) for results that allows healthcare providers to address crucial patient needs, deliver prompt medical attention, and help expedite patient recovery.

In addition to being able to operate the analyzer according to manufacturer's instructions and possessing the phlebotomy skills required to collect the specimen, anyone who does POCT must be able to carry out the quality control and maintenance procedures necessary to ensure that results obtained are accurate. Anyone who performs POCT must meet CLIA qualifications for testing and OSHA guidelines for specimen handling

BLEEDING TIME

Bleeding time is the time required for blood to stop flowing from a standardized puncture on the inner surface of the forearm. The **bleeding time (BT)** test, which evaluates platelet plug formation in the capillaries to detect platelet function disorders and capillary integrity problems, has always been a point-of-care test and does not require special POCT instrumentation. It is used in diagnosing problems with hemostasis and as a presurgical screening test. Although it has largely been replaced by other coagulation tests such as platelet function assays, it is still occasionally ordered, and since accuracy of results depends on technique, it must be performed correctly.

The BT test is performed on the volar (inner) lateral surface of the forearm, using a blood pressure cuff to standardize and maintain a constant pressure. The incision is made with a sterile automated incision device such as the Surgicutt (ITC, Edison, NJ) (Fig. 11-15) or Simplate (bioMerieux, Durham, NC) that control the width and depth of the incision. BT procedure is shown in Procedure 11-3.

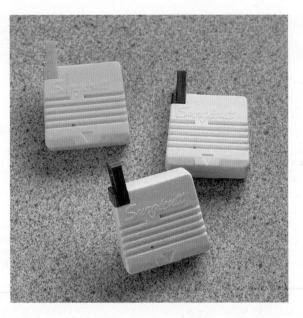

FIGURE 11-15

Closeup of Surgicutt automated bleeding time device. (ITC, Edison, NJ.)

Sources of Error

- Ingestion of aspirin or other salicylate-containing drugs or drugs such as ethanol, dextran, and streptokinase within 2 weeks of the test can abnormally prolong bleeding time.
- Disturbing platelet plug formation will increase the bleeding time.
- Failure to maintain blood pressure at 40 mm Hg will decrease the bleeding time.
- Failure to start the timing as soon as the incision is made will decrease the bleeding time.

Coagulation Monitoring

A number of different coagulation POCT analyzers can be used to monitor patient warfarin and heparin therapy. Examples include the Protime 3 and Hemochron Jr. Signature (ITC, Edison, NJ), CoaguChek (Roche Diagnostics, Indianapolis, IN), which performs CLIA-waived PT and **international normalized ratio (INR)** tests on whole blood from a fingerstick, and the Rapidpoint Coag (Bayer Diagnostics, Tarrytown, NY). These analyzers perform a variety of tests including:

- Protime (PT) and INR
- Activated partial thromboplastin time (APTT or PTT)
- **Activated clotting time (ACT)**
- **Heparin management test (HMT)**

P T

The PT test is used to monitor warfarin (e.g., Coumadin) therapy. Many Coumadin/anti-coagulation clinics use POCT coagulation analyzers such as the Roche CoaguChek to

PROCEDURE 11-3

Bleeding Time Test

Purpose: To perform a bleeding time test

Equipment: Gloves, suitable skin antiseptic, automated bleeding time incision device, blood pressure cuff, timing device, filter paper (#1 Whatman or equivalent), alcohol pads, butterfly bandage or Steri-Strips, waterproof bandage, permanent ink pen

Step	Rationale
1. Identify patient and sanitize hands	Correct ID is vital to patient safety and meaningful test results. Proper hand hygiene plays a major role in infection control by protecting the phlebotomist, patient, and others from contamination. Gloves are sometimes put on at this point. Follow facility protocol
2. Determine whether the patient has taken aspirin or any other salicylate-containing drug within the previous 2 weeks. Advise the patient of the potential for scarring	Salicylates interfere with interpretation of the test by prolonging bleeding time. Although the incision is minor, there is a possibility of scarring
3. Support the patient's arm on a steady surface	Support is required so the patient is comfortable for the duration of the test and doesn't move the arm when the incision is made
4. Select an area on the inner (volar) lateral surface of the forearm, approximately 5 cm distal to the antecubital area and devoid of surface veins, scars, bruises, or edema. It may be necessary to shave the test area lightly if it is covered with a large amount of hair	The lateral aspect is preferred because the medial aspect tends to cause more pain and has a higher incidence of scarring. Scars, veins, bruises, and edema are avoided for accuracy of test results. The area must be devoid of hair for the incision device to make proper contact with the skin before activation
5. Place the blood pressure cuff around the arm	The blood pressure cuff must be in place and ready to be inflated before the incision is made. Applying it before cleaning the site minimizes chance of contaminating the site during application and adjustment
6. Clean the selected area with alcohol and allow to air dry	Cleaning the site with an antiseptic helps avoid contaminating the patient with skin surface bacteria when the incision is made. Letting the site dry naturally permits maximum antiseptic action, prevents contamination caused by wiping, and avoids stinging when the incision is made
7. Put on gloves and prepare equipment	According to the OSHA BBP standard, gloves must be worn during phlebotomy procedures. Preparing equipment while the site is drying saves time

Step	Explanation/Rationale

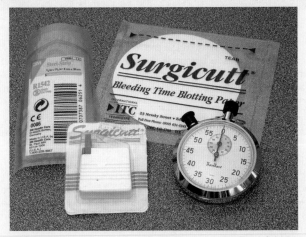

8. Remove the puncture device from its package, being careful not to touch or rest the blade slot on any nonsterile surface	Sterility of the incision device must be maintained for the safety of the patient
9. Inflate the blood pressure cuff to 40 mm Hg	This pressure *must* be maintained throughout the entire procedure for standardization purposes
10. Quickly remove the safety clip and place the puncture device firmly on the lateral aspect of the forearm (without pressing hard) approximately 5 cm below and parallel to the antecubital crease	Time between inflation of the blood pressure cuff and making the incision should be between 30 and 60 seconds for accuracy of results. A horizontal incision parallel to the antecubital crease is recommended

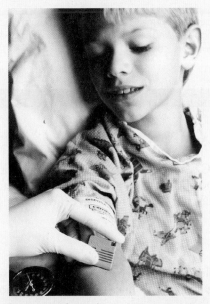

(Courtesy ITC, Edison, N.J.)

(Continued)

PROCEDURE 11-3 *(Continued)*

Step	Explanation/Rationale
11. Depress the trigger while simultaneously starting the timer. Remove the device from the arm as soon as the blade has retracted and discard in sharps container	Timing is critical and must start when the incision is made. Removing the device before the blade retracts can result in injury to the patient or phlebotomist. All sharp objects must be discarded in a sharps container
12. Blot the blood flow at 30 seconds by bringing the filter paper close to the incision and absorbing or "wicking" the blood onto the filter paper without touching the wound	Standardization of timing is necessary for accuracy of results. Touching the wound disturbs platelet plug formation
13. Stop the timer when blood no longer stains the filter paper. (If bleeding persists beyond 15 minutes the test is normally stopped and the result is reported as 15 minutes or greater)	The end point is determined by stoppage of blood flow indicated when no more blood soaks into the paper. Follow facility protocol for stopping the test if the bleeding time is excessive
14. Remove blood pressure cuff, clean the arm, and apply a butterfly bandage or Steri-Strip. Cover with an adhesive bandage. Instruct the patient not to remove the bandage or get the site wet for 24 hours	A butterfly bandage (or Steri-Strip) pulls the sides of the wound together and helps prevent scarring. For proper healing the site should not get wet or be disturbed for 24 hours
15. Record the time to the nearest 30 seconds. Normal: 2–8 minutes depending on method and facility reference ranges	Timing cannot be more precise because blotting only occurs at 30-second intervals
16. Dispose of used and contaminated supplies. Thank and dismiss (outpatient) or leave patient (inpatient)	Wrappers are normally discarded in the regular trash. The blood soaked filter paper is typically discarded in a biohazard container

provide timely laboratory results. Some POCT analyzers allow patients to perform pro-times at home and transmit their results to the physicians' office. The physician can adjust medication over the phone and the patient does not have to make an office visit.

PTT

The APTT /PTT test is used to screen for bleeding disorders prior to surgery, investigate bleeding or clotting disorders, detect clotting factor deficiencies, and to monitor low-dose heparin therapy.

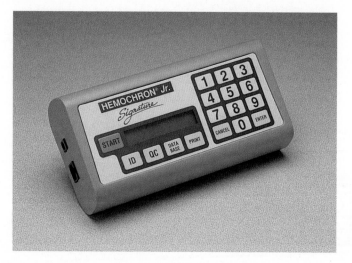

FIGURE 11-16

The Hemochron Jr. Signature analyzer for ACT determinations. (Courtesy International Technidyne Corp., Edison, NJ.)

ACT

The ACT test analyzes activity of the intrinsic coagulation factors and is used to monitor heparin therapy. Heparin is given intravenously to patients who have blood clots or whose blood is apt to clot too easily and as a precaution following certain surgeries. Effects on intravenous heparin administration are immediate but difficult to control. Too much heparin can cause the patient to bleed; therefore, heparin therapy is closely monitored. Once a patient's condition is stabilized, the patient is placed on oral anticoagulant therapy such as Coumadin and is monitored by PT testing.

The ACT test has traditionally been a bedside test; however, timing and mixing was done manually and prone to error. With automated ACT analyzers, the mixing and timing are done automatically. One example is the ITC Hemochron Jr. Signature (Fig.11-16), which is capable of performing the following tests:

- *ACT-LR:* monitors low-to-moderate levels of heparin useful in dialysis and cath lab procedures.
- *ACT+:* monitors moderate-to-high levels of heparin for use in cardiac bypass procedures.
- *APTT:* monitors low-dose heparin anticoagulation.
- *PT:* provides the flexibility to use venous or fingerstick samples. Results are reported as a plasma equivalent value and an INR.
- *Citrate PT:* for PT testing of a whole blood sample collected in sodium citrate. Results are reported as a plasma equivalent value and an INR.

HMT

The HMT is a test for high-dose heparin monitoring needed in catheterization laboratories and during surgery. One HMT point-of-care analyzer, the Rapidpoint Coag (Bayer, Tarrytown, NY) (Fig.11-17), uses one drop of specimen on a credit card-sized test cartridge.

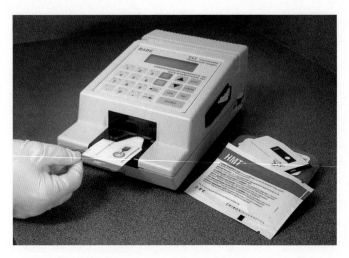

FIGURE 11-17
Rapid Point Coag used for HMT
(Bayer, Tarrytown, NY).

Arterial Blood Gas and Chemistry Panels

Several small, portable, and in some cases hand-held instruments are available that measure panels or groups of commonly ordered stat tests such as blood gases and electrolytes. The body normally maintains these analytes in specific proportions within narrow ranges, and any uncorrected imbalance can quickly lead to death. Consequently, these tests are often ordered in emergency and critical care situations in which immediate response provided by POCT analyzers is vital to the patient's survival.

COMMON POCT CHEMISTRY PANELS

Arterial Blood Gases   Arterial blood gases (ABGs) measured by POCT methods include **pH**, **partial pressure of carbon dioxide** (PCO_2), and **partial pressure of oxygen** (PO_2).

- pH is an abbreviation for potential hydrogen, a scale representing the relative acidity or alkalinity of a solution. The arterial blood pH test is a measure of the body's acid–base balance and indicates a patient's metabolic and respiratory status. The normal range for arterial blood pH is 7.35 to 7.45. Below-normal pH is referred to as acidosis and above-normal pH is referred to as alkalosis.
- The PCO_2 is a measure of the pressure exerted by dissolved CO_2 in the blood plasma and is proportional to the PCO_2 in the alveoli and, therefore, an indicator of how well air is being exchanged between the blood and the lungs. CO_2 levels are maintained within normal limits by the rate and depth of respiration. An abnormal increase in PCO_2 is associated with hypoventilation and a decrease with hyperventilation.
- The PO_2 is a measure of the pressure exerted by dissolved O_2 in the blood plasma and indicates the ability of the lungs to diffuse O_2 through the alveoli into the blood. It is used to evaluate the effectiveness of oxygen therapy.

Electrolytes The most common electrolytes measured by POCT are **sodium (Na^+)**, **potassium (K^+)**, **chloride (Cl^-)**, **bicarbonate ion (HCO_3^-)**, and **ionized calcium (iCa^{2+})**.

- Sodium is the most plentiful electrolyte in the blood. It plays a major role in maintaining osmotic pressure and acid–base balance and in transmitting nerve impulses. Reduced sodium levels are referred to as **hyponatremia**. Elevated levels are referred to as **hypernatremia**.
- Potassium is primarily concentrated within the cells, with very little found in the bones and blood. It is released into the blood when cells are damaged. Potassium plays a major role in nerve conduction, muscle function, acid–base balance, and osmotic pressure. It influences cardiac output by helping to control the rate and force of heart contraction. Presence of a U wave on an electrocardiogram indicates potassium deficiency. Decreased blood potassium is called **hypokalemia**. Increased blood potassium is called **hyperkalemia**.
- Chloride exists mainly in the extracellular spaces in the form of sodium chloride (NaCl) or hydrochloric acid. Chloride is responsible for maintaining cellular integrity by influencing osmotic pressure and acid–base and water balance. Chloride must be supplied along with potassium when correcting hypokalemia.
- Bicarbonate ion plays a role in transporting carbon dioxide (CO_2) to the lungs and in regulating blood pH. HCO_3 is formed in the red blood cells and plasma from CO_2. Hydrogen ion (H^+) is released in the process, causing a decrease in pH, which means that the blood becomes more acid. HCO_3^- moves from the cells to the plasma and is carried to the lungs, where it reenters the cells and releases CO_2 for removal through the walls of the alveoli. Removal of CO_2 by the lungs results in a decrease of H^+ ions and an increase in blood pH. Decreased ventilation (hypoventilation) results in higher CO_2 levels and production of more H^+ ions and can lead to acidosis. Hyperventilation decreases CO_2 levels and can lead to alkalosis.
- Ionized calcium accounts for approximately 45% of the calcium in the blood; the rest is bound to protein and other substances. Only ionized calcium can be used by the body for such critical functions as muscular contraction, cardiac function, transmission of nerve impulses, and blood clotting.

POCT CHEMISTRY ANALYZERS

The hand-held i-STAT (Fig. 11-18) (Abbott Diagnostics, Abbott Park, IL) measures blood gas values for pH, PCO_2, and O_2 and the electrolytes Na^+, K^+, Cl^- and HCO_3^- It can also measure BUN, glucose, Hgb & Hct, and ACT values. This system uses small test cartridges, with separate cartridges for various test capabilities. Other POCT analyzers that measure blood gases and electrolytes are the OPTI CCA (Critical Care Analyzer) (Roche Diagnostics), the Nova Stat Profile Analyzer (Nova Biomedical, Waltham, MA), and the Gem Premier (Instrumentation Laboratories, Lexington, MA).

The Careside analyzer (Fig. 11-19) (Careside, Culver City, CA) has over 40 FDA-cleared tests covering chemistry and coagulation and is a dry film, unit-dose-testing, closed-cartridge-based system. This analyzer is often used in physician offices.

The small, portable IRMA (Fig. 11-20) (Phillips Medical, Inc., St. Paul, MN) measures blood gas values for pH, PCO_2, and PO_2 and the electrolytes Na^+, K^+, and iCa^{2+}. The

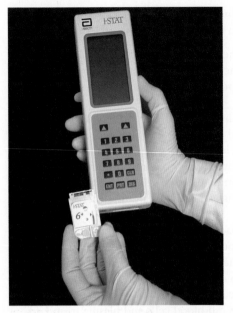

FIGURE 11-18

i-STAT instrument.   (Abbott Diagnostics, Abbott Park, IL.)

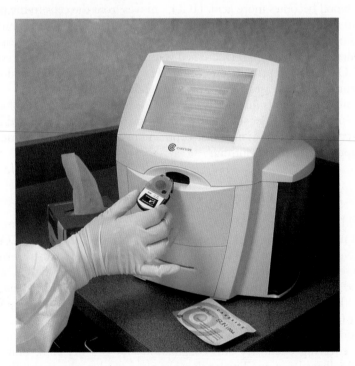

FIGURE 11-19

Careside Point-of-Care instrument.   (Careside, Inc., Culver City, CA.)

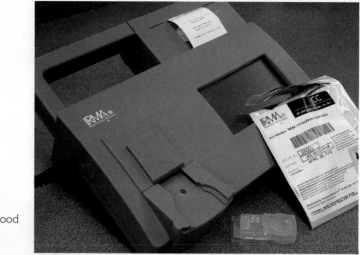

FIGURE 11-20

Portable IRMA (Immediate Response Mobil Analysis) blood chemistry analyzer. (Phillips Medical, Inc., St. Paul, MN.)

IRMA system can also calculate other blood gas parameters such as HCO_3^- and O_2 saturation. A blood analysis is performed by a small cartridge that is inserted into the instrument. The cartridge automatically calibrates itself when it is inserted into the instrument. Once calibration is complete, a small sample of blood is injected into the system's sensor cartridge. The test is performed in less than 2 minutes. The cartridge is then removed from the instrument and discarded in a biohazard container. Results are displayed on a screen and a hard copy printout is generated.

Cardiac Troponin T and I

Cardiac troponin T (TnT) and **troponin I (TnI)** are proteins specific to heart muscle. Blood levels of cardiac TnT begin to rise within 4 hours of the onset of myocardial damage and may stay elevated for up to 14 days. Cardiac TnI levels rise within 3 to 6 hours and return to normal in 5 to 10 days. Measurement of these proteins is a valuable tool in the diagnosis of acute myocardial infarction (AMI) or heart attack. TnT is also measured to monitor the effectiveness of thrombolytic therapy in heart attack patients. Cardiac troponin POCT analyzers include

- The CARDIAC T Rapid Assay (Roche Corporation, Indianapolis, IN), a one-step, whole-blood test for cardiac TnT that uses disposable test kits to provide results in minutes
- The Cardiac STATus from Spectral (Carepoint Cardiac Corporation, Toronto, CAN) and the Triage Meter (Fig.11-21) (Biosite, San Diego, CA) provide results for three cardiac markers, TnI, CK-MB, and myoglobin

Lipid Testing

The Cholestech LDX analyzer (Fig.11-22) (Cholestech, Hayward, CA) can perform cholesterol, triglyceride, low-density lipoprotein (LDL), and high-density lipoprotein (HDL)

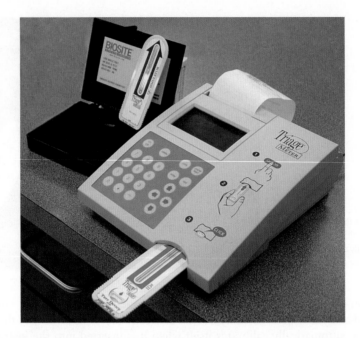

FIGURE 11-21

Triage meter. (Biosite, San Diego, CA.)

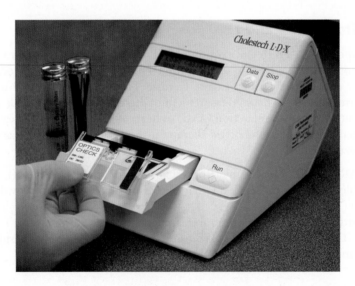

FIGURE 11-22

Cholestech analyzer. (Haywood, CA.)

tests. Blood can be obtained by fingerstick and collected in a lithium heparin capillary tube or by venipuncture. A quantitative result is obtained by visual evaluation of the intensity of a colored bar. A separate cartridge includes alanine transferase (ALT), a liver enzyme that is monitored when patients are on certain lipid-lowering medications. Glucose testing is also available on some cartridges.

B-Type Natriuretic Peptide

B-type natriuretic peptide (BNP) is a cardiac hormone produced by the heart in response to ventricular volume expansion and pressure overload. It is the first objective measurement for congestive heart failure (CHF). BNP levels help physicians differentiate chronic obstructive pulmonary disease (COPD) and congestive heart failure. This facilitates early patient diagnosis and placement into the appropriate care plan. BNP blood concentrations increase with severity of CHF and have been shown to more accurately reflect final diagnosis than echocardiogram ejection fractions. BNP can be determined by the Biosite Triage (Fig. 11-21) meter using a whole-blood EDTA specimen and a special cartridge.

Glucose

Glucose testing is one of the most common POCT procedures and is most often performed to monitor glucose levels of patients with diabetes mellitus. POCT glucose analyzers are small, portable, and relatively inexpensive. Examples include the Advantage HQ (Fig. 11-23) and ACCU-CHEK Inform (Fig. 11-24), both from Roche Diagnostics (Indianapolis, IN), ONE TOUCH (Life Scan, Inc., Milpitas, CA), and the B-Glucose Analyzer (Fig. 11-25) (HemoCue, Inc., Mission Viejo, CA). Most glucose analyzers use whole-blood specimens obtained by routine skin puncture. Some will also accept heparinized venous specimens.

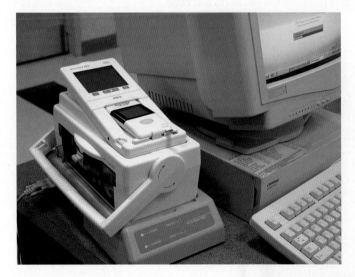

FIGURE 11-23

Advantage HQ Blood Glucose Meter. (Roche Diagnostics, Indianapolis, IN.)

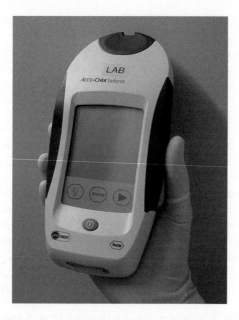

FIGURE 11-24

Advantage Inform.   (Roche Diagnostics, Indianapolis, IN.)

Some analyzers such as the ACCU-CHEK Inform and ONE TOUCH require use of special reagent test strips that come in airtight containers. To prevent deterioration of the strips, the containers must be protected from heat and not left open for more than a few minutes. Some test strip containers have a code number. A code number in the analyzer must be set to match this number. To perform the test, a drop of blood is applied to the test strip that has been inserted into the analyzer. The analyzer determines the level of glucose in the blood, and the result appears on a screen.

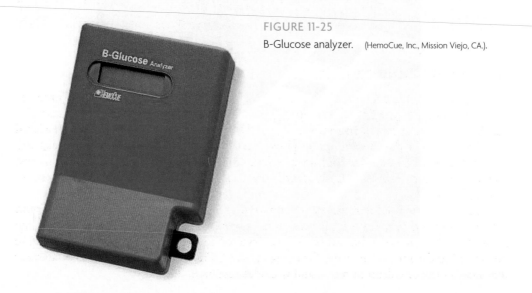

FIGURE 11-25

B-Glucose analyzer.   (HemoCue, Inc., Mission Viejo, CA.).

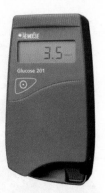

FIGURE 11-26

Glucose 201 system from HemoCue.

(HemoCue, Inc., Mission Viejo, CA.)

The HemoCue B-Glucose Analyzer accepts arterial specimens as well as skin puncture and venous specimens. The test is performed using a microcuvette instead of a test strip. The unit is available with a data management system that allows operator and patient identification to be entered for record retention. The Glucose 201 (Fig. 11-26) is the latest hand-held glucose monitor from HemoCue.

Most analyzers can be connected to computers for downloading of results. The Advantage HQ (Roche) in Figure 11-25 is shown connected to a nursing station computer. This allows transfer of patient results to the laboratory, which can in turn monitor results and quality control (QC). CLSI guidelines recommend that a phlebotomist receive institutional authorization to perform POCT glucose testing only after completing formal training in facility-established procedures, including maintenance and QC.

> **key • point**   QC should be repeated if the analyzer is dropped, the battery is replaced, or patient results or analyzer functioning are questioned.

Glycosylated Hemoglobin

Glycosylated hemoglobin is a diagnostic tool for monitoring diabetes therapy. Three hemoglobins—A_{1a}, A_{1b}, and A_{1c}—are types of Hgb A formed by glycosylation. Because glycosylation occurs at a constant rate during the 120-day life cycle of a red cell, glycosylated Hgb levels reflect the average blood glucose level during the preceding 4–6 weeks and thus can be used to evaluate long-term effectiveness of diabetes therapy. Since this test measures glucose within a red blood cell, levels are more stable than plasma or whole-blood glucose.

Glycosylated hemoglobin values are reported as a percentage of the total hemoglobin within an erythrocyte. Since A_{1c} is present in larger quantity than the others, it is the one measured. One analyzer that measures glycosylated hemoglobin is the FDA-waived A1c NOW (Metrika Inc., Sunnyvale, CA) (Fig. 11-27). The device is a pager-sized analyzer that needs only one drop of blood and provides results in 8 minutes.

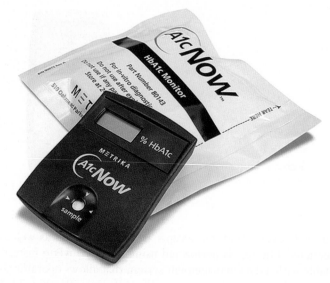

FIGURE 11-27

A1c NOW meter.   (Metrika Inc. Sunnyvale CA.)

Hematocrit

Hematocrit (Hct), also called packed cell volume (PCV), is a measure of the volume of red blood cells in a patient's blood. It is calculated by centrifuging a specific volume of antico-agulated blood and determining the proportion of red blood cells to plasma. Blood is collected in special microhematocrit capillary tubes. The tubes are sealed at one end with clay or a special stopper and placed in a special hematocrit centrifuge. After centrifugation, the results can often be calculated while the tube is still in the centrifuge by lining the tube up with a special chart that is part of the machine and reading results from the chart. The result is expressed as a percentage.

Hcts are often performed in physician office labs (POLs), clinics, and blood donor stations to screen for anemia or as an aid to diagnose and monitor patients with polycythemia.

Hemoglobin

Measurement of hemoglobin (hgb) levels is an important part of managing patients with anemia. A number of POCT analyzers measure hemoglobin. One example is the B-Hemoglobin Analyzer (Fig. 11-28) (HemoCue, Inc., Mission Viejo, CA). It can determine hemoglobin levels in arterial, venous, or capillary blood specimens. A sample of blood is placed in a special microcuvette and inserted into the machine for a reading.

Occult Blood (Guaiac)

Detection of occult (hidden) blood in stool (feces) is an important tool in diagnosing and determining the location of a number of diseases of the digestive tract, including gastric ulcer

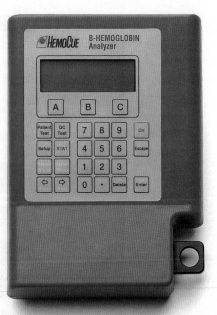

FIGURE 11-28

Hemoglobin Data Management System.   (HemoCue, Inc., Mission Viejo, CA.)

and colon cancer. Most tests that detect fecal blood make use of the peroxidase activity of the hemoglobin molecule to bring about a color change in the specimen being tested. For this reason, a patient's diet should be free of meat and vegetable sources of peroxidase, which may lead to false-positive results. Other sources of false-positive results may be certain drugs, vitamin C, alcohol, and aspirin.

Testing for occult blood in POCT settings typically involves the use of special kits containing cards on which small amounts of feces are placed (Fig. 11-29). The specimen can be collected and tested on-site or the cards sent home with the patient to collect and mail back to the lab. Another type of occult blood test that can be done on-site or sent home with a patient involves a special reagent-impregnated pad that is dropped into the toilet after a bowel movement. A color change on the pad is compared with a result chart.

Pregnancy Testing

Most rapid pregnancy tests detect the presence of **human chorionic gonadotropin (HCG)**, a hormone produced by the placenta that appears in both urine and serum beginning approximately 10 days after conception. Most rapid pregnancy testing is performed on urine. Peak urine levels of HCG occur at approximately 10 weeks of gestation.

A number of manufacturers supply urine pregnancy testing kits. Two examples are the Hybritech Icon II HCG urine assay (Hybritech, Inc., San Diego, CA) and the Quidel Quick Vue One Step (Fig. 11-30). Each manufacturer's kit has unique reagents and timing and testing methods, and most test kits have a built-in control system. It is important to follow directions exactly.

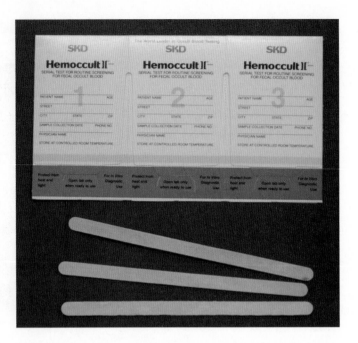

FIGURE 11-29

Hemoccult II occult blood collection cards.   (Coulter, Fullerton, CA.)

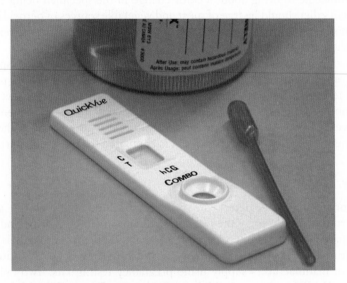

FIGURE 11-30

Quick Vue pregnancy test kit.   (Quidel Corp., San Diego, CA.)

Skin Tests

Some laboratories offer skin testing services, especially for outpatients. Skin tests most often involve the intradermal (within the skin) injection of an allergenic substance (substance that causes an immune response). They are performed to determine if an individual has come in contact with a specific allergen (antigen) and developed antibodies against it. Many disease-producing microorganisms function as allergens, stimulating an antibody response in susceptible individuals. Skin testing can determine an individual's immune status associated with such microorganisms.

EXAMPLES OF SKIN TESTS

- *Tuberculin (TB) test:* Also called PPD test because of the purified protein derivative used in testing; tests for tuberculosis. It is probably the most common skin test
- *Aspergillus test:* Detects hypersensitivity to aspergillus, a type of mold
- *Coccidioidomycosis (cocci) test:* Tests for an infectious fungus disease caused by *Coccidioides immitis*
- *Histoplasmosis (histo) test:* Tests for past or present infection by the fungus *Histoplasma capsulatum*

TUBERCULIN TEST

The tuberculin (TB) test is a skin test that determines if an individual has developed an immune response to *Mycobacterium tuberculosis*, the microbe that causes tuberculosis. An immune response or reaction to the test can occur if someone currently has TB or they have been exposed to it in the past. The procedure for administering a TB test is given in Procedure 11-4.

PROCEDURE 11-4

TB Test Administration

Purpose: Administer a TB skin test

Equipment: Gloves, alcohol pad, tuberculin syringe, 1/2 inch 27-gauge safety needle, TB antigen, permanent ink pen

Step	Rationale
1. Identify patient, explain the procedure, and sanitize hands	Correct ID is vital to patient safety and meaningful test results. Proper hand hygiene plays a major role in infection control by protecting the phlebotomist, patient, and others from contamination. Gloves are sometimes put on at this point. Follow facility protocol

(Continued)

PROCEDURE 11-4 *(Continued)*

Step	Rationale
2. Support the patient's arm on a firm surface and select a suitable site on the volar surface of the forearm, below the antecubital crease	The arm must be supported to minimize movement during test administration. Areas with scars, bruises, burns, rashes, excessive hair, or superficial veins must be avoided as they can interfere with interpretation of the test
3. Clean the site with an alcohol pad and allow it to air dry	Cleaning with antiseptic and allowing it to air dry permits maximum antiseptic action
4. Put on gloves at this point if you have not already done so	Gloves are necessary for safety and infection control
5. Clean the top of the antigen bottle and draw 0.1 mL of diluted antigen into the syringe	The top of the bottle must be clean to prevent contamination of the antigen
6. Stretch the skin taut with the thumb in a manner similar to venipuncture and slip the needle just under the skin at a very shallow angle (approximately 10–15°)	The skin must be taut so the needle will slip into it easily. The antigen must be injected just beneath the skin for accurate interpretation of results
7. Pull back on the syringe plunger slightly to make certain a vein has not been entered	The antigen must not be injected into a vein
8. Slowly expel the contents of the syringe to create a distinct, pale elevation commonly called a bleb or wheal	Appearance of the bleb or wheal is a sign that the antigen has been injected properly

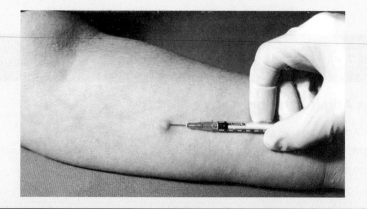

PROCEDURE 11-4 *(Continued)*

Step	Rationale
9. Without applying pressure or gauze to the site, withdraw the needle, activate the safety feature, and discard	Applying pressure could force the antigen out of the site. Gauze might absorb the antigen. Both actions could invalidate test results. Activation of safety features and prompt needle disposal minimizes the chance of an accidental needlestick
10. Ensure that the arm remains extended until the site has time to close. Do not apply a bandage	A bandage can absorb the fluid or cause irritation, resulting in misinterpretation of test results
11. Check the site for a reaction in 48 to 72 hours. This is called "reading" the reaction	Maximum reaction is achieved in 48 to 72 hours. A reaction can be underestimated if read after this time
12. Measure induration (hardness) and interpret result. Do not measure erythema (redness). *Negative:* induration absent or less than 5 mm in diameter *Doubtful:* induration between 5 and 9 mm in diameter *Positive:* induration 10 mm or greater in diameter	A TB reaction is interpreted according to the amount of induration or firm raised area due to localized swelling

key · point A TB test is also called a PPD test after the purified protein derivative used in the test.

Strep Testing

Numerous kits are available for direct detection of group A streptococci on throat swab specimens, for example, the Cards QS Strep A test kit (Quidel Corp.) as shown in Fig. 11-31. Performance of the test normally requires two steps. The first involves nitrous acid or enzymatic extraction of the swab; the second involves a latex agglutination or enzyme immunoassay method of antigen detection. Results are available in minutes.

Urinalysis

A routine urinalysis (UA) consists of a physical and chemical analysis of the specimen as well as microscopic analysis if indicated. A medical laboratory technician or technologist must perform a microscopic analysis.

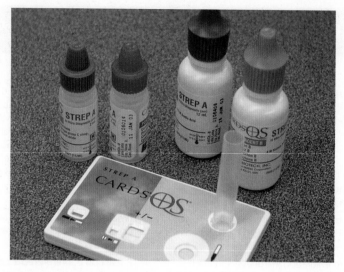

FIGURE 11-31
Cards QS Strep A test kit. (Quidel Corp., San Diego, CA.)

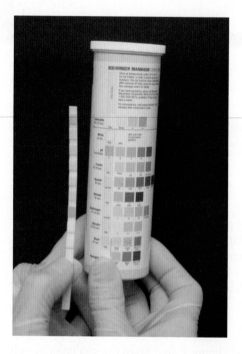

FIGURE 11-32
Technician comparing urine reagent strip with chart on reagent strip container.

Chemical composition is most commonly determined by use of an inert plastic reagent strip containing pads impregnated with reagents that test for the presence of bacteria, blood, bilirubin, glucose, leukocytes, protein, and urobilinogen, as well as measure pH and specific gravity. (Specific gravity can also be measured separately using an instrument called a refractometer.) A chemical reaction resulting in color changes to the strip takes place when the strip is dipped in urine. The results can be determined by comparing the strip visually against a code on the container as shown in (Fig. 11-32) or by inserting the strip into a machine called a reflectance photometer, which reads the strip and prints the results. Reflectance photometers include the Clinitek 200+ (Bayer) and the Chemstrip 101 Urine Analyzer (Roche, Indianapolis, IN), which is a CLIA-waived analyzer.

To ensure the integrity of the strips, they should remain tightly capped in their original containers when not in use, to protect them from the deteriorating effects of light, moisture, and chemical contamination. The containers should also be protected from heat.

STUDY & REVIEW QUESTIONS

1. **When drawing a blood alcohol specimen, it is acceptable to clean the arm with**
   a. Benzalkonium chloride
   b. Isopropyl alcohol
   c. Methanol
   d. Tincture of iodine

2. **Which of the following is the most critical part of blood culture collection?**
   a. Adequately filling two media vials
   b. Antisepsis of the collection site
   c. Selecting the collection site
   d. Timing of the second set of cultures

3. **TDM peak concentration may be defined as the**
   a. Highest concentration of the drug during a dosing interval
   b. Lowest concentration of the drug during a dosing interval
   c. Maximum effectiveness of the drug
   d. Time when the amount of drug entering the body is equal to the amount leaving the body

4. **When performing a glucose tolerance test, the fasting specimen is drawn at 0815 and the patient finishes the glucose beverage at 0820. When should the 1-hour specimen be collected?**
   a. 0915
   b. 0920
   c. 0945
   d. 0950

5. **A bleeding time test detects**
   a. Abnormalities in drug metabolism
   b. Diabetes mellitus
   c. Platelet function disorders
   d. Septicemia

6. **Removing a unit of blood from a patient and not replacing it is used as a treatment for**
   a. ABO Rh incompatibility
   b. Leukemia
   c. Polycythemia
   d. Tuberculosis

7. **Which of the following tests may require special chain-of-custody documentation when the specimen is collected?**
   a. Blood culture
   b. Crossmatch
   c. Drug screen
   d. TDM

8. **What type of specimen is needed for a guaiac test?**
   a. Amniotic fluid
   b. Blood
   c. Feces
   d. Urine

9. **Which of the following tests must have a 9:1 ratio of blood to anticoagulant in the collection tube?**

   a. 2-hour PP   c. Electrolytes

   b. Blood culture   d. Protime

10. **Which of the following specimens is collected in a trace-element-free tube?**

    a. ABGs   c. Lead

    b. BUN   d. Occult blood

11. **Common chemistry tests performed by POCT instruments include**

    a. Hgb and Hct   c. Pt and PTT

    b. Na and K   d. T_4 and TSH

12. **Which of the following is a test that measures packed cell volume?**

    a. HCG   c. INR

    b. Hct   d. TnT

CASE · STUDY · 11-1

Performing a Glucose Tolerance Test

Nancy, a phlebotomist helped Mr. Smith prepare for a glucose tolerance test over the telephone last week. Today Mr. Smith comes in to have his tolerance performed. Nancy asks Mr. Smith if he ate regular, balanced meals for 3 days before today and did not eat, smoke, drink coffee or alcohol, or exercise strenuously for 12 hours before coming in. Mr. Smith answered that he had followed all the directions exactly. Nancy drew the fasting blood at 0815. Mr. Smith was given the drink at 0825.

QUESTIONS

1. How quickly must Mr. Smith completely finish the drink?
2. At what time would Nancy collect the 1-hour specimen?
3. If Mr. Smith's glucose was 300 at 30 minutes is this normal?
4. If Mr. Smith vomits after 45 minutes what should Nancy do?

Bibliography and Suggested Readings

Bishop, M. L., Fody, E. P., & Schoeff, L. (2005). Clinical chemistry: principles, procedures, correlations (3rd ed.). Philadelphia: Lippincott Williams & Wilkins.

Chernecky C. C., Berger B. J., eds. (2004). Laboratory tests and diagnostic procedures (4th ed.). Philadelphia: W. B. Saunders.

Clinical and Laboratory Standards Institute, H45-A2, (2005) Performance of the bleeding time test; approved guideline (2nd ed.). Wayne, PA: CLSI/NCCLS.

Dunne, W.M., Nolte, F.S., & Wilson, M.L. (April 1997). Cumulative techniques and procedures in clinical microbiology, blood culture III. American Society for Microbiology Press.

Fischbach, F. T., & Dunning, M. B. III, eds. (2004). Manual of laboratory & diagnostic tests (7th ed.). Philadelphia: Lippincott Williams & Wilkins.

Joint Commission. (1999). Quality point of care testing: a Joint Commission handbook. Oakbrook Terrace, IL: Joint Commission.

Joint Commission (2002–2003). Comprehensive accreditation manual for pathology and clinical laboratory sciences. Oakbrook Terrace, IL: JCAHO.

Lotspeich-Steininger, C. A., Stiene-Martin, E. A., & Koepke, J. A. (1992). Clinical hematology: principles, procedures, correlations. Philadelphia: J. B. Lippincott.

Morris, L. D., Pont, A., & Lewis, S. M. Use of a new HemoCue system for measuring haemoglobin at low concentrations Clinical & Laboratory Haematology 2001;23:91–96.

National Committee for Clinical Laboratory Standards, T/DM6-A 1997;17(14) (Reaffirmed September 2002). Blood alcohol testing in the clinical laboratory: approved guideline. Wayne, PA: CLSI/NCCLS.

National Committee for Clinical Laboratory Standards, H21-A4 (2003). Collection, transport, and processing of blood specimens for testing plasma-based coagulation assays: approved guideline (4th ed.). Wayne, PA: CLSI/NCCLS.

National Committee for Clinical Laboratory Standards, C38-A (1997). Control of preanalytical variation in trace element determinations: approved guideline. Wayne, PA:.CLSI/NCCLS.

National Committee for Clinical Laboratory Standards, AST4-A2 (2005). Glucose monitoring in settings without laboratory support; approved guideline (2nd ed.). Wayne, PA: CLSI/NCCLS.

National Committee for Clinical Laboratory Standards, C31-A 2 (2001). Ionized calcium determinations; precollection variables, specimen choice, collection, and handling; approved guideline (2nd ed.) Wayne, PA: CLSI/NCCLS.

National Committee for Clinical Laboratory Standards, C30-A2 (2002). Point-of-care blood glucose testing in acute and chronic care facilities; approved guideline (2nd ed.). Wayne, PA: CLSI/NCCLS.

National Committee for Clinical Laboratory Standards, AST2-A. (1999). Point-of-care in vitro diagnostic (IVD) testing: approved guideline. Wayne, PA: CLSI/NCCLS.

National Committee for Clinical Laboratory Standards, H49-A (2004). Point-of-care monitoring of anticoagulation therapy; approved guideline. Wayne, PA: CLSI/NCCLS.

National Committee for Clinical Laboratory Standards, H7-A3 (2000) Procedure for determining packed cell volume by the microhematocrit method; approved standard (3rd ed.). Wayne, PA: CLSI/NCCLS.

National Committee for Clinical Laboratory Standards, H-18A3. (2004). Procedures for the handling and processing of blood specimens: approved guideline. Wayne, PA: CLSI/NCCLS.

National Committee for Clinical Laboratory Standards, T/DM8-A (1999). Urine drug testing in the clinical laboratory; approved guideline. Wayne, PA: CLSI/NCCLS.

Pagana, K. D., Pagana, T. J. (2002). Mosby's manual of diagnostic and laboratory tests (2nd ed.). St. Louis: Mosby.

ARTERIAL PUNCTURE PROCEDURES

key • terms

abducted	brachial artery	L/M
ABGs	collateral circulation	radial artery
Allen test	femoral artery	steady state
arteriospasm	FiO$_2$	ulnar artery

objectives

Upon successful completion of this chapter, the reader should be able to:

1. Define the key terms and abbreviations listed at the beginning of this chapter.

2. State the primary reason for performing arterial punctures and identify the personnel who may be required to perform them.

3. Explain the purpose of collecting arterial blood gas specimens and identify and describe commonly measured ABG parameters.

4. Identify the sites that can be used for arterial puncture, the criteria used for selection of the site, and the advantages and disadvantages of each site.

5. List equipment and supplies needed for arterial puncture.

6. Identify typical required and supplemental requisition information and describe patient assessment and preparation procedures, including the administering of local anesthetic, prior to performing arterial blood gases.

7. Explain the purpose of the modified Allen test, describe how it is performed, define what constitutes a positive or negative result, and give the procedure to follow for either result.

8. Describe the procedure for collecting radial arterial blood gases and the role of the phlebotomist in other site collections.

9. List hazards and complications of arterial puncture, identify sampling errors that may affect the integrity of an arterial sample, and describe the criteria for specimen rejection.

453

An arterial blood specimen is collected anaerobically by directly puncturing an artery with a sharp, short-beveled hypodermic needle or winged infusion set attached to a syringe or other collection device. Arterial blood is the ideal specimen for many analyses because its composition is fairly consistent throughout the body, whereas the composition of venous blood varies relative to the metabolic needs of the areas of the body it serves. However, because arterial puncture is technically more difficult to perform and potentially more painful and hazardous to the patient than venipuncture, arterial specimens are not used for routine blood tests. The primary reason for performing arterial puncture is to obtain blood for evaluation of **arterial blood gases (ABGs)**.

ABGS

ABG evaluation is used in the diagnosis and management of respiratory disease to provide valuable information about a patient's oxygenation, ventilation, and acid–base balance and in the management of electrolyte and acid–base balance in patients with other disorders such as diabetes. Because arterial blood specimens are very sensitive to the effects of preanalytical errors, accurate patient assessment and proper specimen collection and handling are necessary to ensure accurate diagnostic results.

Most instruments used to process ABG specimens directly measure pH, partial pressure of carbon dioxide (PCO_2), and partial pressure of oxygen (PO_2) and calculate bicarbonate (HCO_3), base excess (or deficit), and oxygen (O_2) saturation. Table 12-1 provides an explanation of commonly measured ABG parameters. Many instruments can now also measure

TABLE 12-1	Commonly Measured Arterial Blood Gas (ABG) Parameters	
Parameter	**Normal Range**	**Description**
pH	7.35–7.45	A measure of the acidity or alkalinity of the blood; used to identify a condition as acidosis or alkalosis.
PO_2	80–100 mm Hg	Partial pressure of oxygen. A measure of how much oxygen is dissolved in the blood. Indicates if ventilation is adequate. Decreased oxygen levels in the blood increase the respiration rate and vice versa.
PCO_2	35–45 mm Hg	Partial pressure of carbon dioxide. A measure of how much carbon dioxide is dissolved in the blood. Evaluates lung function. Increased CO_2 levels in the blood increase the respiratory rate and vice versa. *Respiratory* disturbances alter PCO_2 levels.
HCO_3	22–26 mEq/L	Bicarbonate. A measure of the amount of bicarbonate in the blood. Evaluates the bicarbonate buffer system of the kidneys. *Metabolic* disturbances alter HCO_3 levels.
O_2 saturation	97–100%	Oxygen saturation. The percent of oxygen bound to hemoglobin. Determines if hemoglobin is carrying the amount of oxygen it is capable of carrying.
Base excess (or deficit)	(−2) – (+2) mEq/L	A calculation of the nonrespiratory part of acid-base balance based on the PCO_2, HCO_3, and hematocrit.

other critical care analytes such as sodium, potassium, chloride, ionized calcium, glucose, and hemoglobin on the same specimen.

PERSONNEL WHO PERFORM ARTERIAL PUNCTURE

Paramedical personnel (healthcare workers other than physicians) who may be required to perform arterial puncture include nurses, medical technologists and technicians, respiratory therapists, emergency medical technicians, and level II phlebotomists. Personnel who perform ABG procedures are normally certified by their healthcare institutions after successfully completing extensive training involving theory, demonstration of technique, observation of the actual procedure, and performance of arterial puncture under the supervision of qualified personnel. Skills are typically reverified annually.

SITE SELECTION CRITERIA

Several different sites can be used for arterial puncture. The criteria for site selection are

1. Presence of **collateral circulation**, which means that the site is supplied with blood from more than one artery so that circulation can be maintained if one vessel is obstructed or damaged.
2. Artery accessibility and size. The more accessible and larger an artery is, the easier it is to feel and puncture.
3. Tissue surrounding the puncture site. The chosen artery should be in an area that poses little risk of injuring adjacent structures or tissue during puncture, helps fix the artery to keep it from rolling, and allows adequate pressure to be applied to the artery after specimen collection.

In addition, the chosen site should not be inflamed, irritated, edematous, or in close proximity to a wound or hematoma. Sites recently used for arterial puncture should be avoided, if possible.

c a u t i o n   *Never* select a site in a limb with an A–V shunt or fistula. It is a patient's lifeline for dialysis and should not be disturbed; also, venous and arterial blood mix together at the site.

ARTERIAL PUNCTURE SITES

The Radial Artery

The first choice and most commonly used site for arterial puncture is the **radial artery**, located in the thumb side of the wrist (Fig. 12-1). Although smaller than arteries in other sites, it is easily accessible in most patients.

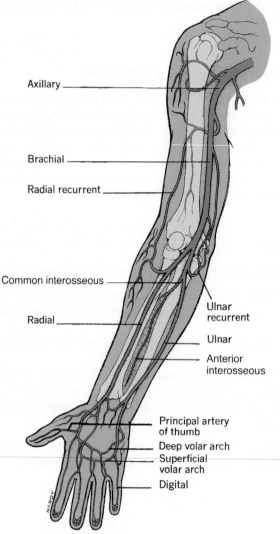

Axillary

Brachial

Radial recurrent

Common interosseous

Radial

Ulnar recurrent

Ulnar

Anterior interosseous

Principal artery of thumb

Deep volar arch

Superficial volar arch

Digital

FIGURE 12-1

Arteries of the arm and hand.

ADVANTAGES

The biggest advantage of using the radial artery is the presence of collateral circulation. Under normal circumstances, both the radial and the **ulnar artery** (see Fig. 12-1), which is located on the opposite side of the wrist from the radial artery, supply the hand with blood. If the radial artery were to be inadvertently damaged as a consequence of arterial puncture, the ulnar artery could supply blood to the hand. For this reason, the ulnar artery is never used for arterial puncture. Collateral circulation can be evaluated by an instrument called a

Doppler ultrasonic flow indicator or by performing the modified Allen test. If collateral circulation is absent, the radial artery should not be punctured.

Another advantage of using the radial artery is that there is less chance of hematoma formation following the procedure, because the radial artery can be easily compressed over the ligaments and bones of the wrist.

> *fyi* The radial artery is named after the radial bone in the lateral aspect (thumb side) of the lower arm, and the ulnar artery is named after the ulna, the large bone in the lower arm on the side opposite the thumb.

DISADVANTAGES

Disadvantages of using the radial artery include the fact that considerable skill is required to puncture it successfully because of its small size, and it may be difficult or impossible to locate on patients with low cardiac output.

The Brachial Artery

The **brachial artery** (see Fig. 12-1) is the second choice for arterial puncture. It is located in the medial anterior aspect of the antecubital fossa near the insertion of the biceps muscle.

ADVANTAGES

Advantages of the brachial artery are that it is large and easy to palpate and puncture. It is sometimes the preferred artery if a large volume of blood needs to be collected. It has adequate collateral circulation, though not as much as the radial artery.

DISADVANTAGES

There are a number of disadvantages to puncturing the brachial artery:

- It is deeper and can be harder to palpate than the radial artery.
- It lies close to a large vein (the basilic) as well as the median nerve, both of which may be inadvertently punctured.
- Unlike the radial artery, there are no underlying ligaments or bone to support compression of the brachial artery, resulting in an increased risk of hematoma formation following the procedure.

> m e m o r y • j o g g e r   The median cutaneous nerve lies medial to the brachial artery, which lies medial to the biceps tendon. The order from lateral to medial can be remembered by the mnemonic TAN, where T stands for tendon, A for artery, and N for nerve.

The Femoral Artery

The **femoral artery** (Fig. 12-2) is the largest artery used for arterial puncture. It is located superficially in the groin, lateral to the pubis bone. Femoral puncture is performed primarily by physicians and specially trained emergency room personnel and is generally used only in emergency situations or when no other sites are available.

ADVANTAGES

The femoral artery is large and easily palpated and punctured. It is sometimes the only site where arterial sampling is possible, especially on patients with low cardiac output.

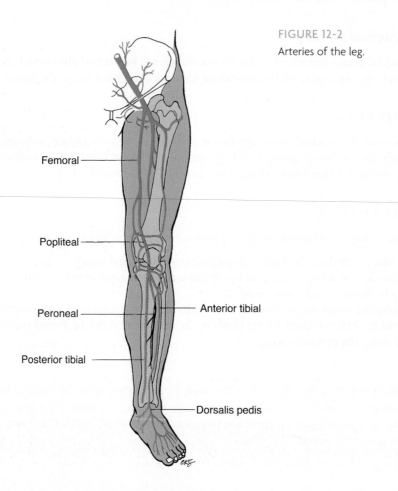

FIGURE 12-2

Arteries of the leg.

Femoral

Popliteal

Peroneal — — Anterior tibial

Posterior tibial

Dorsalis pedis

DISADVANTAGES

Disadvantages of femoral arterial puncture include poor collateral circulation, increased risk of infection because of its location, difficulty in achieving aseptic technique because of the presence of pubic hair, and the possibility of dislodging plaque buildup from the inner artery walls of older patients. In addition, the femoral artery lies close to the femoral vein, which may be inadvertently punctured.

Other Sites

Other sites where arterial specimens may be obtained include the scalp and umbilical arteries in infants and the dorsalis pedis arteries of the adult. The phlebotomist is not normally trained to perform arterial punctures at these locations or to obtain specimens from cannulas, catheters, or other indwelling devices at these or any other locations.

ABG SPECIMEN COLLECTION

Test Requisition

As with any other test, a physician's order is needed before ABG specimens are collected. In addition to normal patient identification information, specific information concerning conditions at the time of collection such as current body temperature, respiratory rate, ventilation status, and **fraction of inspired oxygen (FiO$_2$)**, which for room air is 0.21, or prescribed flow rate in **liters per minute (L/M)** must be documented on the test requisition for meaningful interpretation of results. Required requisition information may vary according to regulatory requirements and institutional policy. Typical ABG requisition information is listed in Box 12-1.

Equipment and Supplies

PERSONAL PROTECTIVE EQUIPMENT

Personal protective equipment (PPE) needed by the blood drawer when collecting arterial specimens includes a fluid-resistant lab coat, gown, or apron; gloves; and face protection because of the possibility of blood spray during arterial puncture.

SPECIMEN COLLECTION EQUIPMENT AND SUPPLIES

ABG specimen collection equipment (Fig. 12-3) includes a safety needle, special heparinized syringe, and cap or other device to plug or cover the syringe after specimen collection to maintain anaerobic conditions.

key • point   Needles for radial ABG collection are typically 22 gauge or smaller, as larger diameter needles may be too large to successfully access the artery.

BOX • 12-1   Typical ABG Requisition Information

Required information:
- Patient's full name
- Medical record or identification number
- Age or date of birth
- Room number or other patient location
- Date and time of test collection
- Fraction of inspired oxygen (FiO_2) or flow rate in liters per minute (L/M)
- Body temperature
- Respiration rate
- Clinical indication for specimen collection (e.g., FiO_2 or mechanical ventilation change)
- Blood drawer's initials
- Requesting physician's name

Supplemental information as required by institutional policy or regulatory agencies:
- Ventilation status (i.e., breathing spontaneously or mechanically supported)
- Method of ventilation (i.e., pressure support) or delivery (i.e., cannula or mask)
- Sampling site and type of procedure (i.e., arterial or capillary puncture or indwelling catheter)
- Patient activity and position
- Working diagnosis or ICD code

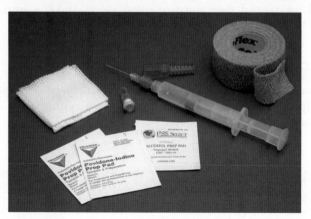

FIGURE 12-3
ABG equipment.

ABG syringes typically contain special filters that vent residual air and seal upon contact with blood, or air bubble removal caps that provide a safe way to remove air bubbles from the specimen. ABG equipment is commonly available in sterile prepackaged kits that contain a heparinized syringe, capping device and safety needle or needle removal device. ABG collection equipment and supplies are listed in Box 12-2.

fyi   ABG specimens are collected in syringes rather than tubes because evacuated tube pressure can affect test results.

Patient Preparation

IDENTIFICATION AND EXPLANATION OF PROCEDURES

The blood drawer must properly identify the patient (see Chapter 8), explain the procedure, and obtain the patient's consent. The patient must be treated in a pleasant, reassuring manner, as blood gas values can be altered by hyperventilation due to anxiety, breath-holding, or crying.

PATIENT PREPARATION AND ASSESSMENT

The patient must be relaxed and in a comfortable position. He or she should be lying in bed or seated comfortably in a chair for a minimum of 5 minutes or until breathing has stabilized. (Outpatients may take longer to stabilize.) Required collection conditions must be verified and documented on the requisition per institution policy. In addition, it should be determined whether or not the patient is on anticoagulant therapy, and if an anesthetic is to be used, it should be confirmed that the patient is not allergic to it.

STEADY STATE

Current body temperature, breathing pattern, and the concentration of oxygen inhaled, affect the amount of oxygen and carbon dioxide in the blood. Consequently, a patient should have been in a stable or **steady state** (i.e., no exercise, suctioning, or respirator changes) for at least 20 to 30 minutes before the blood gas specimen is obtained. This is especially important for patients with abnormal respiratory function such as patients with chronic lung disease. With the exception of certain emergency situations, ABG collection should not be performed until a steady state that meets required collection conditions has been achieved.

MODIFIED ALLEN TEST

It must be determined that the patient has collateral circulation before arterial puncture is performed. The modified **Allen test** is an easy way to assess collateral circulation before collecting a blood specimen from the radial artery. It is performed without the

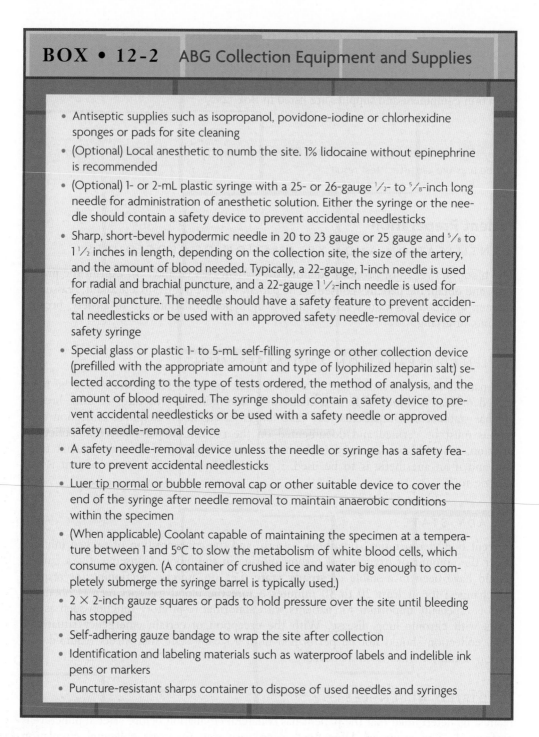

BOX • 12-2 ABG Collection Equipment and Supplies

- Antiseptic supplies such as isopropanol, povidone-iodine or chlorhexidine sponges or pads for site cleaning
- (Optional) Local anesthetic to numb the site. 1% lidocaine without epinephrine is recommended
- (Optional) 1- or 2-mL plastic syringe with a 25- or 26-gauge $^{1}/_{2}$- to $^{5}/_{8}$-inch long needle for administration of anesthetic solution. Either the syringe or the needle should contain a safety device to prevent accidental needlesticks
- Sharp, short-bevel hypodermic needle in 20 to 23 gauge or 25 gauge and $^{5}/_{8}$ to $1^{1}/_{2}$ inches in length, depending on the collection site, the size of the artery, and the amount of blood needed. Typically, a 22-gauge, 1-inch needle is used for radial and brachial puncture, and a 22-gauge $1^{1}/_{2}$-inch needle is used for femoral puncture. The needle should have a safety feature to prevent accidental needlesticks or be used with an approved safety needle-removal device or safety syringe
- Special glass or plastic 1- to 5-mL self-filling syringe or other collection device (prefilled with the appropriate amount and type of lyophilized heparin salt) selected according to the type of tests ordered, the method of analysis, and the amount of blood required. The syringe should contain a safety device to prevent accidental needlesticks or be used with a safety needle or approved safety needle-removal device
- A safety needle-removal device unless the needle or syringe has a safety feature to prevent accidental needlesticks
- Luer tip normal or bubble removal cap or other suitable device to cover the end of the syringe after needle removal to maintain anaerobic conditions within the specimen
- (When applicable) Coolant capable of maintaining the specimen at a temperature between 1 and 5°C to slow the metabolism of white blood cells, which consume oxygen. (A container of crushed ice and water big enough to completely submerge the syringe barrel is typically used.)
- 2 × 2-inch gauze squares or pads to hold pressure over the site until bleeding has stopped
- Self-adhering gauze bandage to wrap the site after collection
- Identification and labeling materials such as waterproof labels and indelible ink pens or markers
- Puncture-resistant sharps container to dispose of used needles and syringes

use of special equipment. If the test result is positive, arterial puncture can be performed on the radial artery. If the result is negative, arterial puncture should not be performed on that arm and the patient's nurse or physician should be notified of the problem. The procedure for the modified Allen test is described in Procedure 12-1.

PROCEDURE 12-1

Modified Allen Test

Purpose: Assess collateral circulation through the ulnar artery

Equipment: None

Step	Rationale/Explanation
1. Have the patient make a tight fist	A tight fist partially blocks blood flow and causes temporary blanching until the hand is opened
2. Using the middle and index fingers of both hands, apply pressure to the patient's wrist, compressing both the radial and ulnar arteries at the same time	Pressure over both arteries is needed to block blood flow. Obstruction of both arteries is necessary to be able to assess blood return when pressure is released
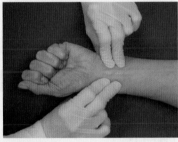	
3. While maintaining pressure, have the patient open the hand slowly. It should appear blanched or drained of color.	Blanched appearance of the hand verifies that blood flow through both arteries is temporarily blocked. The patient must not hyperextend the fingers when opening the hand, as this can cause decreased blood flow and misinterpretation of results
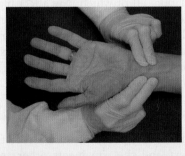	

PROCEDURE 12-1 *(Continued)*

Step	Rationale/Explanation
4. Lower the patient's hand and release pressure on the ulnar artery only	The ulnar artery is released while the radial is still obstructed to determine if it will be able to provide blood flow should the radial artery be injured during ABG collection
5. Assess Results:	
Positive Allen test result: The hand flushes pink or returns to normal color within 15 seconds	A positive test result indicates return of blood to the hand via the ulnar artery and the presence of collateral circulation. If the Allen test result is positive, proceed with ABG collection
Negative Allen test result: The hand *does not* flush pink or return to normal color within 15 seconds	A negative test result indicates inability of the ulnar artery to adequately supply blood to the hand and therefore the absence of collateral circulation. If the Allen test result is negative, the radial artery should not be used and another site must be selected
6. Record the results on the request slip	Verification that the Allen test was performed

ADMINISTRATION OF LOCAL ANESTHETIC

The advent of improved thin-wall needles has made the routine administration of anesthetic prior to arterial puncture unnecessary. However, it may be a reassuring option for some patients, especially children, who are fearful of the procedure. A fearful patient may respond by breath-holding, crying, or hyperventilation, all of which may affect blood gas results. In addition to minimizing or preventing such patient reactions, local anesthesia may also prevent vasoconstriction. The recommended local anesthetic for ABG collection is 1% lidocaine without epinephrine; however, it may cause prolonged bleeding in patients on anticoagulant therapy. The procedure for preparing and administering local anesthetic is described in Procedure 12-2.

Radial ABG Procedure

Puncture of the radial artery can be performed only if it is determined that there is collateral circulation provided by the ulnar artery and the site meets other selection

PROCEDURE 12-2

Preparing and Administering Local Anesthetic

Purpose: Prepare and administer local anesthetic prior to arterial puncture

Equipment: Gloves, 25-26 gauge needle*, 1-mL syringe*, 1% epinephrine-free lidocaine, alcohol wipes, sharps container

*Either the needle or tube holder must have a safety feature to prevent needlesticks.

Step	Explanation/Rationale
1. Verify absence of allergy to anesthetic or its derivatives	Allergy to lidocaine or its derivatives can cause a life-threatening reaction
2. Sanitize hands and put on gloves	Hand hygiene aids in infection control. Gloves provide a barrier to bloodborne pathogen exposure
3. Attach the needle to the syringe	A safety needle (or syringe with a safety device) must be used to reduce the chance of accidental needlestick
4. Clean the stopper of the anesthetic bottle with an isopropyl alcohol wipe	The stopper must be cleaned with an antiseptic to prevent contamination
5. Insert the needle through the bottle stopper and withdraw anesthetic	0.25 to 0.5mL of lidocaine is adequate for most adult applications
6. Carefully replace the needle cap and leave the syringe in a horizontal position	Protects sterility of the needle and prevents contamination and leakage of the anesthetic
7. Clean and air-dry the site	Cleaning the site with antiseptic helps avoid contaminating the patient with skin surface bacteria picked up during needle entry. Letting the site dry naturally permits maximum antiseptic action, prevents contamination caused by wiping, and avoids stinging on needle entry from residual alcohol
8. Insert the needle of the anesthetic syringe into the skin over the proposed arterial puncture site at an angle of approximately 10°	The anesthetic must be injected directly over the puncture site for optimum effect
9. Pull back slightly on the plunger	Verifies that a vein was not inadvertently penetrated. (If blood appears in the syringe, withdraw the needle, discard both needle and syringe, prepare a fresh needle and syringe, and repeat the procedure in a slightly different spot)
10. Slowly expel the contents into the skin forming a raised wheal	Appearance of the wheal verifies proper application of the anesthetic
11. Wait 1 to 2 minutes before proceeding with arterial puncture	It takes 1 to 2 minutes for the anesthetic to take full effect. (The anesthetic wears off in 15 to 20 minutes)
12. Note anesthetic application on the requisition	Use of anesthetic must be documented on the requisition

criteria previously described. The major points of radial ABG procedure are explained as follows:

POSITION THE ARM

Position the patient's arm out to the side, away from the body (abducted) with the palm facing up and the wrist supported. (A rolled towel placed under the wrist is typically used to provide support.) Ask the patient to extend the wrist at approximately a 30° angle to stretch and fix the tissue over the ligaments and bone of the wrist.

LOCATE THE ARTERY

Use the index finger of the nondominant hand to locate the radial artery pulse proximal to the skin crease on the thumb side of the wrist. Palpate the artery to determine its size, direction, and depth.

caution Never use the thumb to palpate, as it has a pulse that can be misleading.

CLEAN THE SITE

Prepare the site by cleaning first with alcohol and then with povidone-iodine or other suitable antiseptic. Allow the site to dry, being careful not to touch it with any unsterile object.

PREPARE EQUIPMENT

Attach the safety needle to the syringe if not preassembled and set the syringe plunger to the proper fill level, if applicable. Put on gloves if they were not put on in step 6 and clean the gloved nondominant finger so that it does not contaminate the site when relocating the pulse before needle entry.

INSERT THE NEEDLE

Pick up and hold the syringe or collection device in the dominant hand as if holding a dart. Uncap and inspect the needle for defects. (Discard and replace it if flawed.) Relocate the artery by placing the index finger of the opposite hand directly over the pulse. Warn the patient of imminent puncture and ask him or her to relax the wrist as much as possible while maintaining its extended position. Direct the needle away from the hand, facing into the arterial blood flow, and insert it bevel up into the skin at a 30 to 45° angle (femoral puncture requires a 90° angle) approximately 5 to 10 mm distal to the index finger that is locating the pulse.

ADVANCE THE NEEDLE INTO THE ARTERY

Slowly advance the needle, directing it toward the pulse under the index finger. When the artery is pierced, a "flash" of blood will appear in the hub of the needle. When the flash appears, stop advancing the needle. Do not pull back on the syringe plunger. The blood will pump into the syringe under its own power unless a needle smaller than 23 gauge is used, in which case a gentle pull on the plunger may be required. Hold the syringe very steady until the desired amount of blood is collected. If the artery is missed, slowly withdraw the needle until the bevel is just under the skin before redirecting it into the artery.

> ⚠ c a u t i o n *Do not* probe. Probing is painful and can cause hematoma or thrombus formation or damage the artery.

WITHDRAW THE NEEDLE AND APPLY PRESSURE

When the desired amount of blood has been obtained, withdraw the needle, immediately place a folded clean dry gauze square over the site with one hand and simultaneously activate the needle safety device with the other hand or place the needle in an approved needle removal safety device. Apply firm pressure to the puncture site for a minimum of 3 to 5 minutes. Longer application of pressure is required for patients on anticoagulant therapy.

> ⚠ c a u t i o n *Never* allow the patient to apply the pressure. A patient may not apply pressure firmly enough. In addition *do not* replace manually holding the site for the required time with the application of a pressure bandage.

REMOVE AIR, CAP SYRINGE, AND MIX SPECIMEN

While applying pressure to the site with one hand, use your free hand to remove the safety needle and discard it in a sharps container. Handle the specimen carefully to avoid introducing air bubbles into it, as they can affect test results. If any air bubbles are present, immediately eject them from the specimen. If the equipment has an air bubble removal cap, follow manufacturer's instructions. Cap the syringe and gently but thoroughly mix the specimen by inversion or rotation to prevent clot formation. Label the specimen and place on ice, if required.

CHECK THE SITE

After applying pressure for 3 to 5 minutes, check the site. The skin below the site should be of normal color and temperature with no evidence of bleeding or swelling. If bleeding, swelling, or bruising is noted, reapply pressure for an additional 2 minutes. Repeat this process if necessary until you are certain bleeding has stopped.

> ⚠ c a u t i o n Never leave a patient if the site is still bleeding. If bleeding doesn't stop within a reasonable time, notify the patient's nurse or physician of the problem.

If the site appears normal, clean the povidone-iodine from the site with an alcohol prep pad, wait 2 minutes, and check it again. Next check the pulse distal to the site. If the pulse is absent or faint, alert the patient's nurse or physician immediately, because a thrombus may be blocking blood flow. If the site appears normal and the pulse is normal, apply a pressure bandage and make a notation as to when the bandage may be removed.

WRAP-UP PROCEDURES

Label the specimen before leaving the patient's bedside. Dispose of used equipment properly. Remove gloves and face protection and wash hands. Thank the patient.

TRANSPORTATION AND HANDLING

Transport the specimen according to laboratory protocol and deliver to the laboratory ASAP. According to CLSI, ABG specimens collected in plastic syringes can be transported at room temperature provided the specimen will be analyzed within 30 minutes. If the patient has an elevated leukocyte or platelet count the specimen should be analyzed within 5 minutes of collection. If a delay in analysis is expected, specimens should be collected in glass syringes and cooled as soon as possible by placing on ice. Specimens for electrolyte testing in addition to ABG evaluation should not be cooled as it affects potassium levels. Such specimens should be transported and tested ASAP. The complete procedure for collection of radial ABGs is shown in Procedure 12-3.

PROCEDURE 12-3

Radial ABG Procedure

Purpose: To obtain an ABG specimen from the radial artery by syringe

Equipment: Gloves, antiseptic prep pads, heparinized blood gas syringe, cap and appropriate needle, gauze pads, self-adhesive bandaging material, permanent ink pen, coolant if applicable, sharps container

Step	Explanation/Rationale
1. Review and accession test request	The requisition must be reviewed for completeness of information (See Chapter 8 Venipuncture Procedure step 1) and required collection conditions such as oxygen delivery system, and FiO_2 or L/M
2. Approach, identify, and prepare patient	Correct patient approach, identification, and preparation are essential. (See Chapter 8 Venipuncture Procedure step 2.) Explaining the procedure in a calm and reassuring manner encourages cooperation and reduces apprehension. (Hyperventilation due to anxiety, breath-holding, or crying can alter test results)

Step	Explanation/Rationale
3. Check for sensitivities to latex and other substances	Increasing numbers of individuals are allergic to latex, antiseptics, and other substances
4. Assess steady state, verify collection requirements, and record required information	Required collection conditions must be met and must not have changed for 20 to 30 minutes prior to collection. Test results can be meaningless or misinterpreted and patient care compromised if required collection conditions have not been met. The patient's temperature, respiratory rate, and FiO_2 affect blood gas results and must be recorded along with other required information
5. Sanitize hands and put on gloves	Proper hand hygiene plays a major role in infection control, protecting the phlebotomist, patient, and others from contamination. Gloves provide a barrier to bloodborne pathogen exposure. Gloves may or may not be put on at this point, depending on hospital protocol
6. Assess collateral circulation	Collateral circulation must be verified by either the modified Allen test or Doppler ultrasonic flow indicator or both. Proceed if result is positive; choose another site if negative
7. Position arm, ask patient to extend wrist	The arm should be abducted, with the palm up and the wrist extended approximately 30° to stretch and fix the soft tissues over the firm ligaments and bone. (Avoid hyperextension as it can eliminate a palpable pulse)
8. Locate the radial artery and clean the site	The index finger is used to locate the radial artery pulse proximal to the skin crease on the thumb side of the wrist, and palpate it to determine size, depth, and direction. An arterial puncture site is typically cleaned with alcohol, followed by povidone-iodine, and must not be touched again until ready to access the artery
9. (Optional) Administer local anesthetic	(See Procedure 12-2) Document anesthetic application on requisition
10. Prepare equipment and clean gloved nondominant finger	Assemble ABG equipment and set the syringe plunger to the proper fill level, if applicable. Put on gloves if you have not already done so, and clean the nondominant finger so that it does not contaminate the site when relocating the pulse before needle entry
11. Pick up equipment and uncap and inspect needle	The syringe is held in the dominant hand as if holding a dart. The needle must be inspected for defects and replaced if any are found
12. Relocate radial artery and warn patient of imminent puncture	The artery is relocated by placing the index finger of the nondominant hand directly over the pulse. The patient is warned to prevent a startle reflex, and asked to relax the wrist to ensure smooth needle entry

(Continued)

PROCEDURE 12-3 *(Continued)*

Step	Explanation/Rationale
13. Insert the needle at a 30° to 45° angle, slowly direct it toward the pulse, and stop when a flash of blood appears	A needle inserted at a 30–45° angle, 5 to 10 mm distal to the finger that is over the pulse should contact the artery directly under that finger. When the artery is entered, a flash of blood normally appears in the needle hub or syringe. (If a needle smaller than 23-gauge is used it may be necessary to pull gently on the syringe to obtain blood flow)

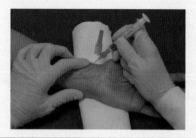

Step	Explanation/Rationale
14. Allow the syringe to fill proper level	Blood will normally fill the syringe under its own to the power, which is an indication that the specimen is indeed arterial blood (see exception in step 13)
15. Place gauze, remove needle, activate safety feature, and apply pressure	A clean folded gauze square is placed over the site so firm manual pressure can be applied by the phlebotomist immediately after needle removal and for 3 to 5 minutes thereafter. The needle safety device must be activated as soon as possible per manufacturer instructions to prevent chance of accidental needlestick
16. Remove and discard syringe needle	For safety reasons, the specimen must not be transported with the needle attached. The needle must be removed and discarded in the sharps container with one hand while site pressure is applied with the other
17. Expel air bubbles, cap syringe, mix and label specimen	Air bubbles in the specimen can affect test results and must be expelled per manufacturer's instructions. The specimen must be capped to maintain anaerobic conditions, mixed thoroughly by inversion or rotating to prevent clotting, labeled properly for identification purposes, and if applicable, placed in coolant to protect analytes from effects of cellular metabolism

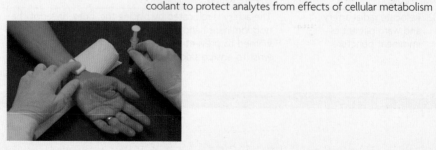

Step	Explanation/Rationale
18. Check patient's arm and apply bandage	The site is checked for swelling or bruising. If none is noted, any povidone-iodine is cleaned from the site to prevent irritation. The site is checked again after 2 more minutes, and the pulse is checked distal to the site to confirm normal blood flow. (The patient's nurse or physician is to be notified immediately if the pulse is weak or absent.) If pulse and site are normal, a pressure bandage is applied and the time it should be removed is noted
19. Dispose of used and contaminated materials, remove gloves, and sanitize hands	Used and contaminated items must be disposed of per facility protocol. Gloves must be removed and hands sanitized as an infection control precaution
20. Thank patient, and transport specimen to the lab ASAP	Thanking the patient is courteous and professional. Prompt delivery of the specimen to the lab protects specimen integrity

ABG Collection from Other Sites

Collection of ABGs from brachial, femoral, and other sites is similar to the procedure for radial ABGs. Because phlebotomists are not normally trained to collect specimens from these sites, specific procedures are not given in this text. Phlebotomists may, however, be asked to provide the equipment and assist in labeling and transporting specimens collected from these sites by others (e.g., an emergency room physician).

HAZARDS AND COMPLICATIONS ASSOCIATED WITH ARTERIAL PUNCTURE

As with any invasive procedure, there are hazards and complications associated with arterial puncture. Examples include the following:

Arteriospasm

Pain or irritation caused by needle penetration of the artery muscle and even patient anxiety can cause a reflex (involuntary) contraction of the artery referred to as an **arteriospasm**. The condition is transitory but may make it difficult to obtain a specimen. To help minimize the chance of arteriospasm reassure the patient by fully explaining the procedure and its purpose and answer questions to help relieve patient anxiety.

Discomfort

Some discomfort is generally associated with arterial puncture, even with use of a local anesthetic. Extreme pain during arterial puncture may indicate nerve involvement, and the procedure should be terminated.

Infection

Infection can result from improper site preparation or contamination of the site prior to specimen collection. Proper antiseptic preparation of the site and avoiding activities that can contaminate the site prior to specimen collection minimizes the chance of infection.

Hematoma

Blood is under considerable pressure in the arteries and is initially more likely to leak from an arterial puncture site than from a venipuncture site. However, arterial puncture sites tend to close more rapidly because of the elastic nature of the arterial wall. Elasticity tends to decrease with age, increasing the probability of hematoma formation in older patients. The probability of hematoma formation is also greater in patients receiving anticoagulant therapy. Precise needle insertion and proper pressure applied by the phlebotomist following needle withdrawal is essential to minimize the chance of hematoma formation.

Numbness

Numbness of the hand or wrist can result from nerve irritation or damage due to error in technique such as improper redirection of the needle when the artery is missed.

Thrombus Formation

Injury to the intima or inner wall of the artery can lead to thrombus or clot formation. A thrombus may grow until it blocks the entire lumen of the artery, obstructing blood flow and impairing circulation. A thrombus can also be the source of an embolus that results in a thrombus, clot, or embolism appearing in another area of the body.

Vasovagal Response

A vasovagal response, faintness or loss of consciousness related to hypotension caused by a nervous system response (increased vagus nerve activity) to abrupt pain or trauma, can occur during arterial puncture. If a patient feels faint or faints during arterial puncture, remove the needle immediately, activate the safety device, hold pressure over the site, and follow syncope procedures discussed in Chapter 9.

SAMPLING ERRORS

A number of factors can affect the integrity of a blood gas sample and lead to erroneous results. These factors include the following:

Air Bubbles

If air bubbles are not immediately or completely expelled from the sample, oxygen from the air bubbles can diffuse into the sample, and CO_2 can escape from the sample, changing test results.

Delay in Analysis

Blood cells continue to metabolize or consume oxygen and nutrients and produce acids and carbon dioxide at room temperature. If the specimen remains at room temperature for more than 30 minutes, the pH, blood gas, and glucose values will not accurately reflect the patient's status. Processing the specimen as soon as possible after it is obtained helps ensure the most accurate results.

Improper Mixing

Inadequate or delayed mixing of the sample can lead to clotting, making the sample unacceptable for testing. Undetected microclots can lead to erroneous results.

Improper Syringe

Use only syringes especially designed for ABG procedures. The use of regular plastic syringes will lead to erroneous values. Use of commercially available ABG kits can eliminate this source of error.

Obtaining Venous Blood by Mistake

Markedly inaccurate ABG values will result if a venous sample is obtained by mistake. Normal arterial blood is bright cherry red in color. Venous blood is a darker bluish-red color. However, it is sometimes difficult to distinguish between arterial and venous blood in poorly ventilated patients because their arterial blood may appear as dark as venous blood. The best way to be certain that a specimen is arterial is if the blood pulses into the syringe. In some instances, such as low cardiac output, a specimen may need to be aspirated. In these cases it is hard to be certain that the specimen is truly arterial.

Use of Improper Anticoagulant

Heparin is the acceptable anticoagulant for blood gas specimens. Oxalates, EDTA, and citrates may alter results, especially pH.

Use of Too Much or Too Little Heparin

Too much heparin in the syringe can result in acidosis of the specimen and cause erroneous results. Too little heparin can result in clotting of the specimen. Use of commercially available kits containing preheparinized syringes can eliminate this source of error.

CRITERIA FOR ABG SPECIMEN REJECTION

ABG specimens that have been improperly collected, handled, or transported can produce erroneous results that can negatively affect patient care. Consequently, specimens with obvious problems will be rejected by laboratory personnel. Examples of typical criteria used to reject ABG specimens for analysis are shown in Box 12-3.

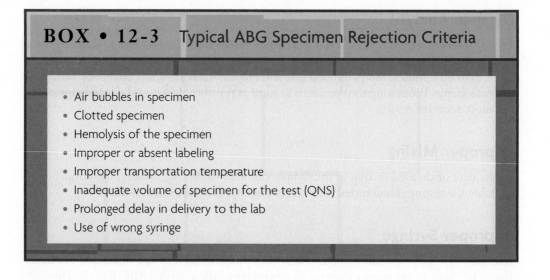

BOX • 12-3 Typical ABG Specimen Rejection Criteria

- Air bubbles in specimen
- Clotted specimen
- Hemolysis of the specimen
- Improper or absent labeling
- Improper transportation temperature
- Inadequate volume of specimen for the test (QNS)
- Prolonged delay in delivery to the lab
- Use of wrong syringe

STUDY & REVIEW QUESTIONS

1. **The primary reason for performing arterial puncture is to**
   a. Determine hemoglobin levels
   b. Evaluate blood gases
   c. Measure potassium levels
   d. Obtain calcium values

2. **The first choice location for performing arterial puncture is the**
   a. Brachial artery
   b. Ulnar artery
   c. Femoral artery
   d. Radial artery

3. **ABG equipment includes all of the following *except***
   a. Povidone-iodine prep pad
   b. Heparinized syringe
   c. Syringe cap
   d. Tourniquet

4. **Commonly measured ABG parameters include**
   a. pH
   b. PCO_2
   c. O_2 saturation
   d. All of the above

5. **A phlebotomist has a request to collect an ABG specimen while the patient is breathing room air. When the phlebotomist arrives to collect the specimen the patient is still on a ventilator. What should the phlebotomist do?**
   a. Call the phlebotomy supervisor and ask what to do
   b. Collect the specimen and write the ventilator setting on the requisition
   c. Consult with the patient's nurse
   d. Take the patient off the ventilator and draw the specimen

6. **The purpose of the modified Allen test is to determine**
   a. Blood pressure in the radial artery
   b. The presence of collateral circulation
   c. The coagulation time of the arteries
   d. Whether the patient is absorbing oxygen

7. **Which of the following is an acceptable angle of needle insertion for radial ABGs?**
   a. 10°
   b. 20°
   c. 45°
   d. 90°

8. **Which of the following complications are associated with arterial puncture?**
   a. Arteriospasm
   b. Hematoma
   c. Infection
   d. All of the above

9. **All of the following can cause erroneous ABG values *except***

   a. Air bubbles in the sample
   b. Cooling a specimen with a high white blood count
   c. Delay in analysis exceeding 30 minutes
   d. Improper mixing

10. **What would cause you to suspect that a thrombus formed in the radial artery while you were collecting an ABG specimen from it?**

   a. A hematoma forms at the site
   b. The patient complains of extreme pain
   c. The pulse distal to the site is weak or absent
   d. There is no way to tell

CASE • STUDY • 12-1

ABG Collection Complications

A phlebotomist has a requisition to collect an ABG specimen from a patient in the cardiac care unit (CCU). The phlebotomist identifies the patient and records required requisition information. The patient has an IV in the left arm in the area of the wrist so the phlebotomist chooses the right arm. The patient is having difficulty breathing and appears quite restless and agitated. The phlebotomist performs the modified Allen test. The result is positive. The phlebotomist attempts puncture of the radial artery. The patient moves his arm as the needle is inserted and it misses the artery. The phlebotomist redirects the needle several times and finally hits the artery. The blood pulses into the syringe but is dark reddish blue in color. The phlebotomist completes the draw, removes the needle, holds pressure over the site, and at same time activates the needle safety device, removes the needle, and caps the syringe, being careful not to introduce air bubbles into it. Then, after holding pressure for 5 minutes and cleaning the povidone-iodine from the site, the phlebotomist checks the pulse distal to the site. The pulse is barely discernable.

QUESTIONS

1. What should the phlebotomist do next?
2. What might be affecting the pulse?
3. How might the patient have contributed to the problem?
4. How might the phlebotomist's technique have contributed to the problem?
5. Can the phlebotomist be certain that the specimen is arterial?

Bibliography and Suggested Readings

Bishop, M., Fody, E., & Schoeff, L. (2005). Clinical chemistry, principles, procedures, correlations (5th ed.). Philadelphia: Lippincott Williams & Wilkins.

Burtis, C., & Ashwood, E., (2001). Tietz fundamentals of clinical chemistry (3rd ed.). Philadelphia: W. B. Saunders.

National Committee for Clinical Laboratory Standards H11-A4. (September 2004). Procedures for the collection of arterial blood specimens: approved standard (4th ed.). Wayne, PA: CLSI/NCCLS.

University of Iowa website. Introduction to interpreting arterial blood gases for medical students. http://www.int-med.uiowa.edu/education/abg.htm

NONBLOOD SPECIMENS AND TESTS

key·terms

AFP	iontophoresis	sputum
amniotic fluid	midstream	suprapubic
buccal swab	NP	sweat chloride
catheterized	O&P	synovial fluid
CSF	occult blood	24-hour urine
clean catch	pericardial fluid	UA
C&S	peritoneal fluid	UTI
FOBT	pleural fluid	
gastric analysis	serous fluid	
H. pylori		

objectives

Upon successful completion of this chapter, the reader should be able to:

1. Define the key terms and abbreviations listed at the beginning of the chapter.
2. Describe nonblood specimen labeling and handling.
3. Name and describe the various urine tests, specimen types, and collection and handling methods.
4. Identify and describe the types of nonblood specimens other than urine, and explain why these specimens are tested.
5. Describe collection and handling procedures for nonblood specimens other than urine.
6. Identify tests performed on various nonblood specimens other than urine.

Although blood is the type of specimen most frequently analyzed in the medical laboratory, various other body substances are also analyzed. The phlebotomist may be involved in obtaining the specimen (e.g., throat swab collection); test administration (e.g., sweat chloride collection); instruction (e.g., urine collection); processing (accessioning and preparing the specimen for testing); or merely labeling or transporting the specimens to the lab.

NONBLOOD SPECIMEN LABELING AND HANDLING

Proper labeling helps avoid delays in testing that could compromise patient care. As a minimum, nonblood specimens should be labeled with the same identifying information as blood specimens. Most institutions also require labeling to include the type and/or source of the specimen. Follow facility protocol.

key • point Phlebotomists are often asked to transport specimens to the lab that have been collected by other healthcare personnel. It is important for the phlebotomist to verify proper labeling before accepting a specimen for transport.

Nonblood specimens have various handling requirements. The phlebotomist must be familiar with these requirements to protect the integrity of the specimen and help ensure accurate test results. In addition, all body substances are potentially infectious, and standard precautions must be observed when handling them.

NONBLOOD BODY FLUID SPECIMENS

Nonblood body fluids are liquid or semiliquid substances produced by the body and found in the intracellular and interstitial spaces and within various organs (e.g., the bladder) and body spaces (e.g., joints).

Urine

Urine is the most frequently analyzed nonblood body fluid. Analysis of urine can aid in monitoring wellness, diagnosis and treatment of urinary tract infections, and detection and monitoring of metabolic disease and the effectiveness or complications of therapy. Accuracy of results depends on the method of collection, type of container used, transportation and handling of the specimen, and timeliness of testing.

caution If urine specimens are not tested in a timely fashion, urine components can change. For example, cellular elements decompose, bilirubin breaks down to biliverdin, and bacteria multiply, leading to erroneous test results.

Collection of inpatient urine specimens is typically handled by nursing personnel. Outpatient urine specimen collection, however, is often handled by phlebotomists. The phlebotomist must be able to explain urine collection procedures to a patient without causing him or her embarrassment. Verbal instructions must be followed by written instructions, preferably with illustrations. In outpatient areas, written instructions are often posted on the wall in the restroom designated for patient urine collections. The type of specimen preferred for many urine studies is the first urine voided (passed naturally from the bladder or urinated) in the morning, because it is the most concentrated. However, the type of specimen and the method of urine collection vary depending on the type of test ordered. The most common urine tests, types of urine specimens requested, and various collection methods follow.

COMMON URINE TESTS

Routine Urinalysis (UA)   A routine **urinalysis (UA)** test typically includes the physical, chemical, and microscopic analysis of a urine specimen.

- Physical analysis involves macroscopic observation and notation of color, clarity, and odor, as well as measurements of volume and specific gravity (SG) or osmolality. (SG and osmolality indicate urine concentration.)
- Chemical analysis detects the presence of bacteria, blood, white blood cells, protein, glucose, and other substances. Analysis is commonly performed using a plastic strip (often called a dipstick) that contains pads impregnated with test reagents. The strip is dipped into the urine and color reactions that take place on the pads are compared to a color chart, usually found on the label of the reagent strip container. Special timing is involved in reading the results, which are reported in the manner indicated on the comparison chart. Results are typically reported using the terms *trace, 1+, 2+,* and so on to indicate the degree of a positive result, and *negative (neg)* or (−) when no reaction is noted. Machines are available that read the strips automatically (see the discussion of point-of-care testing in Chapter 11). The strip is used once and discarded.
- Microscopic analysis identifies urine components such as cells, crystals, and microorganisms by examining a sample of urine sediment under a microscope. To obtain the sediment, a measured portion of urine is centrifuged in a special plastic tube. After centrifugation, the supernatant, or top portion of the specimen, is discarded. A drop of the remaining sediment is placed either on a glass slide and covered with a small square of glass called a coverslip or in a special chamber. It is then examined under the microscope by a laboratory technologist or technician. There are also machines that perform this function.

Routine UA specimens should be collected in clear, dry, chemically clean containers with tight-fitting lids. If a culture and sensitivity (C&S) is also ordered on the specimen, the container should be sterile. Urine specimens should be transported to the lab promptly. Specimens that cannot be transported or analyzed promptly can be held at room temperature and protected from light for up to 2 hours. Specimens held longer should be refrigerated. Specimens that require both UA and C&S testing should be refrigerated if immediate processing is not possible.

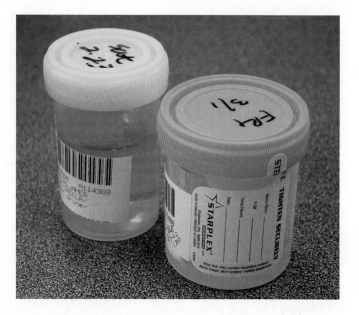

FIGURE 13-1

Urine specimens collected in
sterile containers for C&S testing.

A regular voided specimen is acceptable for routine urinalysis. However, to avoid contamination of the specimen by genital secretions, pubic hair, and bacteria surrounding the urinary opening, the ideal procedure for collecting a specimen for routine urinalysis is referred to as **midstream** collection. (See Urine Collection Methods for regular voided and midstream collection methods).

Urine Culture and Sensitivity A urine **culture and sensitivity (C&S)** test may be requested on a patient with symptoms of **urinary tract infection (UTI)**. The culture involves placing a measured portion of urine on special nutrient media that encourages the growth of microorganisms, incubating it for 18 to 24 hours, checking it for growth, and identifying any microorganisms that grow. If a microorganism is identified, a sensitivity or antibiotic susceptibility test is performed to determine which antibiotics will be effective against the microorganism. Urine for C&S testing must be collected in a sterile container (Fig. 13-1), following midstream **clean-catch** (see Collection Methods) procedures to ensure that the specimen is free of contaminating matter from the external genital areas.

caution Specimens for C&S and other microbiologic studies should be transported to the lab and processed immediately. If a delay in transportation or processing is unavoidable, the specimen should be refrigerated.

Urine Cytology Studies Cytology studies on urine are performed to detect cancer, cytomegalovirus, and other viral and inflammatory diseases of the bladder and other structures of the urinary system. Cells from the lining of the urinary tract are readily shed into the urine, and a smear containing them can easily be prepared from urinary sediment or filtrate. The smear is stained by the Papanicolaou (PAP) method and examined under a microscope for the presence of abnormal cells. A fresh clean-catch specimen is required for the test. Ideally, the specimen should be examined as soon after collection as possible. If a delay is unavoidable, the specimen can be preserved by the addition of an equal volume of 50% alcohol. Follow facility protocol.

Urine Drug Screening   Urine drug screening is performed to detect illicit recreational drug use, use of anabolic steroids to enhance performance in sports, and unwarranted use of prescription drugs; to monitor therapeutic drug use to minimize withdrawal symptoms; and to confirm a diagnosis of drug overdose. With the exception of alcohol, urine is preferred for drug screening since many drugs can be detected in urine but not blood.

Screening tests are typically performed in groups based on drug classifications or families (see Chapter 11, Table 11-2). A random sample in a chemically clean, covered container is required for the test. Specimens containing blood cells or having a high or low urine pH (highly alkaline or highly acid) or a low specific gravity will yield erroneous results and will require recollection of the specimen. (For additional information see Forensic Specimens in Chapter 11.)

Urine Pregnancy Testing   Pregnancy can be confirmed by testing urine for the presence of human chorionic gonadotropin (HCG), a hormone produced by cells within the developing placenta that appears in serum and urine approximately 8 to 10 days after conception or fertilization. Although a random urine specimen can be used for testing, the first morning specimen is preferred because it is typically more concentrated and would therefore have the highest HCG concentration. HCG also appears in the urine of patients with melanoma, tumors of the ovaries or testes, and certain types of cancer including breast, lung, and renal.

Other Urine Tests   Numerous chemistry tests, including electrophoresis, tests for heavy metals (e.g., copper and lead), myoglobin clearance, creatinine clearance, and porphyrins, can be performed on urine specimens. Many of these tests require a pooled timed specimen such as a 24-hour collection.

TYPES OF URINE SPECIMENS

Random   Random urine specimens can be collected at any time. They are used primarily for routine urinalysis and screening tests. Random refers only to the timing of the specimen and not the method of collection.

Timed   Some tests require individual urine specimens collected at specific times. Others require the collection and pooling of urine throughout a specific time period. Some of the most frequently encountered timed urine tests are as follows.

First Morning/8-Hour Specimen

A first morning/8-hour urine specimen (also called a first voided, overnight, or early morning specimen) is usually collected immediately upon awakening in the morning after approximately 8 hours of sleep. This type of specimen normally has a higher specific gravity, which means that it is more concentrated than a random specimen. For this reason, first morning specimens are often requested to confirm results of random specimens and specimens with low specific gravity.

Tolerance Test Specimen

Tolerance tests typically require collection of urine at specific times. The traditional standard glucose tolerance test (GTT) requires individual urine specimens collected serially at specific times that correspond with the timing of blood collection, such as fasting, 1/2 hour, 1 hour, and so on. Timing of the specimens is important in the interpretation of test results. For this reason, the specimens must be collected as close to the requested time as possible, and the label of the specimen should include the time of collection and the type of specimen (e.g., fasting, 1/2 hour).

24-Hour Specimen

A **24-hour urine** specimen is collected to allow quantitative analysis of a urine analyte. Collection and pooling of all urine voided in the 24-hour period is critical. The best time to begin a 24-hour collection is when the patient wakes in the morning, typically between 6 and 8 AM. Collection of the specimen requires a large, clean, preferably wide-mouth container capable of holding several liters (Fig. 13-2). A special collection device that fits over the toilet

FIGURE 13-2

Two styles of 24-hour urine specimen collection containers.

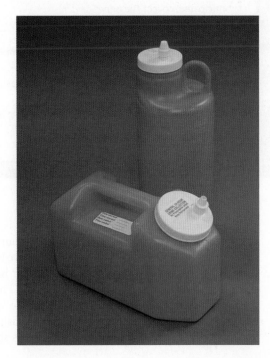

PROCEDURE 13-1

24-Hour Urine Collection Procedure

Purpose: To provide instruction in how to properly collect a 24-hour urine specimen

Equipment: Requisition, specimen label, 24-hour urine container, preservative (if applicable), disposable ice chest (if required), copy of written instructions

Step	Explanation/Rationale
1. Void into toilet as usual upon awakening	The bladder must be empty when timing starts. Urine voided is from the previous time period
2. Note the time and date on the specimen label, place it on the container, and begin timing	Timing (which should ideally start between 6 and 8 AM) is important. If urine is collected for a longer or shorter period, results will be inaccurate. The label should be affixed to the container and not the lid
3. Collect all urine voided for the next 24 hours	Results are based on the total amount of urine produced in 24 hours
4. Refrigerate the specimen throughout the collection period if required	Most specimens (except urate tests) require refrigeration to maintain analyte integrity. The specimen container should be kept cool in a disposable ice chest placed in the bath tub, for example
5. When a bowel movement is anticipated, collect the urine specimen before it, not after	Prevents fecal contamination of the specimen
6. Drink a normal amount of fluid unless instructed to do otherwise	Prevents dehydration and facilitates specimen collection
7. Void one last time at the end of the 24 hours	This specimen must be added to the container
8. Seal the container, place it in a portable cooler, and transport it to the laboratory ASAP	Cooling and prompt delivery help protect the integrity of the specimen

and looks somewhat like an upside down hat is sometimes provided to the patient to make collection of the specimen easier. Some 24-hour specimens require the addition of a preservative prior to collection. Others, such as creatinine clearance, must be kept refrigerated throughout collection. Information on proper handling of the specimen can be obtained by consulting the laboratory procedure manual. The label of the specimen, in addition to standard patient identification, must state that the specimen is a 24-hour specimen, the type of preservative added to the container (if applicable), and any precautions associated with it. The procedure for 24-hour urine collection is shown in Procedure 13-1.

Double-Voided Specimen

A double-voided urine specimen is one that requires first emptying the bladder and then waiting a specified amount of time (typically 30 minutes) before collecting the specimen. It is most commonly used to test urine for glucose and ketones. A fresh double-voided-specimen is thought to more accurately reflect the blood concentration of the analyte tested, whereas a specimen that has been held in the bladder for an extended period may not.

URINE COLLECTION METHODS

Regular Voided Specimen A regular voided urine collection requires no special patient preparation and is collected by having the patient void (urinate) into a clean urine container.

Midstream Specimen A midstream urine collection is performed to obtain a specimen that is free of genital secretions, pubic hair, and bacteria surrounding the urinary opening. To collect a midstream specimen, the patient voids the initial urine flow into the toilet. The urine flow is interrupted momentarily and then restarted, at which time a sufficient amount of urine is collected into a specimen container. The last of the urine flow is voided into the toilet.

Midstream Clean-Catch Specimen Midstream clean-catch urine is collected in a sterile container and yields a specimen that is suitable for microbial analysis or culture and sensitivity testing. Clean-catch procedures are necessary to ensure that the specimen is free of contaminating matter from the external genital areas. Special cleaning of the genital area is required before the specimen is collected. The cleaning methods vary somewhat depending upon whether the patient is male or female. A phlebotomist must be able to explain the proper procedure to both male and female patients. Clean-catch urine collection procedure for females is described in Procedure 13-2. The procedure for males is described in Procedure 13-3.

Catheterized Specimen A **catheterized** urine specimen is collected from a sterile catheter inserted through the urethra into the bladder. A catheterized specimen is collected when a patient is having trouble voiding or is already catheterized for other reasons. Catheterized specimens are sometimes collected on babies to obtain a specimen for C&S, on female patients to prevent vaginal contamination of the specimen, and on bedridden patients when serial specimen collections are needed.

Suprapubic Specimen A **suprapubic** urine specimen is collected by inserting a needle directly into the urinary bladder and aspirating (withdrawing by suction) the urine directly from the bladder into a sterile syringe. The specimen is then transferred into a sterile urine container or tube. The procedure normally requires use of local anesthetic and is performed by a physician. If the patient has a catheter, the specimen can be collected from the catheter by a nurse using a sterile needle and syringe. Suprapubic collection is used for samples for microbial analysis or cytology studies. It is sometimes used to obtain uncontaminated samples from infants and young children.

PROCEDURE 13-2

Clean-Catch Urine Collection Procedure for Women

Purpose: To instruct a female in how to properly collect a clean-catch urine specimen

Equipment: Requisition, specimen label, sterile urine container, special sterile antiseptic wipes, and copy of written instructions

Step	Rationale
1. Wash hands thoroughly	Aids in infection control and helps avoid contamination of the site while cleaning
2. Remove the lid of the container, being careful not to touch the inside of the cover or the container	The lid and container must remain sterile for accurate interpretation of results
3. Stand in a squatting position over the toilet	Facilitates cleaning and downward flow of urine
4. Separate the folds of skin around the urinary opening	Allows proper cleaning of the area
5. Cleanse the area on either side and around the opening with the special wipes, using a fresh wipe for each area and wiping from front to back. Discard used wipes in the trash or toilet	Antiseptic solution in the wipe removes bacteria from area. Front to back motion carries bacteria away from the site
6. While keeping the skin folds separated, void into the toilet for a few seconds	Separation of the folds maintains site antisepsis. Voiding the first portion of urine into the toilet washes away the antiseptic and microbes remaining in the urinary opening
7. Touching only the outside and without letting it touch the genital area, bring the urine container into the urine stream until a sufficient amount of urine (30–100 mL) is collected	Bringing the urine container into the stream without touching the genital area helps ensure sterility of the specimen. An adequate amount of urine is needed to perform the test
8. Void the remainder of urine into the toilet	Only 30–100 mL of urine is needed for the test
9. Cover the specimen with the lid provided, touching only the *outside* surfaces of the lid and container	The specimen must be covered to maintain sterility and protect others from exposure to contents
10. Clean any urine on the outside of the container with an antiseptic wipe	Aids in infection control
11. Wash hands	Aids in infection control
12. Hand specimen to phlebotomist or place where instructed if already labeled	Follow facility protocol

PROCEDURE 13-3

Clean-Catch Urine Collection Procedure for Men

Purpose: To instruct a male in how to properly collect a clean-catch urine specimen

Equipment: Requisition, specimen label, sterile urine container, special sterile antiseptic wipes, and copy of written instructions

Step	Rationale
1. Wash hands thoroughly	Aids in infection control and helps avoid contamination of the site while cleaning
2. Remove the lid of the container, being careful not to touch the inside of the cover or the container	The lid and container must remain sterile for accurate interpretation of results
3. Wash the end of the penis with the special wipe (or soapy water), beginning at the urethral opening and working away from it in a circular motion (the foreskin of an uncircumcised male must first be retracted). Repeat the procedure with a clean wipe	The foreskin must be retracted to allow thorough cleaning of the penis. Antiseptic solution in the wipe removes bacteria from the area. Wiping away from the urinary opening carries microbes away from the site
4. Keeping the foreskin retracted, if applicable, void into the toilet for a few seconds	Keeping the foreskin retracted maintains site antisepsis. Voiding the first portion of urine into the toilet washes away the antiseptic and microbes remaining in the urinary opening
5. Touching only the outside and without letting it touch the penis, bring the urine container into the urine stream until a sufficient amount of urine (30–100 mL) is collected	Bringing the urine container into the stream without touching the penis helps ensure sterility of the specimen. An adequate amount of urine is needed to perform the test
6. Void the remainder of urine into the toilet	Only 30–100 mL urine is needed for the test
7. Cover the specimen with the lid provided, touching only the *outside* surfaces of the lid and container	The specimen must be covered to maintain sterility and protect others from exposure to contents
8. Clean any urine spilled on the outside of the container with an antiseptic wipe	Aids in infection control
9. Wash hands	Aids in infection control
10. Hand specimen to phlebotomist or place where instructed if already labeled	Follow facility protocol

Pediatric Urine Collection   A plastic urine collection bag with hypoallergenic skin adhesive is used to collect a urine specimen from an infant or small child who is not yet potty trained. The patient's genital area is cleaned and dried before the bag is taped to the skin. The bag is placed around the vagina of a female and over the penis of a male. A diaper is placed over the collection bag. The patient is checked every 15 minutes until an adequate specimen is obtained. The bag is then removed, sealed, labeled, and sent to the lab as soon as possible. A 24-hour specimen can be obtained by using a special collection bag with a tube attached that allows the bag to be emptied periodically.

Amniotic Fluid

Amniotic fluid is the clear, almost colorless-to-pale yellow fluid that fills the membrane (amnion or amniotic sac) that surrounds and cushions a fetus in the uterus. It is preferably collected after 15 weeks of gestation (pregnancy) and is obtained by transabdominal amniocentesis, a procedure that involves inserting a needle through the mother's abdominal wall into the uterus and aspirating approximately 10 mL of fluid from the amniotic sac.

Amniotic fluid can be analyzed to detect genetic disorders such as Down syndrome, identify hemolytic disease resulting from blood incompatibility between the mother and fetus, and determine gestational age. However, the most common reasons for testing amniotic fluid are to detect problems in fetal development (particularly neural tube defects such as spina bifida) and assess fetal lung maturity.

Genetic disorders can be detected by chromosome studies done on fetal cells removed from the fluid, although the procedure has for the most part been replaced by studies on chorionic villi or placental tissue because it can be obtained earlier in the gestational period than amniotic fluid. Hemolytic disease can be detected by measuring bilirubin levels.

Although ultrasonography has become the accepted means of estimating gestational age, amniotic fluid creatinine levels have been used to estimate gestational age because levels are related to fetal muscle mass.

Problems in fetal development can be detected by measuring **alpha-fetoprotein (AFP)**, an antigen normally present in the human fetus that is also found in amniotic fluid and maternal serum. (AFP is also present in certain pathological conditions in males and nonpregnant females.) Abnormal AFP levels may indicate problems in fetal development such as neural tube defects. AFP testing is initially performed on maternal serum and abnormal results are confirmed by amniotic fluid AFP testing. Because normal AFP levels are different in each week of gestation, it is important that the gestational age of the fetus be included on the specimen label.

Fetal lung maturity can be assessed by measuring the amniotic fluid levels of substances called phospholipids that act as surfactants to keep the alveoli of the lungs inflated. Results are reported as a lecithin-to-sphingomyelin (L/S) ratio. Lungs are most likely immature if the L/S ratio is less than 2. Amniotic fluid testing to assess fetal lung maturity may be ordered on or near the patient's due date and is often ordered STAT when the fetus is in distress.

Amniotic fluid is normally sterile and must be collected in a sterile container. The specimen should be protected from light to prevent breakdown of bilirubin and delivered to the laboratory ASAP. Specimens for chromosome analysis must be kept at room temperature. However, specimens for some chemistry tests must be kept on ice. Follow laboratory protocol.

Cerebrospinal Fluid

Cerebrospinal fluid (CSF) is a clear, colorless liquid that circulates within the cavities surrounding the brain and spinal cord. CSF has many of the same constituents as blood plasma. Specimens are obtained by a physician; most often through lumbar (spinal) puncture. The primary reason for collecting CSF is to diagnose meningitis. Routine tests performed on spinal fluid include cell counts, chloride, glucose, and total protein. Other tests are performed if indicated. CSF is generally collected in three special sterile tubes numbered in order of collection. Laboratory protocol dictates which tests are to be performed on each particular tube, unless indicated by the physician. Normally, the first tube is used for chemistry and immunology tests, the second tube for microbiology studies, and the third tube for cell counts. CSF should be kept at room temperature, delivered to the lab stat, and analyzed immediately.

Gastric Fluid/Gastric Analysis

Gastric fluid is stomach fluid. A **gastric analysis** examines stomach contents for abnormal substances and measures gastric acid concentration to evaluate stomach acid production. A basal tube gastric analysis involves aspirating a sample of gastric fluid by means of a tube passed through the mouth and throat (oropharynx) or nose and throat (nasopharynx) into the stomach following a period of fasting. This sample is tested to determine acidity prior to stimulation. After the basal sample has been collected, a gastric stimulant, most commonly histamine or pentagastrin, is administered intravenously and several more gastric samples are collected at timed intervals. All specimens are collected in sterile containers. The role of the phlebotomist in the procedure is to assist in labeling specimens and draw blood specimens for serum gastrin (a hormone that stimulates gastric acid secretion) determinations.

Nasopharyngeal Secretions

Nasopharyngeal (NP) refers to the nasal cavity and pharynx. NP secretions are cultured to detect the presence of the microorganisms that cause diphtheria, meningitis, pertussis (whooping cough), and pneumonia. NP specimens are collected using a sterile Dacron or cotton-tipped flexible wire swab. The swab is inserted gently into the nose and passed into the nasopharynx. There it is gently rotated, then carefully removed, placed into transport medium, labeled, and delivered to the lab.

Saliva

Saliva (fluid secreted from glands in the mouth) is increasingly being used to monitor hormone levels and detect alcohol and drug abuse because it can be collected quickly and easily in a noninvasive manner. In addition, detection of drugs in saliva indicates recent drug use. Numerous kits are available for collecting and testing saliva specimens. Many are point-of-care tests. Saliva specimens for hormone tests, however, are typically frozen to ensure stability and sent to a laboratory for testing.

Semen

Semen (seminal fluid) is the sperm-containing thick yellowish white fluid discharged during male ejaculation. It is analyzed to assess fertility or to determine the effectiveness of sterilization following vasectomy. Semen specimens are collected in sterile containers and must be kept warm and delivered to the lab immediately.

key • point A semen specimen should not be collected in a condom. Condoms often contain spermicides (substances that kill sperm) that invalidate test results.

Serous Fluid

Serous fluid is a pale yellow watery fluid found between the double-layered membranes that enclose the pleural, pericardial, and peritoneal cavities. It lubricates the membranes and allows them to slide past one another with minimal friction. The fluid is normally present in small amounts, but volumes increase when inflammation or infection is present or when serum protein levels decrease.

fyi Accumulation of excess serous fluid in the peritoneal cavity is called ascites (a-si' tez).

Serous fluids can be aspirated for testing purposes or when increased amounts are interfering with normal function of associated organs. A physician performs the procedure. Fluid withdrawn for testing is typically collected in EDTA tubes if cell counts or smears are ordered, oxalate or fluoride tubes for chemistry tests, and sterile containers for cultures. The type of fluid should be indicated on the specimen label. Serous fluids are identified according to the body cavity of origin as follows:

- **Pleural fluid**: aspirated from the pleural cavity surrounding the lungs
- **Peritoneal fluid**: aspirated from the abdominal cavity
- **Pericardial fluid**: aspirated from the pericardial cavity that surrounds the heart

Sputum

Sputum is mucus or phlegm that is ejected from the trachea, bronchi, and lungs through deep coughing. Sputum specimens are sometimes collected in the diagnosis or monitoring of lower respiratory tract infections such as tuberculosis (TB).

key • point The TB microbe is called an acid-fast bacillus (AFB), and the sputum test for TB is called an AFB culture.

First morning specimens are preferred, as secretions tend to collect in the lungs overnight and a larger volume of specimen can be produced. The patient must first remove dentures if applicable, then rinse the mouth and gargle with water to minimize contamination with mouth flora and saliva. The patient then brings up the sputum through deep coughing into a special sterile container.

> **key·point** The patient must cough up material from deep in the respiratory tract and not simply spit into the container.

Specimens are transported at room temperature and require immediate processing upon arrival in the laboratory to maintain specimen quality.

Sweat

Sweat is analyzed for chloride content in the diagnosis of **cystic fibrosis**, predominantly in children and adolescents under the age of 20. Cystic fibrosis is a disorder of the exocrine glands that affects many body systems, but primarily the lungs, upper respiratory tract, liver, and pancreas. Patients with cystic fibrosis have abnormally high levels (2 to 5 times normal) of chloride in their sweat, which can be measured by the **sweat chloride** test. The test involves transporting pilocarpine (a sweat-stimulating drug) into the skin by means of electrical stimulation from electrodes placed on the skin, a process called **iontophoresis**. The forearm is the preferred site, but the leg or thigh may be used on infants or toddlers. Sweat is collected, weighed to determine the volume, and analyzed for chloride content.

Sweat specimens can also be used to detect illicit drug use. Sweat is collected on patches placed on the skin for extended periods of time, then tested for drugs.

Synovial Fluid

Synovial fluid is a clear, pale yellow, viscous fluid that lubricates and decreases friction in moveable joints. It normally occurs in small amounts but increases when inflammation is present. It can be tested to identify or differentiate arthritis, gout, and other inflammatory conditions. It is typically collected in three tubes; an EDTA or heparin tube for cell counts, identification of crystals, and smear preparation; a sterile tube for culture and sensitivity; and a nonadditive tube for macroscopic appearance, chemistry, and immunology tests and to observe clot formation.

OTHER NONBLOOD SPECIMENS

Buccal Swabs

Collection of a **buccal** (cheek) **swab** is a less invasive, painless alternative to blood collection for obtaining cells for DNA analysis. The phlebotomist collects the sample by gently massaging the mouth on the inside of the cheek with a special swab. DNA is later extracted from cells on the swab.

Bone Marrow

Because it is the site of blood cell production, bone marrow is sometimes aspirated and examined to detect and identify blood diseases. A bone marrow biopsy may be performed at the same time. To obtain bone marrow, a physician inserts a special large-gauge needle into the bone marrow in the iliac crest (hip bone) or sternum (breast bone). Once the bone marrow is penetrated, a 10 mL or larger syringe is attached to the needle to aspirate 1.0 to 1.5 mL of specimen. A laboratory hematology technologist is typically present and makes special slides from part of the first marrow aspirated. Additional syringes may be attached to collect marrow for other tests such as chromosome studies or bacterial cultures. Part of the first sample may be placed in an EDTA tube for other laboratory studies. Remaining aspirate is sometimes allowed to clot and placed in formalin or other suitable preservative and sent to histology for processing and examination. In an alternate method, blood and particles from the EDTA tube are filtered through a special paper. The filtered particles are then folded in the paper and placed in formalin. If a bone marrow biopsy is collected at the same time, the cylindrical core of material obtained is touched lightly to the surface of several clean slides before being placed in a special preservative solution. The slides are air dried and later fixed with methanol and stained with Wright's stain in the hematology department. The biopsy specimen and several slides are sent to the histology department for processing and evaluation. The remaining slides including biopsy touch slides are sent to the hematology department for staining and evaluation under the microscope.

Breath Samples

Breath samples are collected and analyzed for hydrogen content in one type of lactose tolerance test and to detect the presence of *Helicobacter pylori (H. pylori)*, a type of bacteria that secretes substances that damage the lining of the stomach, causing chronic gastritis that can lead to peptic ulcer disease.

C-UREA BREATH TEST

A common test used to detect *H. pylori* is the **C-urea breath test**. This test is based on the fact that *H. pylori* bacteria produce urease, an enzyme that breaks down urea but is not normally present in the stomach. To perform the test, a baseline breath sample is collected, after which the patient drinks a special substance that contains synthetic urea. The synthetic urea contains a form of carbon called carbon-13. If *H. pylori* organisms are present, the urease they produce will breakdown the synthetic urea and in the process release carbon dioxide (CO_2) that contains carbon-13. The CO_2 will be absorbed into the bloodstream and exhaled in the patient's breath. The patient breathes into a special Mylar balloon or other collection device at specified intervals. The breath specimens are analyzed for carbon-13 content. If carbon-13 is found in amounts higher than those in the baseline sample, there are *H. pylori* bacteria in the stomach.

HYDROGEN BREATH TEST

The hydrogen breath test is thought to be the most accurate lactose tolerance test. The patient must not have taken antibiotics for at least 2 weeks before the test and is instructed to avoid certain foods for 24 hours prior to the test. The patient must be fasting the day of the test and is asked to refrain from vigorous exercise and smoking for 30 minutes prior to and during the test. On the day of the test a baseline breath sample is taken by having the patient exhale into a special bag or device. Then the patient is given a drink that contains a measured amount of lactose (typically 25 g for adults). Additional breath samples are collected at regular intervals, typically, every 30 minutes for up to 3 hours, depending on the amount of hydrogen detected in the samples. Increased hydrogen levels in the breath samples indicate increased lactose in the intestinal tract, most likely due to inability to metabolize lactose.

Feces (Stool)

Examination of feces (stool) is helpful in the evaluation of gastrointestinal disorders. Stool specimens can be evaluated for the presence of intestinal parasites and their eggs (**ova** and **parasites**, or **O&P**), checked for fat and urobilinogen content, cultured to detect the presence of pathogenic bacteria, and tested for the presence of **occult** (hidden) **blood** using the **guaiac test**.

Stool specimens are normally collected in clean, dry containers that should be sealed and sent to the laboratory immediately after collection. Special containers with preservative are available for ova and parasite collection (Fig. 13-3). Preserved specimens can usually be kept at room temperature. Large gallon containers, similar to paint cans, are used for 24-, 48-, and 72-hour stool collections for fat and urobilinogen; these specimens must normally be refrigerated throughout the collection period. Consult the facility procedure manual for test-specific collection and handling requirements.

Special test cards, such as Hematest (Miles Inc., Elkhart, IN) and Hemoccult (Smith-Kline Diagnostics, San Jose, CA), are often given to outpatients to collect stool specimens for **fecal occult blood testing (FOBT)**. The patient is usually instructed to have a meat-

FIGURE 13-3

Ova and parasite specimen containers.

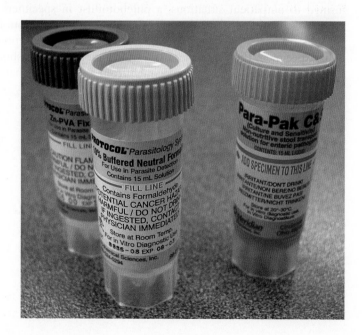

free diet for 3 days prior to the test. Patients are then instructed to collect separate specimens for 3 successive days. Cards can be mailed or brought to the lab after collection.

Hair

Samples of hair are sometimes collected for trace and heavy metal analysis and the detection of drugs of abuse. Use of hair samples for drug testing is advantageous because hair is easy to obtain and cannot be easily altered or tampered with. Hair shows evidence of chronic drug use rather than recent use. Although use of hair for drug testing is on the rise, lack of standardization in this area has held up widespread acceptance.

Throat Swabs

Throat swab specimens are most often collected to aid in the diagnosis of streptococcal (strep) infections. Nursing staff usually collect throat swab specimens on inpatients. Phlebotomists commonly collect throat culture specimens on outpatients. A throat culture is typically collected using a special kit containing a sterile polyester-tipped swab in a covered transport tube containing transport medium (Fig. 13-4). The procedure for throat culture specimen collection is shown in Procedure 13-4. Throat swabs for rapid strep tests are collected in a similar manner.

Tissue Specimens

Tissue specimens from biopsies may also be sent to the laboratory for processing. Most tissue specimens arrive at the laboratory in formalin or suitable solution and need only be accessioned and sent to the proper department. However, with more biopsies being performed in outpatient situations, a phlebotomist in specimen processing may encounter specimens that have not yet been put into the proper solution. It is important for the phlebotomist to check the procedure manual to determine the proper handling for any unfamiliar specimen. (For example, tissues for genetic analysis should *not* be put in formalin.) Improper handling can ruin a specimen from a procedure that is, in all probability, expensive, uncomfortable for the patient, and not easily repeated.

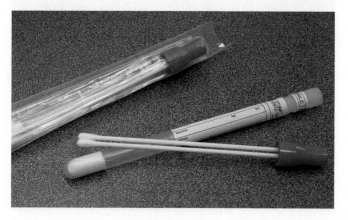

FIGURE 13-4

Throat swab and transport tube.

PROCEDURE 13-4

Throat Culture Specimen Collection

Purpose: To provide instruction in how to properly collect a throat culture specimen

Equipment: Requisition, specimen label, sterile container with swab and transport medium

Step	Rationale
1. Wash hands and put on gloves. The phlebotomist may wish to wear a mask and goggles. Follow facility protocol	Aids in infection control. Throat culture collection will often cause the patient to have a gag reflex or cough
2. Open container and remove swab in an aseptic manner	Sterility of the swab must be maintained for accurate interpretation of results
3. Stand back or to the side of the patient	Helps avoid droplet contact if the patient coughs
4. Instruct the patient to tilt back the head and open the mouth wide	Allows adequate evaluation of the collection site and ease in collection of the specimen
5. Direct light onto the back of the throat using a small flashlight or other light source	Illuminates areas of inflammation, ulceration, exudation, or capsule formation
6. Depress the tongue with a tongue depressor and ask the patient to say "ah"	Depressing the tongue helps avoid touching other areas of the mouth and contaminating the sample during collection. Saying "ah" raises the uvula (soft tissue hanging from the back of the throat) out of the way
7. Swab both tonsils, the back of the throat, and any areas of ulceration, exudation, or inflammation, being careful not to touch the swab to the lips, tongue, or uvula	Standard protocol that ensures sampling of the problem area. Touching other areas of the mouth can contaminate the swab with microbes from the oral cavity and not the throat. Touching the uvula can cause a gag reflex
8. Maintain tongue depressor position while removing the swab; then discard it	Keeping the tongue depressor in place until the swab is removed prevents the tongue from contaminating the swab
9. Place the swab back in the transport tube, embed in medium, and secure cover. (Follow instructions to crush ampule and release medium first, if applicable)	The transport medium keeps the microbes alive until they can be cultured in the laboratory
10. Label specimen	Prompt labeling is essential to ensure correct specimen identification
11. Remove gloves and sanitize hands	Proper glove removal and hand decontamination prevents the spread of infection
12. Arrange transport or deliver to the laboratory as soon as possible	Timely processing is necessary to prevent over-growth of normal flora

STUDY & REVIEW QUESTIONS

1. Additional information typically required on a nonblood specimen label includes the
   a. Billing code
   b. Party to be charged
   c. Physician.
   d. Specimen type

2. Which type of urine specimen is used to detect UTI?
   a. 2-hour
   b. 24-hour
   c. Clean catch
   d. Midstream

3. Which of the following statements describes proper 24-hour urine collection?
   a. Collect the first morning specimen, start the timing, and collect all urine for the next 24 hours, except the first specimen voided the following morning
   b. Collect the first morning specimen, start the timing, and collect all urine for the next 24 hours, including the first specimen voided the following morning
   c. Discard the first morning specimen, start the timing and collect all urine for the next 24 hours except the first specimen voided the following morning
   d. Discard the first morning specimen, start the timing and collect all urine for the next 24 hours including the first specimen voided the following morning

4. Which nonblood specimen is most frequently analyzed in the lab?
   a. CSF
   b. Pleural fluid
   c. Synovial fluid
   d. Urine

5. Which of the following fluids is associated with the lungs?
   a. Gastric
   b. Peritoneal
   c. Pleural
   d. Synovial

6. A procedure called iontophoresis is used in the collection of what specimen?
   a. CSF
   b. Saliva
   c. Sweat
   d. Synovial fluid

7. Saliva specimens can be used to detect
   a. Alcohol
   b. Drugs
   c. Hormones
   d. All of the above

8. Which test typically requires a refrigerated stool specimen?
   a. Fecal fat
   b. Guaiac
   c. Occult blood
   d. Ova and parasites

9. **A breath test can be used to detect organisms that cause**
   a. Meningitis
   b. Peptic ulcers
   c. TB
   d. Whooping cough

10. **Serous fluids come from between membranes that line the**
    a. Amnion
    b. Joints
    c. Spinal cavity
    d. Ventral body cavities

CASE · STUDY · 13-1
24-Hour Urine Specimen Collection

A patient arrives at an outpatient lab with a 24-hour urine specimen. The specimen container is properly labeled and appears to hold a normal volume of urine. In speaking with the patient, however, the phlebotomist learns that the patient did not include the final morning specimen because he woke up several hours past the 24-hour collection deadline.

QUESTIONS

1. Should the phlebotomist accept the specimen? Why or why not?
2. Should the specimen have been accepted if the patient *had* included the specimen that was several hours late? Why or why not?
3. What can be done to ensure that future 24-hour collections are handled properly?

Bibliography and Suggested Readings

Bishop, M., Fody, P., & Schoeff, L. (2005). Clinical chemistry (5th ed.). Philadelphia: Lippincott Williams & Wilkins.

Burtis, C. & Ashwood, E. (2001). Tietz, fundamentals of clinical chemistry (5th ed.). Philadelphia: W. B. Saunders.

Fischbach, F. (2004). A manual of laboratory & diagnostic tests (7th ed.). Philadelphia: Lippincott Williams & Wilkins.

Harmening, D. (2002). Clinical hematology and fundamentals of hemostasis (4th ed.). Philadelphia: F. A. Davis.

National Committee for Clinical Laboratory Standards, C-34-A2. (2000; reaffirmed Sept. 2005). Sweat testing: sample collection and quantitative analysis, approved guideline (2nd ed.). Wayne, PA: CLSI/NCCLS.

National Committee for Clinical Laboratory Standards, GP16-A2. (2001). Urinalysis and collection, transportation, and preservation of urine specimens, approved guideline (2nd ed.). Wayne, PA: CLSI/NCCLS.

Linne, J. & Ringsrud, K. (1999). Clinical laboratory science, the basics and routine techniques (4th ed.). St. Louis: Mosby.

COMPUTERS AND SPECIMEN HANDLING AND PROCESSING

key•terms

accession number	hardware	output
aerosol	HPC	password
aliquot	icon	PDA
bar code	ID code	preanalytical
central processing	input	QNS
CPU	interface	RAM
centrifuge	LAN	ROM
cursor	LIS	software
data	menu	storage
DOT	mnemonic	terminal
enter key	network	USB drive
FAA		

objectives

Upon successful completion of this chapter, the reader should be able to:

1. Define the key terms and abbreviations listed at the beginning of this chapter.
2. Describe components and elements of a computer, identify general computer skills, and define associated computer terminology.
3. Trace the flow of specimens through the laboratory with an information management system.
4. Define how bar codes are used in healthcare and list information found on a bar code computer label.
5. Describe routine and special specimen handling procedures for laboratory specimens.
6. List time constraints and exceptions for delivery and processing of specimens.
7. Identify OSHA required protective equipment worn when processing specimens.
8. Describe the steps involved in processing the different types of specimens and list the criteria for specimen rejection.

COMPUTERIZATION IN HEALTHCARE

Computers have become an essential tool in healthcare. Various types of computer hardware and software are being used to manage **data** (information collected for analysis or computation), monitor patient vital signs, and most recently, aid in diagnosis. Consequently, computer literacy is a required skill in all areas of healthcare. To be considered "computer literate," an individual must be able to do the following:

1. Know basic computer terminology (Table 14-1)
2. Understand the computer and the functions it performs
3. Perform basic operations to complete required tasks
4. Demonstrate willingness to adapt to the changes computers bring to our lives

Computers range in size from large supercomputers to personal computers (PCs) with a CPU tower to very convenient, **hand-held PCs (HPCs)** and **personal digital assistants (PDAs)**. Hand-held models are ideal for patient identification using bar code systems and paperless collection of data because they can go anywhere the patient may be.

Computer Networks

A computer **network** is a group of computers that are all linked for the purpose of sharing resources, which offers healthcare organizations a great advantage for coordinating data. In

TABLE 14-1	Common Computer Terminology
Term	**Definition**
Accession number	A unique number generated when the test request is entered into the computer
CPU	Central processing unit
Cursor	Flashing indicator on the monitor
Data	Information collected for analysis or computation
Hardware	Equipment used to process data
Icon	Image that signifies a computer application (program or document)
ID code	A unique code used to identify a person for purposes of tracking
Input	Data entered into the computer
LIS	Laboratory information system
Logging on	Entering as a user on the system via a password
Mnemonic	Memory-aiding code or abbreviation
On-line	The computer is connected to the system and is operational
Output	Processed information generated by the computer
Password	Secret word or phrase used to enter the system
Peripherals	All additional equipment attached to the CPU
RAM	Random access memory; temporary storage of data in the memory of the CPU
ROM	Read-only memory; contains instruction for operation of the computer installed by the manufacturer
Software	Coded instructions required to control the hardware in the processing of data
Storage	A place for keeping data, outside the computer it is called secondary storage
Verify	To confirm or check for correctness of input

a computer network, individual computer stations are called *nodes*. The network interconnection allows all the computers to have access through a special node called a server to each other's information or to a large database of information on a mainframe at a remote site. The computers can be connected by coaxial cables, fibers optics, standard telephone lines, the Ethernet, and wireless radiowave connections. These systems are also known as **local area networks (LANs)**.

Networking can take the form of simple interoffice connections or complex systems between several organizations in different cities or across continents. A good example of a large and complex system is the Internet, in which computers all over the world can access multiple sites and unlimited information. The advantage of networking for businesses, such as healthcare institutions, is its efficiency. The immediate access it provides speeds up processing, increases productivity, and reduces costs.

The Internet has greatly expanded access and sharing of information. At this time, a limited number of major manufacturers of laboratory analyzers have the capability to connect their computer via the healthcare facility's internet with an analyzer in their customer's laboratory for purposes of monitoring the instrument's status and troubleshooting. This Web connection provides real-time intervention for those occasions when an analyzer malfunctions by decreasing down time and increasing efficiency.

Computer Components

When operating any type of computer, the user will employ the three basic components of any system. These components provide a means to input information, a way to process information, and a method to output information.

INPUT

There are several ways to **input** or enter data into a computer. The most common way is to use a keyboard, much like a typewriter keyboard with additional keys for computer functions. Other methods of input include a light pen designed to read information on the computer screen; a "touchscreen" using a finger or pen for input; scanners programmed to read figures, letters, and bar codes; and a mouse or glidepad (a touch-sensitive pad).

PROCESS

After information has been input, it is processed through a component called the **central processing unit (CPU)**. The CPU is made up of many electrical components and microchips and has three elements. It is the thinking part of the computer that does comparisons and calculations and makes decisions. When you enter new data, the information will be stored in memory until the CPU can obey the command. Memory may be of two types: **random-access memory (RAM)** and **read-only memory (ROM)**. RAM (main memory) serves as temporary storage for data that will be lost when the computer is shut off. If the information needs to be kept for a later date, the operator must transfer it to secondary storage in the form of a hard drive, USB device, floppy disk, or compact disk (CD). ROM storage, installed by the manufacturer, instructs the computer to carry out operations requested by the user.

OUTPUT

Output describes the processed information or data generated by the computer to be received by the user or someone in another location. Just as there are several ways to input information, there are several means by which processed data can be received. One of the most common ways is through a printer. When data are printed on paper, they are said to be "hard copy." Another output device is the computer screen or other nonpermanent media displaying the data as it is entered and during processing.

Elements of the Computer

Three elements make up computer systems. These elements are called hardware, software, and storage.

Hardware is the equipment that is used to process data and includes the CPU and peripherals (all additional equipment attached to the CPU) used for the input or output of information. Examples of hardware peripherals are keyboards, computer screens, bar code readers, scanners, PDAs, HPCs, facsimile machines, printers, and modems that are used to transfer data to other computers. A computer screen and keyboard combination is called a **"terminal"** (Fig. 14-1); these are necessary peripherals for most computers. Portable computers (laptops and hand-helds) have their display and keypad built into the device.

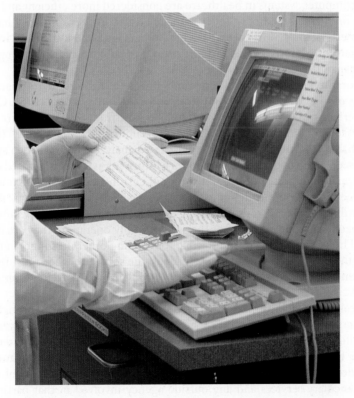

FIGURE 14-1

A computer terminal in the specimen-processing area of the laboratory.

Software is the programming (coded instructions) required to control the hardware in processing of data. Two basic types exist: systems software and applications software. Systems software controls the normal operation of the computer and is the operating system that communicates between the hardware and the applications. Applications software refers to programs prepared by software companies or in-house programmers to perform specific tasks required by users. Software applications come in five basic types: spreadsheets, communication systems, database systems, word processing, and graphics. Packages that perform more than one application, such as word processing, spreadsheet, and database, are called integrated software. The advantage of integrating applications is that it allows the different functions to be merged easily in one document.

Storage (preserving information) outside the CPU is necessary because RAM, as mentioned above, is limited temporary storage that will be lost when the computer is turned off. Storage outside the CPU is called secondary storage. Examples of permanent secondary storage devices for documents and programs are floppy disks, external hard drives, zip drives, **Universal Serial Bus (USB) drives**, CDs, and DVDs.

Computers and the Laboratory

As stated above, computers are accurate processors of information at incredible speeds. For this reason, computer systems in healthcare are considered more efficient and cost-effective than relying on manual methods. Today some analyzers in the laboratory have a sophisticated computer system that has been designed to manage patient data and **interface** (connect for the purpose of interaction) with the main hospital intranet and through phone lines back to their manufacturer's headquarters.

In the laboratory, multiple computers can connect to each other and share data. There are two types of interfaces used in **laboratory information systems (LIS)**. One is a unidirectional interface, which means data only go one way, from the analyzer to the LIS computer. The second interface is bidirectional, meaning data can upload (transfer from analyzer to LIS) or download (transfer from LIS to analyzer) between two systems. Competition between companies that sell laboratory information systems is based on the ease of input, the format of output, and the availability of customized software. Extensive research goes into selecting the right computer system for specific laboratory needs. After selecting a vendor, it will take several months to bring a system online (make it operational). Usually one or two people are put in charge of the system's daily operation; they are called "system managers." These individuals are responsible for training other personnel in the laboratory and keeping them updated as changes are made to the software. They must readily develop troubleshooting skills as they solve day-to-day problems that develop after the system is installed.

Today's healthcare facility may be totally integrated (connected) through networking of computers and a common software system. Some point-of-care analyzers used outside the main laboratory can be interfaced with data management systems, which in turn connect to the LIS. This means, for example, that patient information can be acquired and downloaded from the nursing unit, accumulated in a central database and shared with ancillary services and any outside agency involved in that particular patient's care. In the future, a totally integrated system will have an "electronic chart" and will make a paperless facility possible.

fyi   Intranets (networks within companies) connect multiple LIS systems, and the Internet (network outside companies) connects them to the world.

General Computer Skills

General skills that the phlebotomist must learn, regardless of what LIS is used, involve the following.

Logging on. A person who is allowed to access a computer system is given a username and **password.** The password uniquely identifies that person and allows him or her to become a system user. The process of entering a username and password to gain access to the system is called "logging on." When the log-on sequence is completed, a **menu** is displayed listing the options from which the user may choose. For security and authorization purposes, most systems are designed to allow users unique access to different menus or programs.

Cursor movement. After logging on, a flashing indicator on the screen, called the **cursor,** indicates the starting point for input. When entering patient information in a LIS, the cursor will automatically reset itself at the correct point for data input after the **Enter key** has been pressed.

Using icons. Access to documents and software programs can be initiated by using the mouse to click on a small representative image called an icon that opens a document or launches a software program.

Entering data. After necessary information has been input, the Enter key must be pressed for information to be processed. If an error in spelling or selection is made, it can easily be deleted by backspacing before pressing the Enter key. If the wrong information is entered, however, it is still possible to correct errors.

Correcting errors. This procedure is necessary to correct mistakes that are detected after the Enter key has been pressed. The procedure to delete errors is program-dependent and must be learned with each system. Some LIS programs use order verification, an additional step in the process, to allow a review of the information before it is accepted.

Verifying data. After all patient information has been entered, it will appear on the monitor screen as a complete order. At this point, the user can review the information again and can choose to modify, delete, or accept it. When all orders have been entered, the user can request an inquiry of the orders as another check.

Making order inquiries. Selecting "order inquiry" allows the user to retrieve any or all of the test orders associated with a patient.

Canceling orders. If, after entering an order, a user finds that it is incorrect, he or she can request that the computer delete or cancel it.

Laboratory Information Systems

The objectives of the LIS are to file results, accumulate statistics to determine workload, generate report forms, and monitor quality assurance and quality control in the laboratory.

The advantages of using a LIS are improved accuracy in testing, reduced clerical and billing errors, flexible delivery options for reports, and increased efficiency.

fyi There are multiple vendors and types of laboratory information systems on the market at this time. Those with more than 1000 installation sites include Cerner Corporation/Cerner Citation/Cerner DHT, Misys, and Medical Information Technology, Inc. (Meditech).

Each type of information system allows users to define their own parameters for terms and conditions that make the system unique to that facility. Several programs within the system allow the users to do specific tasks, seemingly at the same time, such as (1) admit patients, (2) request test orders, (3) print labels, (4) enter results, (5) inquire about results, and (6) generate reports.

ID CODE

In laboratory settings, users are given an **ID code,** a unique identification and a password. Passwords must be kept strictly confidential because they enable access to the LIS. The security associated with ID code determines what system functions can be accessed. An ID code is also logged with every transaction on the system, allowing the system manager to identify the person performing each transaction and for the purpose of accruing workload. ID codes are not always confidential because it is not always possible for phlebotomists to verify their own collections. A data entry clerk may verify all collections and must have access to the list of ID codes so that he or she can associate the proper phlebotomist with each draw.

ICONS

The Cerner Millenium LIS uses **icons** or images (as in the Windows MS operating system for PCs) to request the appropriate program or function necessary to enter data. Other laboratory information systems may use a menu of **mnemonic** (memory-aiding) codes or a abbreviation for selecting a function.

For example, in the Cerner Millenium Laboratory Information System a phlebotomist would select the "dept order entry" icon. This requisition entry program can be called by many different names, but it is basically the same procedure for any of the systems. During this data entry phase, an **accession number** is given to each requested order. This number is generated by the LIS when the specimen request is entered into the computer and will be identified with the specimen as long as it is in the laboratory.

To create labels and collection lists for the phlebotomist to use in collecting the appropriate samples, it is necessary to select another icon to "label reprint" individual labels if not done at time of order entry. The "collection list" icon can be used to print labels for specimen collection. After collection has been accomplished, the phlebotomist returns to the laboratory and verifies the collection through another application, "specimen log-in." Other

FIGURE 14-2

A computerized label generated when the requisition order is entered.   (Cerner Corp., Kansas City, MO.)

programs in the lab system that the phlebotomist might use are "order result viewer" to search for lab orders or results and "request a chart" to print or send a patient's report via fax.

A mnemonic code to identify the type and volume of tube required is always printed whenever a label is generated (Fig.14-2). For example, if the phlebotomist knows that a complete blood count is ordered and the code on the label reads 5.0 mL LAV, he or she knows what tube type to choose and the amount of blood to draw. This demonstrates one of the benefits of computerized label generation; the label aids the phlebotomist in acquiring the proper specimen in a timely fashion. The steps an LIS uses for processing a typical specimen, from arrival in the lab through reporting of results, are shown in Figure 14-3.

BAR CODES

A **bar code** is a parallel array of alternately spaced black bars and white spaces representing a code. The code may represent numbers or letters. Some of the uses of bar codes in

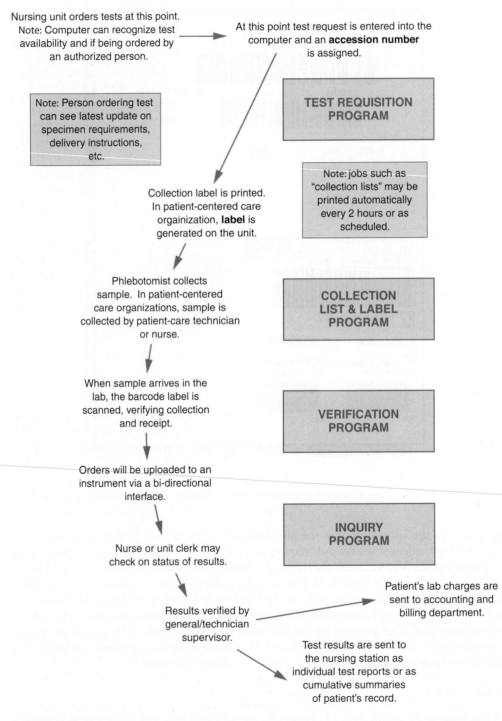

Nursing unit orders tests at this point. Note: Computer can recognize test availability and if being ordered by an authorized person.

At this point test request is entered into the computer and an **accession number** is assigned.

TEST REQUISITION PROGRAM

Note: Person ordering test can see latest update on specimen requirements, delivery instructions, etc.

Collection label is printed. In patient-centered care orgainization, **label** is generated on the unit.

Note: jobs such as "collection lists" may be printed automatically every 2 hours or as scheduled.

Phlebotomist collects sample. In patient-centered care organizations, sample is collected by patient-care technician or nurse.

COLLECTION LIST & LABEL PROGRAM

When sample arrives in the lab, the barcode label is scanned, verifying collection and receipt.

VERIFICATION PROGRAM

Orders will be uploaded to an instrument via a bi-directional interface.

INQUIRY PROGRAM

Nurse or unit clerk may check on status of results.

Patient's lab charges are sent to accounting and billing department.

Results verified by general/technician supervisor.

Test results are sent to the nursing station as individual test reports or as cumulative summaries of patient's record.

FIGURE 14-3

Example of a work flow chart.

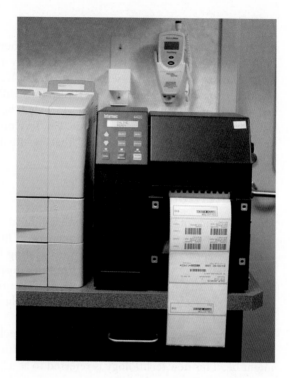

FIGURE 14-4

Bar code label printer at the nursing station.

healthcare include identification of patients (bar code ID bands), supply inventory, specimen identification, and pharmaceutical drug name, dose, and route. Many laboratory analyzers use bar code technology for specimen identification. A bar code label, produced by the LIS on a bar code label printer as seen in (Fig.14-4), is applied to the collected specimens, making specimen processing in the laboratory more efficient. HPC systems are being used to read patient ID bar code bands and generate the labels used for specimen collection at the patient's bedside. One system that performs this function is the BD.id System from Becton Dickinson (Franklin Lakes, NJ). While at the patient's bedside, the wireless HPC scanner identifies the patient, displays the collection tubes needed, the order of draw, and the person who is performing the phlebotomy. After collection, the HPC prints labels for only the specimens collected, with the actual time of collection and the collector's ID printed on the label.

key • point Computer technology makes sharing of information so easy that patient confidentiality can be violated. Congress took steps to eliminate confidentiality violation by enacting the HIPAA (see Chapter 1), which is designed to protect the privacy and security of patient information by standardizing the electronic transfer of data and providing guidelines for sharing protected health information (PHI). This Act affects everyone involved in healthcare: patients, physicians and other healthcare personnel, healthcare organizations, vendors, and insurance companies.

INTERFACING

Computers and their ability to talk to each other are important components in effective communication in healthcare. The Connectivity Industry Consortium (CIC) was recently established to ensure that any point-of-care (POC) analyzer could talk to any LIS, thereby standardizing all data management tools. This will make it possible for healthcare workers to ensure that all POC testing they perform will be transferred to the computer and become part of the patient's chart. A guideline was developed by POC analyzer manufacturers, LIS vendors, and healthcare providers that resulted in the CLSI/NCCLS Point-of-Care Connectivity, Approved Standard.

Computerization Trends

Current trends in healthcare indicate that clinical laboratory operations will continue to decentralize, and that POC testing will increase. The need for complete networking becomes even more apparent as remote laboratory testing facilities increase in numbers. Large reference laboratories, totally separate from the hospital, will need to download results from automated instruments into patient charts or centralized databases. Bar code label systems for the identification of patients and their samples, medications, and supplies will decrease the risk of human error.

With the further development of microchip technology in POC analyzers, testing of patient specimens is being moved from the traditional laboratory to anywhere the patient might be. This new technology is referred to as a "lab-on-a-chip." Additionally, researchers are using the computer's ability to aggregate and analyze massive amounts of medical data. The outcome of this "artificial intelligence" will continue to revolutionize medicine.

SPECIMEN HANDLING

As part of the computerization network that connects many aspects of patient care, the laboratory network tracks patient specimens from the time they are collected until the results are reported. The quality of those results, however, depends upon proper handling of the specimen in the **preanalytical** (prior to analysis) phase, which includes all the steps taken before the actual testing of the sample. It has been estimated that 46 to 68% of all laboratory errors occur prior to analysis. Specimen handling is a critical part of this phase. Proper handling from the time a specimen is collected until the test is performed helps ensure that results obtained on the specimen accurately reflect the status of the patient. Improper handling is a preanalytical error (Box 14-1) that can render the most skillfully obtained specimen useless or affect the analyte (substance undergoing analysis) in a way that causes erroneous (invalid) or misleading test results, which in turn cause delayed or incorrect care for the patient.

🔑 key • point Preanalytical errors are those factors that are introduced into the specimen before and during collection, transport, processing, or storage that alter patient test results.

BOX • 14-1   Possible Sources of Preanalytical Error

Before Collection

- Age of patient
- Altitude
- Dehydrated patient
- Duplicate test orders
- Exercise
- Gender of patient
- Inadequate fast
- Incomplete requisition
- Medications
- Patient stress
- Pregnancy
- Smoking
- Strenuous exercise
- Treatments (e.g., intravenous medications, radioisotopes)
- Wrong test ordered

At Time of Collection

- Misidentified patient
- Antiseptic not dry
- Expired tube
- Failure to properly invert additive tubes
- Faulty technique
- Improper vein selection
- Inadequate volume of blood
- Inappropriate use of plasma separator tube (PST) or serum separator tube (SST)
- Incorrect collection tube
- Incorrect needle position
- Incorrect needle size
- Mislabeled tube
- Mixing tubes too vigorously
- Nonsterile site preparation
- Patient position
- Prolonged tourniquet application
- Underfilled tube
- Wrong collection time

During Specimen Transport

- Agitation-induced hemolysis
- Delay in transporting
- Exposure to light
- Failure to follow temperature requirements
- Transport method (e.g., hand vs. pneumatic tube)

During Specimen Processing

- Contamination (e.g., dust or glove powder)
- Delay in processing or testing
- Delay in fluid separation from cells
- Evaporation
- Failure to centrifuge specimen according to test requirements
- Failure to separate fluid from cells

(Continued)

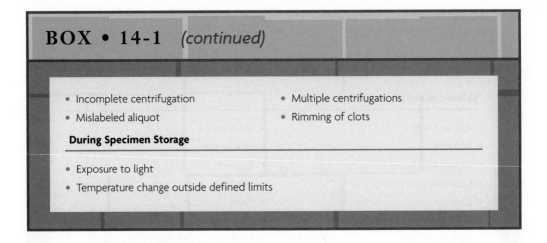

BOX • 14-1 *(continued)*

- Incomplete centrifugation
- Mislabeled aliquot

During Specimen Storage

- Exposure to light
- Temperature change outside defined limits

- Multiple centrifugations
- Rimming of clots

Unfortunately, it is not always easy to tell when a specimen has been handled improperly. Therefore, to ensure delivery of a quality specimen for analysis, it is imperative that all phlebotomists be adequately instructed in this area so that established policies and procedures are followed. In addition, to protect the phlebotomist and others from accidental exposure to potentially infectious substances, all specimens should be handled according to the standard precautions guidelines outlined in Chapter 3.

Routine Handling

MIXING TUBES BY INVERSION

Additive tubes require 3 to 8 gentle inversions (Fig. 14-5) as soon as they are drawn. The required number of inversions depends upon the type of additive (see Chapter 7, Additive Tubes). Gentle inversion helps to evenly distribute the additive while minimizing the chance of hemolysis. Vigorous mixing can cause hemolysis and should be avoided. Examples of tests that cannot be performed on hemolyzed specimens include potassium, magnesium, and most enzyme tests. Inadequate mixing of anticoagulant tubes leads to microclot formation, which can cause erroneous test results, especially for hematology studies. Inadequate mixing of gel separation tubes may prevent the additive from functioning properly, and clotting may be incomplete. Nonadditive tubes do not require mixing.

TRANSPORTING SPECIMENS

It is important to handle and transport blood specimens carefully. Rough handling and agitation can hemolyze specimens, activate platelets, and affect coagulation tests as well as break tubes. Tubes should be transported stopper up to reduce agitation, aid clot formation in serum tubes, and prevent contact of the tube contents with the tube stopper. Blood in contact with tube stoppers can be a source of specimen contamination and contributes to **aerosol** (a fine mist of the specimen) formation during stopper removal.

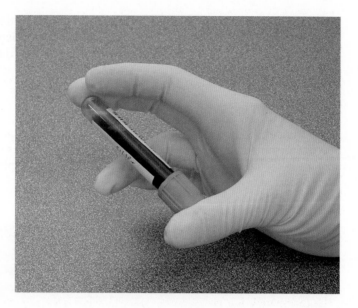

FIGURE 14-5
Mixing of anticoagulated tube.

Blood specimen tubes are typically placed in plastic bags for transportation to the laboratory. CLSI/NCCLS and OSHA guidelines require specimen transport bags to have a biohazard logo, a liquid-tight closure, and a slip pocket for paperwork. Nonblood specimens should be transported in leak-proof containers with adequately secured lids. All specimens transported through pneumatic tube systems should be protected from shock and sealed in zipper-type plastic bags to contain spills (see Fig. 14-6). Specimens sent to off-site locations

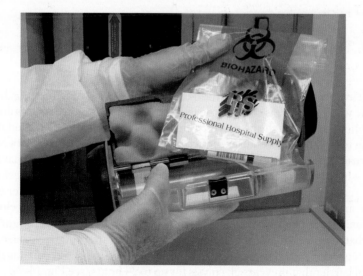

FIGURE 14-6
Specimen prepared for transport through pneumatic tube system.

by courier or mail systems must be packaged and transported according to **Department of Transportation (DOT)** and the **Federal Aviation Administration (FAA)** regulations. In addition, special care should be taken to protect specimens from the effects of extreme heat or cold.

DELIVERY TIME LIMITS

All specimens should be transported to the laboratory without delay. Ideally, routine blood specimens should arrive at the laboratory within 45 minutes of collection. Specimens that require it should be centrifuged to separate the serum or plasma from the cells within 1 hour of arrival.

> **key • point** CLSI/NCCLS guideline H18-A3 sets the maximum time limit for separating serum and plasma from the cells at 2 hours from time of collection unless there is evidence that a longer contact time will not affect the accuracy of the test result. Less time is recommended for some tests such as those for cortisol and potassium.

Prompt delivery and separation minimizes the effects of metabolic processes such as glycolysis. Unless chemically prevented by an additive such as sodium fluoride, glycolysis continues in a blood specimen, lowering glucose levels until the serum or plasma is physically separated from the cells. Cellular metabolism also affects other analytes such as aldosterone, calcitonin, enzymes, and phosphorus.

> **key • point** Glycolysis by erythrocytes and leukocytes in blood specimens can falsely lower glucose values at a rate of up to 200 mg/L per hour.

Prompt delivery is easily achieved with an on-site lab, as in a hospital setting, but it is not always possible when specimens come to the lab from off-site locations, such as doctors' offices and nursing homes. Although specimens from these sites are typically picked up and transported to the testing site by a courier service on a regular basis, the time between collection and delivery can easily exceed 2 hours. Consequently, off-site locations often have a small processing area where blood specimens that require it can be centrifuged (see Specimen Processing) and the serum or plasma separated and transferred to a suitable container for transport. Nonadditive and gel-barrier serum tubes such as SSTs must be completely clotted prior to centrifugation. Heparin gel-barrier tubes such as PSTs can be centrifuged right away. Specimens in gel barrier tubes do not require manual separation after they have been centrifuged, because the separator gel lodges between the fluid and the cells during centrifugation, becoming a physical barrier that prevents glycolysis for up to 24 hours (see Fig. 14-7).

Hematology test specimens drawn in lavender or purple stopper (EDTA) tubes and specimens for other tests performed on whole blood should never be centrifuged. Applicable

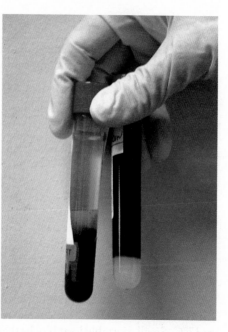

FIGURE 14-7

Hemogard SSTs. (Becton Dickinson, Franklin Lakes, NJ.) *Right,* before being centrifuged. *Left,* after being centrifuged.

temperature requirements for all specimens should be maintained until they are turned over to the courier service.

TIME LIMIT EXCEPTIONS

"Stat" or "medical emergency" specimens take priority over all other specimens and should be transported, processed, and tested immediately. Examples of other exceptions to time limits include the following:

- Blood smears made from EDTA specimens must be prepared within 1 hour of collection to preserve the integrity of the blood cells and prevent artifact formation due to prolonged contact with the anticoagulant.
- EDTA tube specimens for CBCs should be analyzed within 6 hours but are generally stable for 24 hours at room temperature. CBC specimens collected in microcollection containers should be analyzed within 4 hours.
- EDTA specimens for erythrocyte sedimentation rate (ESR) determinations must be tested within 4 hours at room temperature or within 12 hours if refrigerated.
- EDTA specimens for reticulocyte counts are stable up to 6 hours at room temperature and up to 72 hours if refrigerated.
- Glucose test specimens drawn in sodium fluoride tubes are stable for 24 hours at room temperature and up to 48 hours when refrigerated at 2 to 8°C.
- Prothrombin time (PT) results on unrefrigerated and uncentrifuged specimens are reliable for up to 24 hours after collection. Partial thromboplastin time (PTT) test specimens require analysis within 4 hours of collection regardless of storage conditions.

Special Handling

When blood leaves the body it is exposed to the effects of temperature and light that can negatively affect analytes. Those significantly affected require special handling to protect them.

key • point   It is important to know the following temperatures related to specimen handling:

- Body temperature: 37°C
- Room temperature: 15–30°C
- Refrigerated temperature: 2–10°C
- Frozen temperature: −20°C or lower (some specimens require −70°C or lower)

BODY TEMPERATURE SPECIMENS

Some specimens will precipitate or agglutinate if allowed to cool below body temperature. These specimens need to be transported at or near the normal body temperature of 37°C. In addition, most of these specimens require collection in a tube that has been prewarmed to 37°C. Small, portable heat blocks that are kept in a 37°C incubator until needed are available for transporting body-temperature specimens. The heat blocks hold this temperature for approximately 15 minutes after removal from the incubator. Temperature-sensitive specimens that can withstand temperatures slightly higher than 37°C can be wrapped in an activated heel warmer for transport (Fig. 14-8).

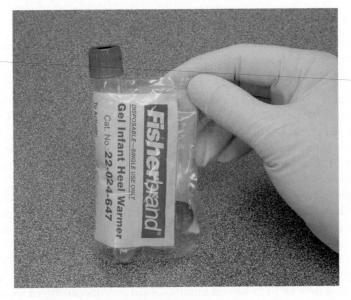

FIGURE 14-8

Specimen wrapped in an activated heel warmer for transfer.

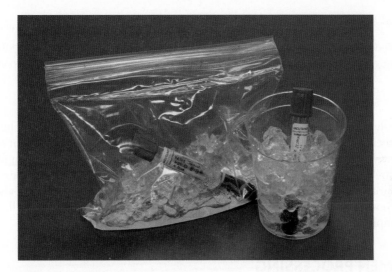

FIGURE 14-9
Specimen immersed in crushed ice and water slurry.

CHILLED SPECIMENS

Some metabolic processes that can affect test results continue in the specimen after collection. Chilling the specimen slows down metabolic processes and protects analytes. Blood specimens that require chilling should be completely immersed in a slurry of crushed ice and water (Fig. 14-9) and either tested immediately or refrigerated upon arrival in the laboratory. Large cubes or chunks of ice without water added do not allow adequate cooling of the entire specimen. Contact with a solid piece of ice can freeze parts of the specimen, resulting in hemolysis and possible analyte breakdown. See Table 14-2 for examples of tests that require a chilled specimen.

TABLE 14-2	Examples of Specimens That Require Special Handling	
Keep at 37°C	**Chill in Crushed Ice Slurry**	**Protect from Light**
Cold agglutinin	Adrenocorticotropic hormone (ACTH)	Bilirubin
Cryofibrinogen	Acetone	Carotene
Cryoglobulins	Angiotensin-converting enzyme (ACE)	Red cell folate
	Ammonia	Serum folate
	Catecholamines	Vitamin B_2
	Free fatty acids	Vitamin B_6
	Gastrin	Vitamin B_{12}
	Glucagon	Vitamin C
	Homocysteine	Urine porphyrins
	Lactic acid	Urine porphobilinogen
	Parathyroid hormone (PTH)	
	pH/blood gas (if indicated)	
	Pyruvate	
	Renin	

> **caution**   Some specimens are negatively affected by chilling. For example, potassium levels artificially increase if the specimen is chilled. When a potassium test is ordered with other analytes that require chilling, it should be collected in a separate tube.

LIGHT-SENSITIVE SPECIMENS

Some analytes are broken down by light, resulting in falsely decreased values. The most common of these is bilirubin, which can decrease by up to 50% after 1 hour of light exposure.

An easy way to protect a blood specimen from light is to wrap it in aluminum foil (Fig. 14-10). Light-blocking amber-colored microcollection containers are available for collection of infant bilirubin specimens. Amber containers for urine specimen collection are also available. Light-blocking secondary specimen transport containers are available as well. Table 14-2 lists examples of specimens that require protection from light.

SPECIMEN PROCESSING

Some off-site drawing stations have processing areas where specimens are centrifuged and separated from the cells to protect analyte stability before being sent to the testing site. Most large laboratories have a specific area, commonly called **central processing** or triage (screening and prioritizing area), where specimens are received and prepared for testing. Here the specimens are identified, logged/accessioned, sorted by department and type of processing required, and evaluated for suitability for testing.

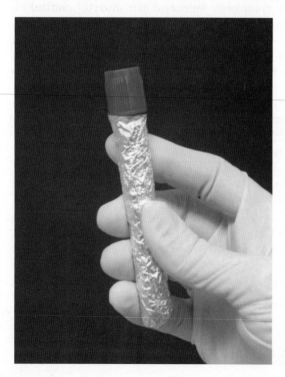

FIGURE 14-10

Specimen wrapped in aluminum foil to protect it from light.

c a u t i o n   OSHA regulations require those who process specimens to wear protective equipment (PE). PE includes gloves, fully closed fluid-resistant lab coats or aprons, and protective face gear such as mask and goggles with side shields, or chin-length face shields.

Specimen Suitability

Suitable specimens are required for accurate laboratory results. Unsuitable specimens must be rejected for testing and new specimens obtained. The most frequently cited reason for rejection of chemistry specimens is hemolysis, followed by insufficient amount of specimen, or **QNS** (quantity not sufficient). The most frequent reason for rejection of hematology specimens is clotting. Some suitability requirements depend on the individual tests ordered. Some rejection criteria, such as hemolysis, may not be identified until processing has begun or even completed. In the case of hematology specimens, hemolysis may not be noticed until after testing is complete and the specimen has separated while sitting in a specimen rack. Individual labs have specific policies concerning rejected specimens. Examples of specimen rejection criteria are listed in Box 14-2. Generally, rejected specimens are not discarded until the ordering physician or nursing unit has been notified.

Once suitability requirements are met, specimens that do not require further processing, such as hematology and urinalysis specimens are promptly distributed to the testing area or department. Specimens for tests that require serum or plasma samples must be centrifuged.

Centrifugation

A **centrifuge** (Fig.14-11) is a machine that spins the blood tubes at a high number of revolutions per minute (rpm). The centrifugal force created causes the cells and plasma or serum to separate (Fig. 14-12). Specimens for tests that require serum or plasma samples must be centrifuged.

TUBES AWAITING CENTRIFUGATION

Stoppers should remain on tubes awaiting centrifugation. Removing the stopper from a specimen can cause loss of CO_2 and an increase of pH, leading to inaccurate results for tests such as pH, CO_2, and acid phosphatase. In addition, leaving the stopper off exposes the specimen to evaporation and contamination. Sources of contamination can be as simple as a drop of sweat, which interferes with electrolyte results, or powder from gloves, which may interfere with calcium determinations (some powders contain calcium). Evaporation leads to inaccurate results because of concentration of analytes.

k e y • p o i n t   Stoppers should also be left on tubes during centrifugation to prevent contamination, evaporation, **aerosol** (fine spray) formation, and pH changes.

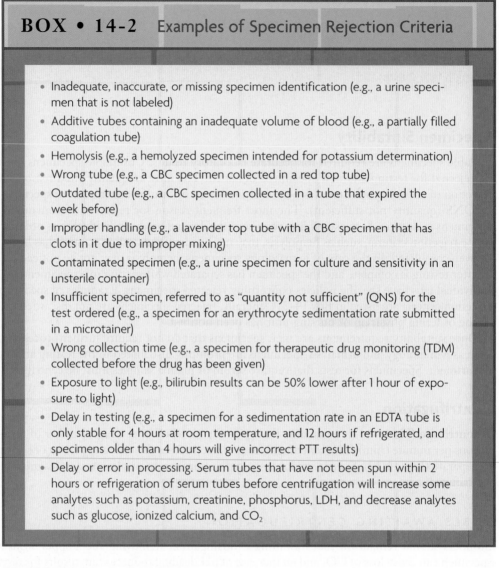

BOX • 14-2 Examples of Specimen Rejection Criteria

- Inadequate, inaccurate, or missing specimen identification (e.g., a urine specimen that is not labeled)
- Additive tubes containing an inadequate volume of blood (e.g., a partially filled coagulation tube)
- Hemolysis (e.g., a hemolyzed specimen intended for potassium determination)
- Wrong tube (e.g., a CBC specimen collected in a red top tube)
- Outdated tube (e.g., a CBC specimen collected in a tube that expired the week before)
- Improper handling (e.g., a lavender top tube with a CBC specimen that has clots in it due to improper mixing)
- Contaminated specimen (e.g., a urine specimen for culture and sensitivity in an unsterile container)
- Insufficient specimen, referred to as "quantity not sufficient" (QNS) for the test ordered (e.g., a specimen for an erythrocyte sedimentation rate submitted in a microtainer)
- Wrong collection time (e.g., a specimen for therapeutic drug monitoring (TDM) collected before the drug has been given)
- Exposure to light (e.g., bilirubin results can be 50% lower after 1 hour of exposure to light)
- Delay in testing (e.g., a specimen for a sedimentation rate in an EDTA tube is only stable for 4 hours at room temperature, and 12 hours if refrigerated, and specimens older than 4 hours will give incorrect PTT results)
- Delay or error in processing. Serum tubes that have not been spun within 2 hours or refrigeration of serum tubes before centrifugation will increase some analytes such as potassium, creatinine, phosphorus, LDH, and decrease analytes such as glucose, ionized calcium, and CO_2

CENTRIFUGE OPERATION

It is crucial that tubes be "balanced" in a centrifuge. That means equal-size tubes with equal volumes of specimen must be placed opposite one another in the centrifuge. An unbalanced centrifuge may break specimen tubes, ruining specimens and causing the contents to form aerosols. The lid to the centrifuge should remain closed during operation and should not be opened until the rotor has come to a complete stop. A properly functioning modern centrifuge will not allow the user to open the lid prematurely.

A specimen should never be centrifuged more than once. Repeated centrifugation can cause hemolysis and analyte deterioration and alter test results. In addition, once the serum or plasma has been removed, the volume ratio of plasma to cells changes.

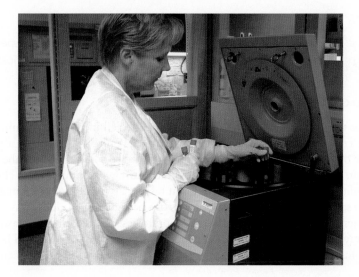

FIGURE 14-11

Specimen processor loading a centrifuge.

FIGURE 14-12

Sodium citrate tubes. *Left,* after being centrifuged. *Right,* before being centrifuged.

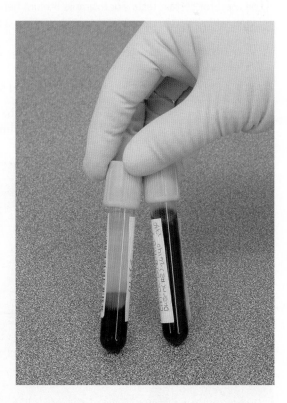

⚠ **c a u t i o n**   Because a centrifuge generates heat during operation, specimens requiring chilling should be processed in a temperature-controlled refrigerated centrifuge.

CENTRIFUGING PLASMA SPECIMENS

Specimens for tests performed on plasma that are collected in tubes containing anticoagulants may be centrifuged without delay. For example, Figure 14-13 shows a prothrombin time (protime or PT) specimen collected in a light-blue top sodium citrate tube that was immediately spun down using a StatSpin Express 2 centrifuge. Although most chemistry tests have been traditionally performed on serum, stat tests are typically collected in green top heparin tubes to save time, since plasma specimens can be centrifuged right away as opposed to serum specimens that must clot first. Some laboratories use heparinized plasma instead of serum for many chemistry tests to simply reduce turn-around time (TAT). PSTs or other heparin-containing gel tubes are available to maintain specimen stability after centrifugation.

⚠ **c a u t i o n**   There are different heparin formulations, and some of them cannot be used for certain tests. For example lithium heparin cannot be used for lithium levels, ammonium heparin cannot be used for ammonia levels, and sodium heparin cannot be used for sodium levels.

CENTRIFUGING SERUM SPECIMENS

Specimens for tests performed on serum must be completely clotted before they are centrifuged. If clotting is not complete when a specimen is centrifuged, latent fibrin formation

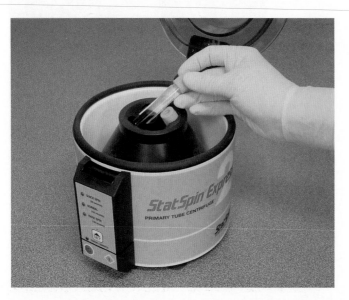

FIGURE 14-13

Prothrombin specimen after centrifugation in a StatSpin Express.

may clot the serum and interfere with the performance of the test. Complete clotting normally takes 30 to 60 minutes at room temperature (22–25°C). Specimens from patients on anticoagulant medication, such as heparin or warfarin (i.e., Coumadin), specimens from patients with high white blood counts, and chilled specimens may take longer to clot. Serum separator tubes and other tubes containing clot activators usually clot within 30 minutes provided they are mixed properly immediately after collection. Thrombin tubes normally clot in 5 minutes. There are also several commercially available clot activators that can be added to the tube after the specimen is drawn.

STOPPER REMOVAL

Some testing machines sample specimens directly through the tube stopper. Most of the time, however, the stopper has to be removed to obtain the serum or plasma needed for testing. Stoppers can be removed using commercially available stopper removal devices or by use of robotics. If a removal device or robotic is not used, the processor should be wearing a full-length face shield or the tube should be held behind a splash shield when the stopper is removed. Either way, the stopper should be covered with a gauze or tissue to catch blood drops or aerosol that may be released as it is removed. Some tubes (such as the Becton Dickinson Hemogard tubes) have stoppers that are specially designed to contain spray (see Fig. 14-14). To prevent or minimize aerosols or blood spray, all tube stoppers should be pulled straight up and off and not "popped" off using a thumb roll technique.

ALIQUOT PREPARATION

An **aliquot** is a portion of a specimen used for testing. Aliquots of specimens are sometimes created when multiple tests are ordered on a single specimen and the tests are performed on different instruments or in different areas of the testing department. Aliquots are prepared by transferring a portion of the specimen into one or more tubes labeled with the same ID information as the specimen tube.

FIGURE 14-14

Example of a Hemogard closure tube.   (Becton Dickinson, Franklin Lakes, NJ.)

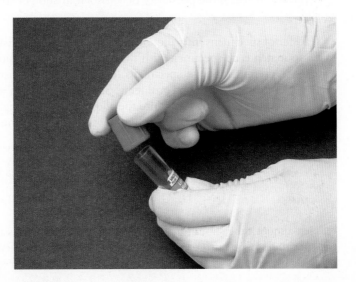

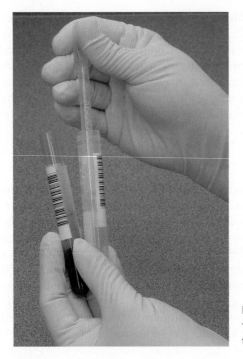

FIGURE 14-15

Transferring a sample from collection tube to aliquot tube.

According to OSHA, "All procedures involving blood or potentially infectious materials shall be performed in such a manner as to minimize splashing, spraying, splattering, and generation of droplets of these substances." Consequently, disposable transfer pipettes should be used when transferring serum or plasma into aliquot tubes (Fig. 14-15).

c a u t i o n   Pouring the serum or plasma into aliquot tubes is not recommended because it increases the possibility of aerosol formation or splashing.

Transfer of specimens into aliquot tubes has an inherent risk of error. Great care must be taken to match each specimen with the corresponding aliquot tube to avoid misidentified samples. Different types of specimens (e.g., serum and plasma) for separate tests on the same patient can also present problems. Serum and plasma are virtually indistinguishable once they have been transferred into the aliquot tubes, so it is important to match the specimen with the aliquot tube of the requested test as well as the patient.

c a u t i o n   Never put serum and plasma, or plasma from specimens with different anticoagulants in the same aliquot tube.

Each aliquot tube should be covered or capped as soon as it is filled. Some tests require the specimen to be refrigerated or frozen for analyte stability, especially if testing is to be delayed. It is important to consult the procedure manual for specific instructions.

STUDY & REVIEW QUESTIONS

1. **Peripherals on a computer include all of the following *except* a**
   a. Bar code reader
   b. Scanner
   c. Modem
   d. CPU

2. **Logging on to most computer systems requires the use of a/an**
   a. Accession number
   b. Bar code reader
   c. Modem
   d. Password

3. **After arriving in the laboratory, all specimens are immediately**
   a. Centrifuged to stop glycolysis
   b. Logged or accessioned
   c. Refrigerated until delivered to the appropriate department
   d. Uploaded to an instrument for analysis

4. **All of the following are found on a lab-generated computer label except**
   a. Accession number
   b. Department for testing
   c. Patient identification
   d. Patient diagnosis

5. **Bar coding in healthcare is used for all of the following except**
   a. Bidirectional interfacing
   b. Drug administration
   c. Labeling and supply inventory
   d. Physical location of the patient

6. **Which of the following specimens should be protected from light?**
   a. BUN
   b. CBC
   c. Bilirubin
   d. Glucose

7. **The machine used to separate the serum or plasma from blood cells in the sample is called a/an**
   a. Autolet.
   b. Centrifuge
   c. Glucometer
   d. Hemostat

8. **After obtaining a specimen for a cold agglutinin test, the blood must be transported**
   a. As "stat"
   b. Away from light
   c. In ice slurry
   d. At body temperature

9. **All of the following are required personal protective equipment when processing specimens except**
   a. A chin-length face shield
   b. A fully closed, fluid-resistant lab coat
   c. Fluid-resistant shoe cover
   d. Disposable gloves

10. **Which of the following blood specimens should be transported in an ice slurry?**

    a. BUN and creatinine

    b. Cold agglutinin and bilirubin

    c. Glucose and electrolytes

    d. Homocysteine and rennin

11. **Perspiration contamination can falsely elevate**

    a. Amylase

    b. Calcium

    c. Chloride

    d. Magnesium

12. **Which of the following specimens would most likely be accepted for testing?**

    a. CBC collected in a lavender top tube

    b. Potassium specimen that is hemolyzed

    c. Protime specimen in a partially filled tube

    d. Specimen lacking an identification label

13. **According to CLSI guidelines, serum for most tests should be removed from the cells within**

    a. 30 minutes

    b. 60 minutes

    c. 90 minutes

    d. 120 minutes

14. **Which of the following specimens can be centrifuged immediately?**

    a. Bilirubin collected in a red top tube

    b. CBC collected in a lavender top

    c. Creatinine collected in an SST

    d. Electrolytes collected in a PST

CASE · STUDY · 14-1

Missing Results

Nurse Susan collected blood for blood urea nitrogen (BUN) and creatinine tests on patient Mr. Jones in bed 201 at 9:30 AM, and sent the specimen to the lab. At 10:30, Susan calls the lab and states she is not able to find Mr. Jones' results in the computer. The technologist, Frank, tells Susan he does not have a specimen with that name on it; however, he did run a BUN and creatinine on patient Betty Smith in bed 202 drawn at 9:30 AM by Susan. Susan says there could not have been an error because she labeled the specimen with the only label she found on the bar-coded label printer at the time.

QUESTIONS

1. What do you think has happened to Mr. Jones' specimen?
2. Why does the lab have results on Mrs. Smith?
3. What steps should Susan take to get the results on Mr. Jones?
4. What is to be done with the results on Mrs. Smith?

sted Readings

ary 2002). 10th annual information systems buyers guide. King of
oratory.

lkirk, J. L., & Fody, E. P. (2005). Clinical chemistry: principles,
5th ed.). Philadelphia: Lippincott Williams & Wilkins.

. R., (2001). Tietz, fundamentals of clinical chemistry (5th ed.).
lers.

9). Intranet technology seeping into laboratories.

on. (2001). Hazardous materials regulations; Title 49, Code of Federal
85.

nical Laboratory Standards, POCT1. (2001). Point of care connectivity,
e, PA: CLSI/NCCLS.

nical Laboratory Standards, H3-A5. (December 2003). Procedures for
ic blood specimens by venipuncture (4th ed.). Wayne, PA: CLSI/

nical Laboratory Standards, H4-A5. (2004). Procedures and devices for
ic capillary blood specimens by venipuncture,. approved standard-(5th
ICCLS.

nical Laboratory Standards, H18-A3. (2004). Procedures for the han-
lood specimens, approved guideline. Wayne, PA: CLSI/NCCLS.

ual of laboratory and diagnostic tests (7th ed.). Philadelphia: Lippincott

diagnostic and management of laboratory methods (19th ed.). Philadel-

ortability and Accountability Act. (August 17, 2000). Federal Register.
ccreditation of Healthcare Organizations (JCAHO). (2001). 2001 Ac-
spitals. Oakbrook Terrace, IL: JCAHO.

alth Administration. (2001). Occupational exposure to bloodborne
d other sharps injuries; final rule. 29 CFR 1910. Federal Register

Institute. (April 2001). Reference manual.

abdominal cavity: Body space between the diaphragm and the pelvis that houses the abdominal organs such as the stomach, liver, pancreas, gallbladder, spleen, and kidneys.

abducted: Away from the body; the position of the patient's arm for arterial blood gas collection.

ABGs: Arterial blood gases.

ABO blood group system: Four blood types, A, B, AB, and O, based on the presence or absence of two antigens identified as A and B.

accession number: A number generated by the LIS when the specimen request is entered into the computer.

accession: To record in the order received.

acid citrate dextrose (ACD): An additive used in the collection of blood specimens for immunohematology tests such as DNA testing and human leukocyte antigen (HLA) phenotyping used in paternity evaluation and to determine transplant compatibility, respectively. Acid citrate prevents coagulation by binding calcium, and dextrose acts as a red blood cell nutrient and preservative by maintaining red cell viability.

acidosis: A dangerous condition in which the pH of the blood is abnormally low (acidic).

ACT: Activated clotting time.

activated partial thromboplastin time (APTT or PTT): Test used to evaluate intrinsic coagulation pathway function and monitor heparin therapy.

additive: A substance (other than the tube stopper or coating) such as an anticoagulant, antiglycolytic agent, separator gel, preservative, or clot activator placed within a tube.

adipose: Denoting fat.

aerobic: With air.

aerosol: A fine mist of the specimen.

AFP: Alpha-fetoprotein.

agglutinate: Clump together; as in the antigen–antibody reaction between red blood cells of two different blood types.

agranulocytes: WBCs that lack granules or have extremely fine granules that are not easy to see.

AHCCCS: Arizona Healthcare Cost Containment System.

airborne precautions: Precautions used in addition to standard precautions for patients known or suspected to be infected with microorganisms transmitted by airborne droplet nuclei.

airborne transmission: Transmission of disease by dispersal of evaporated droplet nuclei containing an infectious agent.

aliquot: A portion of a specimen used for testing.

alkalosis: A dangerous condition in which the pH of the blood is abnormally high (alkaline).

Allen test: A simple, noninvasive test to assess collateral circulation before collecting a blood specimen from the radial artery.

alpha-fetoprotein (AFP): An antigen normally present in the human fetus that is also found in amniotic fluid and maternal serum. It is also present in certain pathologic conditions in males and nonpregnant females.

alveoli: Tiny air sacs in the lungs where the exchange of oxygen and carbon dioxide takes place.

amniotic fluid: Clear, almost colorless to pale-yellow fluid that fills the membrane (amnion or amniotic sac) that surrounds and cushions a fetus in the uterus.

anabolism: A constructive process by which the body converts simple compounds into complex substances needed to carry out the cellular activities of the body.

anaerobic: Without air.

analyte: A general term for a substance undergoing analysis.

anatomic position: The position of standing erect, arms at the side, with eyes and palms facing forward. When describing the direction or the location of a given point of the body, medical personnel normally refer to the body as if the patient were in the anatomic position, regardless of actual body position.

anatomy: The structure of an organism, or the science of the structural composition of living organisms. In humans, the structural composition of the body.

anchor: To secure firmly, as in holding a vein in place by pulling the skin taut with the thumb.

anemia: An abnormal reduction in the number of RBCs in the circulating blood.

antecubital fossa: The area of the arm that is anterior to (in front of) and below the bend of the elbow, where the major veins for venipuncture are located.

antecubital veins: Major superficial veins located in the antecubital fossa.

anterior: Pertaining to or referring to the front of the body; also called ventral.

antibody: Protein substance manufactured by the body in response to a foreign protein or antigen and directed against it.

anticoagulant: A substance that prevents blood from clotting.

antigen: A substance that causes the formation of antibodies that are directed against it.

antiglycolytic agent: A substance that prevents glycolysis, the breakdown or metabolism of glucose (blood sugar) by blood cells. The most common antiglycolytic agent is sodium fluoride.

antimicrobial removal device (ARD): Blood culture bottle containing a resin that removes antimicrobials (antibiotics) from a blood specimen.

antimicrobial therapy: Use of antibiotics to kill or inhibit the growth of microorganisms.

antiseptics: Substances used for skin cleaning that inhibit the growth of bacteria.

aorta: The largest artery in the body, arising from the left ventricle of the heart and approximately 1 inch (2.5 cm) in diameter.

APC: Ambulatory patient classification.

ARD: Antimicrobial removal device.

arm/wrist band: Two other names for identification band/bracelet.

arrhythmia: Irregularity in the heart rate, rhythm, or beat.

arterial line (A-line or Art-line): A catheter that is placed in an artery. It is most commonly placed in a radial artery; it is typically used to provide accurate and continuous measurement of a patient's blood pressure, to collect blood gas specimens and other blood specimens, and for the administration of drugs such as dopamine.

arterialize: Increase arterial composition of capillary blood by warming the site to increase blood flow.

arteries: Blood vessels that carry blood away from the heart.

arterioles: The smallest branches of arteries, which join with the capillaries.

arteriospasm: A reflex (involuntary) contraction of the artery that can be caused by pain or irritation during needle penetration of the artery muscle or result from patient anxiety during arterial puncture.

arteriovenous (AV) shunt: Permanent, surgical fusion of an artery and a vein. It is typically created to provide access for dialysis; also called AV fistula or graft.

ASAP: As soon as possible.

assault: An act or threat causing another to be in fear of immediate battery.

atria (singular, atrium): The upper receiving chambers on each side of the heart.

atrioventricular (AV) valves: The valves at the entrance to the ventricles.

autologous donation: Donating blood for one's own use.

avascular: Without blood or lymph vessels.

axons: Threadlike fibers that carry messages away from the nerve cell body.

bacteremia: Bacteria in the blood.

bar code: A series of black stripes and white spaces of varying widths that correspond to letters and numbers.

barrel: A term for the cylindrical body of a syringe with graduated markings in either milliliters (mL) or cubic centimeters (cc).

basal state: Refers to the resting metabolic state of the body early in the morning after fasting for a minimum of 12 hours.

basilic vein: Large vein on the inner side of the antecubital area that is the last choice vein for venipuncture.

basophils (basos): Normally the least numerous WBC, they release histamine and heparin, which enhance the inflammatory response; identified by their large dark-blue-staining granules that often obscure a typically "s"-shaped nucleus.

battery: Intentional harmful or offensive touching or use of force on a person without consent or legal justification.

BBP: Bloodborne pathogen.

bedside manner: The behavior of a healthcare provider toward or as perceived by a patient.

bevel: The point of a needle that is cut on a slant for ease of skin entry.

bicarbonate ion (HCO$_3^-$): An ion that plays a role in transporting carbon dioxide (CO_2) in the blood to the lungs and in regulating blood pH. HCO_3^- is formed in the red blood cells and plasma from CO_2.

bilirubin: A product of the breakdown of red blood cells.

biohazard: Short for biological hazard; anything potentially harmful to health.

biosafety: Term used to describe the safe handling of biologic substances that pose a risk to health.

bleeding time (BT): Test that measures the time required for blood to stop flowing from a standardized puncture on the inner surface of the forearm.

blood film/smear: A drop of blood spread thinly on a microscope slide.

blood pressure: A measure of the force (pressure) exerted by the blood on the walls of blood vessels.

bloodborne pathogen (BBP): Term applied to infectious microorganisms in blood or other body fluids.

Bloodborne Pathogens (BBP) Standard: OSHA regulations designed to protect employees with potential occupational exposure to pathogens found in blood or other body fluids or substances.

body cavities: Large, hollow spaces in the body that house the various organs.

body plane: A flat surface resulting from a real or imaginary cut through a body in the normal anatomic position.

body substance isolation (BSI): Type of infection control precautions that preceded standard precautions and differed from universal precautions by requiring glove use when contacting any moist body substance.

brachial artery: Artery located in the medial anterior aspect of the antecubital fossa near the insertion of the biceps muscle; the second choice for arterial puncture.

bradycardia: Slow heart rate; less than 60 beats per minute.

breach of confidentiality: Failure to keep privileged medical information private.

bronchae (singular, bronchus): Two airways that branch off of the lower end of the trachea and lead into the lungs; one branch each into the left and right lungs.

BT: Bleeding time test.

B-type natriuretic peptide (BNP): Cardiac hormone produced by the heart in response to ventricular volume expansion and pressure overload.

buccal swabs: Swabs of material collected from the inside of the cheek.

buffy coat: The layer of WBCs and platelets that forms between the red blood cells and plasma when anticoagulated blood settles or is centrifuged.

bullet: Name for a microcollection container.

bursae (singular, bursa): Small synovial fluid-filled sacks in the vicinity of joints that ease friction between joint parts or tendons and bone.

butterfly: Another term for a winged infusion set.

C&S: Culture and sensitivity.

calcaneus: Medical term for heel bone.

calcium (Ca): A mineral that is essential to the clotting process and also needed for proper bone and tooth formation, nerve conduction, and muscle contraction.

CAP: College of American Pathologists.

capillaries: Microscopic, one-cell thick vessels that connect the arterioles and venules forming a bridge between the arterial and venous circulations.

carbaminohemoglobin: Carbon dioxide combined with hemoglobin.

cardiac cycle: One complete contraction and subsequent relaxation of the heart.

cardiac output: Volume of blood pumped by the heart in 1 minute; averaging 5 liters per minute.

cardiac troponin I (TnI): A protein specific to heart muscle.

cardiac troponin T (TnT): Heart muscle-specific protein; elevated longer than TnI.

carryover: Cross-contamination or transfer of additive from one tube to the next.

cartilage: A type of hard, nonvascular connective tissue.

catabolism: The process by which complex substances are broken down into simple ones, including the digestion of food.

catheterized: Term used to describe a urine specimen collected from a sterile catheter inserted through the urethra into the bladder.

causative agent: The pathogen responsible for causing an infection; also called the infectious agent.

CBGs: Capillary blood gases (CBGs); blood gas determinations performed on arterialized capillary specimens.

celite: An inert clay that enhances the coagulation process.

Celsius: A temperature scale on which melting point is 0° and boiling point is 100°. Normal body temperature expressed in Celsius is 37°; also known as the Centigrade scale.

Centers for Disease Control and Prevention (CDC): A division of the U.S. Public Health Service charged with the investigation and control of disease with epidemic potential.

Centigrade: *see* Celsius.

central nervous system (CNS): The brain and spinal cord.

central processing: Screening and prioritizing area where specimens are received and prepared for testing.

central vascular access device (CVAD): Indwelling line; tubing inserted into a main vein or artery used primarily for administering fluids and medications, monitoring pressures, and drawing blood.

central venous catheter (CVC): A line inserted into a large vein such as the subclavian and advanced into the superior vena cava, proximal to the right atrium. The exit end is surgically tunneled under the skin to a site several inches away in the chest; also called central venous line.

centrifuge: A machine that spins the blood tubes at a high number of revolutions per minute.

cephalic vein: The second-choice antecubital vein for venipuncture, located in the lateral aspect of the antecubital fossa.

cerebrospinal fluid (CSF): Clear, colorless liquid that circulates within the cavities surrounding the brain and spinal cord; it has many of the same components as plasma.

certification: Evidence that an individual has mastered fundamental competencies in a particular technical area.

chain of custody: Special strict protocol for forensic specimens that requires detailed documentation tracking the specimen from the time it is collected until the results are reported.

chain of infection: A number of components or events that when present in a series lead to an infection.

chloride (Cl⁻): Electrolyte responsible for maintaining cellular integrity by influencing osmotic pressure and acid–base and water balance.

chordae tendineae: Thin threads of tissue that attach the atrioventricular valves to the walls of the ventricles to help keep them from flipping back into the atria.

circadian: Biologic rhythms or variations having a 24-hour cycle.

circulatory system: System that consists of the cardiovascular system (heart, blood, and blood vessels) and the lymphatic system (lymph, lymph vessels, and nodes) and is the means by which oxygen and nutrients are carried to the cells and carbon dioxide and other wastes are carried away from them.

civil action: Legal actions in which the alleged injured party sues for monetary damages.

Cl⁻: Chloride.

clay sealant: A type of sealer used for closing the end of a microhematocrit tube.

clean catch: Method of obtaining a urine sample so that it is free of contaminating matter from the external genital area.

CLIA '88: Clinical Laboratory Improvement Amendments of 1988.

clot activator: A substance that enhances the coagulation process.

CLSI: Clinical and Laboratory Standards Institute, formerly NCCLS.

CMS: Center for Medicare and Medicaid Services.

coagulation cascade: Sequential activation of the coagulation factors.

coagulation: The blood-clotting process.

collateral circulation: An area supplied with blood from more than one artery so that circulation can be maintained if one vessel is obstructed.

combining form: A word root combined with a vowel.

combining vowel: A vowel (frequently an "o") that is added between two word roots or a word root and a suffix to make pronunciation easier.

common pathway: Coagulation pathway involving the conversion of prothrombin to thrombin, which splits fibrinogen into the fibrin that entraps blood cells and creates the fibrin clot.

communicable: Able to spread from person to person, as a disease.

communication barriers: Biases or personalized filters that are major obstructions to verbal communication.

compatibility: Ability to be mixed together with favorable results, as in blood transfusions.

competencies: Educational standards for phlebotomy programs.

concentric circles: Circles with a common center; starting from the center and moving outward in ever-widening circles.

confidentiality: The ethical cornerstone of professional behavior; the practice of regarding information concerning a patient as privileged and not to be disclosed to anyone without the patient's authorization.

contact precautions: Precautions used in addition to standard precautions when a patient is known or suspected to be infected or colonized with epidemiologically important microorganisms that can be transmitted by direct contact with the patient or indirect contact with surfaces or patient-care items.

contact transmission: Transfer of an infectious agent to a susceptible host through direct or indirect contact. *see* **direct** and **indirect contact transmission.**

continuum of care: A holistic, coordinated system for healthcare services.

coronary arteries: Arteries that branch off of the aorta just beyond the aortic semilunar valve that deliver blood to the heart muscle.

CPD: Citrate-phosphate-dextrose, an additive used in collecting units of blood for transfusion. Citrate prevents clotting by chelating calcium, phosphate stabilizes pH, and dextrose provides cells with energy and helps keep them alive.

CPT: Current procedural terminology codes.

CPU: Central processing unit.

cranial cavity: Body space that houses the brain.

criminal action: Legal recourse for offenses committed against the law that can lead to imprisonment of the offender.

crossmatch: A test to determine suitability of mixing donor and recipient blood.

CSF: Cerebrospinal fluid.

culture and sensitivity (C&S): Microbiology test that includes placing a specimen on special nutrient media that encourages the growth of microorganisms, identifying any that grow, and then performing sensitivity/antibiotic susceptibility testing to identify antibiotics that will be effective against them.

C-urea breath test: A test used to detect *H. pylori* bacteria based on the fact that the bacteria produce urease, an enzyme that breaks down urea and is not normally present in the stomach.

cursor: Flashing indicator on the computer screen.

CVAD: Central vascular access device.

CVC: Central venous catheter.

cyanotic: Marked by cyanosis or bluish in color from lack of oxygen.

cystic fibrosis: Disorder of the exocrine glands that affects many body systems but primarily the lungs, upper respiratory tract, liver, and pancreas. Patients with cystic fibrosis have abnormally high levels (2 to 5 times normal) of chloride in their sweat.

data: Information collected for analysis or computation.

defendant: In a lawsuit, a person or persons against whom the complaint is filed.

delta check: Comparison of current results of a lab test with previous results for the same test on the same patient.

dendrites: Structures that carry messages to the nerve cell body.

deposition: A process in which one party questions another under oath while a court reporter records every word.

dermis: Corium or true skin; a layer composed of elastic and fibrous connective tissue.

diapedesis: Process by which WBCs slip through the walls of the capillaries into the tissues.

diaphragm: The dome-shaped muscle that separates the abdominal cavity from the thoracic cavity.

diastole: The relaxing phase of the cardiac cycle.

diastolic pressure: Pressure in the arteries during relaxation of the ventricles.

differential (diff): A test in which the number, type, and characteristics of blood cells are determined by examining a stained blood smear under a microscope.

direct-contact transmission: Transfer of an infectious agent to a susceptible host through close or intimate contact such as touching or kissing.

directional terms: Medical terms that describe the relationship of an area or part of the body with respect to the rest of the body or body part.

discard tube: Also called "clear tube"; a tube used to collect and discard approximately 5 mL of blood to prevent IV or tissue fluid contamination of a specimen.

discovery: Formal process in litigation that involves taking depositions and interrogating parties involved.

disinfectants: Substances or solutions that are used to remove or kill microorganisms on surfaces and instruments.

distal: Farthest from the center of the body, origin, or point of attachment.

diurnal: Happening daily.

DNAR: Do not attempt resuscitation.

DNR: Do not resuscitate.

"Do Not Use" list: A list of dangerous abbreviations, symbols, and acronyms that must be included on this list by every organization accredited by JCAHO.

dorsal: Posterior or pertaining to the back.

dorsal cavities: Internal spaces located in the back of the body.

DOT: Department of Transportation.

DRGs: Diagnosis-related groups.

droplet precautions: Precautions used in addition to standard precautions for patients known or suspected to be infected with microorganisms transmitted by droplets (particles larger than 5 μm in size) generated when a patient talks, coughs, or sneezes and during certain procedures such as suctioning.

droplet transmission: Transfer of an infectious agent to the mucous membranes of the mouth, nose, or conjunctiva of the eyes via infectious droplets (particles 5 μm in diameter or larger) generated by talking, coughing, sneezing or during procedures such as suctioning.

drug screening: The practice of testing employees' or athletes' urine or blood to screen for illicit or illegal drugs.

due care: The level of care that a person of ordinary intelligence and good sense would exercise under the given circumstances.

edema: Swelling due to abnormal accumulation of fluid in the tissues.

EDTA: Ethylenediaminetetraacetic acid, an anticoagulant that prevents coagulation by binding or chelating calcium and is used for hematology studies because it preserves cell morphology and inhibits platelet clumping.

electrocardiogram (ECG or EKG): An actual record of the electrical currents that correspond to each event in heart muscle contraction.

electrolytes: Substances such as potassium or sodium that conduct electricity when dissolved in water.

EMLA: A eutectic (easily melted) mixture of local anesthetics.

endocardium: The thin inner layer of the heart.

endocrine glands: Glands that secrete hormones directly into the bloodstream.

endocrine: Refers to a gland that secretes directly into the bloodstream.

engineering controls: Devices such as sharps disposal containers and needles with safety features that isolate or remove a bloodborne pathogen hazard from the workplace.

Enter key: Button on keyboard for data input.

Environmental Protection Agency (EPA): A federal agency that regulates the disposal of hazardous waste.

eosinophils (eos): WBCs that ingest and detoxify foreign protein, helping turn off immune reactions; they increase with allergies and pinworm infestations and are identified by their beadlike, bright orange-red-staining granules.

EPA: Environmental Protection Agency.

epicardium: The thin outer layer of the heart

epidermis: The outermost and thinnest layer of the skin.

epiglottis: A thin, leaf-shaped structure that covers the entrance of the larynx during swallowing.

epithelial: Consisting of epithelium.

epithelium: The avascular layer of cells that forms the epidermis and the surface layer of mucous and serous membranes.

erythema: Redness.

erythrocytes: Red blood cells (RBCs); anuclear, disk-shaped blood cells whose main function is to carry oxygen from the lungs to the tissue cells and transport carbon dioxide away from the cells to the lungs.

esophagus: Tube that carries food and liquid from the throat to the stomach.

ethanol: Ethyl or grain alcohol.

ETOH: Abbreviation for ethanol or blood alcohol.

evacuated tube system (ETS): A closed system in which the patient's blood flows directly into a collection tube through a needle inserted into a vein.

evacuated tubes: Type of tubes used in blood collection that have a premeasured vacuum and are color-coded to denote the additive inside.

exocrine glands: Glands that secrete substances through ducts.

exsanguinate: To remove all blood.

exsanguination: Blood loss to a point where life cannot be sustained.

external respiration: Exchange of respiratory gases in the lungs.

external: On or near the surface of the body; superficial.

extrasystoles: Extra heart beats before the normal beat.

extravascular: Outside the blood vessels.

extrinsic pathway: Coagulation pathway initiated by the release of thromboplastin from injured tissue.

FAA: Federal Aviation Administration.

fallopian tubes: Duct that carries ova from the ovaries to the uterus.

FAN: Fastidious antimicrobial neutralization.

fastidious antimicrobial neutralization (FAN): Blood culture bottle that contains activated charcoal that neutralizes antibiotics in a blood specimen.

fasting: No food or drink except water for approximately 12 hours.

feather: Thinnest area of a properly made blood smear where a differential is performed.

fecal occult blood test: A test that detects hidden (occult) blood in stool (feces).

femoral artery: Large artery located superficially in the groin, lateral to the pubis bone, which is the largest artery used for arterial puncture.

fibrillations: Rapid, uncoordinated contractions.

fibrin degradation products (fibrin split products): Fragments remaining from the breakdown of fibrin.

fibrin: A filamentous protein formed by the action of thrombin on fibrinogen.

fibrinogen: Also called factor I; a protein found in plasma that is essential for clotting of blood.

fibrinolysis: Stage 4 of hemostasis; a process that results in removal or dissolution of a blood clot once healing has occurred.

FiO₂: Fraction of inspired oxygen, as in oxygen therapy.

fire tetrahedron: The latest way of looking at the chemistry of fire in which the chemical reaction that produces fire is added as a fourth component to the traditional fire triangle components of fuel, heat, and oxygen.

flanges: Extensions on the sides of an evacuated tube holder that aid in tube placement and removal.

flea: Small metal bar that is inserted into the tube after collection of a capillary blood gas specimen to aid in mixing the anticoagulant by means of a magnet.

FOBT: Fecal occult blood test.

fomites: Inanimate objects such as countertops and computer keyboards that can harbor material containing infectious agents.

forensic specimen: Specimen collected for legal reasons.

formed elements: Cellular portion of the blood.

fraud: Deceitful practice or false portrayal of facts by either words or conduct.

frontal plane: Divides the body vertically into front and back portions; also called coronal plane

FUO: fever of unknown origin

galactosemia: Inherited disorder caused by lack of the enzyme needed to convert the milk sugar galactose into glucose needed by the body for energy.

gallbladder: Accessory organ to the digestive system.

gametes: Sex cells.

gastric analysis: A test that examines stomach contents for abnormal substances and measures gastric acid concentration to evaluate stomach acid production.

gastrointestinal (GI) tract: The passageway that extends from the mouth to the anus through the pharynx, esophagus, stomach, and small and large intestines.

gatekeeper: Primary physician who serves as the patient's advocate and advises the patient on healthcare needs.

gauge: A number that relates to the diameter of the lumen of a needle.

germ cells: Gametes or sex cells.

germicide: An agent that kills pathogenic microorganisms.

glomerulus: A tuft of capillaries that filter water and dissolved substances including wastes from the blood.

GLPs: Good Laboratory Practices.

glucose tolerance test (GTT): A test used to diagnose carbohydrate metabolism problems.

glycolysis: The breakdown or metabolism of glucose (blood sugar) by blood cells.

glycosylated hemoglobin: Increased in RBCs of patients with diabetes mellitus and used as a retrospective index of glucose control over time.

gonads: Glands that manufacture and store gametes and produce hormones that regulate the reproductive process.

gram: The basic unit of weight in the metric system; approximately equal to a cubic centimeter or milliliter of water.

granulocytes: WBCs with easily visible granules.

great saphenous vein: The longest vein in the body, located in the leg.

GTT: Glucose tolerance test.

guaiac test: A test for hidden blood in feces; also called occult blood test.

hardware: Computer equipment used to process data.

Hazardous Communication (HazCom) Standard: Abbreviation for the OSHA Hazardous Communication Standard that requires employers to maintain documentation on all hazardous chemicals.

HazCom: OSHA Hazardous Communication standard.

HBV: Hepatitis B virus; the virus that cause hepatitis B.

HCG: Human chorionic gonadotropin.

HCO₃⁻: Bicarbonate ion.

HDN: Hemolytic disease of the newborn.

Healthcare Infection Control Practices Advisory Committee: A federal organization established in 1991 that advises the CDC on updating guidelines regarding prevention of nosocomial infection.

heart rate: Number of heartbeats per minute, which is normally around 72 beats per minute.

Helicobacter pylori: Bacterial species that secretes substances that damage the lining of the stomach and cause chronic gastritis that can lead to peptic ulcer disease.

hematocrit (Hct): Percentage by volume of red blood cells in whole blood.

hematoma: A swelling or mass of blood (often clotted) such as that caused by blood leaking from a blood vessel during or following venipuncture.

hematopoiesis: *see* **hemopoiesis**

hemoconcentration: A decrease in the fluid content of the blood with a subsequent increase in nonfilterable large molecule- or protein-based blood components such as red blood cells.

hemoglobin (Hgb or Hb): An iron-containing pigment in RBCs that enables them to transport oxygen and carbon dioxide and also gives them their red color.

hemolysis: Damage or destruction of RBCs and release of hemoglobin into the fluid portion of a specimen, causing the serum color to range from pink (slight hemolysis) to red (gross hemolysis).

hemolytic disease of the newborn (HDN): Destruction of RBCs of an Rh-positive fetus by Rh antibodies produced by an Rh-negative mother that cross the placenta into the fetal circulation.

hemolyzed: The condition of serum or plasma that has hemoglobin from broken RBCs in it.

hemopoiesis: Production and development of blood cells and other formed elements, normally in the bone marrow.

hemostasis: Process by which the body stops the leakage of blood from the vascular system after injury; also known as the coagulation process.

hemostatic plug: Blood clot formed from blood cells and platelets trapped in a network of fibrin strands.

heparin lock: A catheter or cannula with a stopcock or cap with a diaphragm to provide access for administering medication or drawing blood.

heparin management test (HMT): A test for high-dose heparin monitoring needed in catheterization laboratories and during surgery.

heparin: Anticoagulant that prevents clotting by inhibiting thrombin formation.

HICPAC: Healthcare Infection Control Practices Advisory Committee.

HIPAA: Health Insurance Portability and Accountability Act.

histologic/histological: Pertaining to the microscopic structure of tissue.

HMOs: Health maintenance organizations.

HMT: Heparin management test.

homeostasis: The "steady state" (state of equilibrium or balance) of the internal environment of the body maintained through feedback and regulation in response to internal and external changes.

hormones: Powerful chemical substances that affect many body processes.

hospice: A type of care for patients who are terminally ill.

HPC: handheld PC.

H. pylori: *Helicobacter pylori.*

hub: The end of the needle that attaches to the blood collection device; also the threaded end of a tube holder where the needle attaches.

human chorionic gonadotropin (HCG or hCG): Hormone that appears in both urine and serum beginning approximately 10 days after conception. HCG is the substance detected in pregnancy tests.

human immunodeficiency virus (HIV): The virus that causes acquired immunodeficiency syndrome (AIDS).

hyperglycemia: A condition in which the blood sugar (glucose) level is high, as in diabetes mellitus.

hyperkalemia: High blood potassium concentration.

hypersecretion: Secreting too much.

hypodermic needle: The type of needle used with the syringe system.

hypoglycemia: Condition in which the blood sugar (glucose) level is decreased.

hypokalemia: Low blood potassium level.

hyponatremia: Low sodium levels in the blood.

hypernatremia: High sodium levels in the blood.

hyposecretion: Secreting too little.

hypothyroidism: Disorder characterized by insufficient levels of thyroid hormones.

iatrogenic: An adjective used to describe an adverse condition brought on by the effects of treatment.

ICD-9-CM: International Classification of Diseases, Ninth Revision, Clinical Modification.

icons: Images used to request the appropriate program or function on a computer.

icteric: A term meaning "marked by jaundice"; used to describe serum, plasma, or urine specimens that have an abnormal deep yellow to yellow-brown color due to high bilirubin levels.

icterus: Also called jaundice; a condition characterized by a high bilirubin (a product of the breakdown of red blood cells) level in the blood, leading to deposits of yellow bile pigment in the skin, mucous membranes, and sclera (whites of the eyes), giving the patient a yellow appearance.

ID band/bracelet: Identification band/ bracelet.

ID card: Clinic-issued patient identification document.

ID code: Unique identification for users.

IDS: Integrated healthcare delivery system.

immune: Protected from or resistant to a particular disease or infection because of the development of antibody against a particular vaccination or recovery.

implanted port: A small chamber attached to an indwelling line that is surgically implanted under the skin in the upper chest or arm.

indirect contact transmission: Transmission of an infectious agent that occurs when a susceptible host touches contaminated objects such as patient bed linens, clothing, or wound dressings.

indwelling line: Another name for central venous catheter (CVC).

infant respiratory distress syndrome (IRDS): A respiratory condition in a premature infant caused by a deficiency of surfactant that causes the alveoli to collapse.

infection: Invasion of the body by a pathogenic microorganism, resulting in injurious effects or disease.

infectious agent: The pathogen responsible for causing an infection; also called the causative agent.

inferior: Beneath, lower, or away from the head; also called caudal.

inflammation: Tissue reaction to injury, such as redness or swelling.

informed consent: Implies voluntary and competent permission for a medical procedure, test, or medication.

input: To enter data into a computer.

INR: International normalized ratio.

integument: Covering or skin.

integumentary system: The skin and its appendages, including the hair and nails; also referred to as the largest organ of the body.

interatrial septum: The partition that separates the right and left atria.

interface: Connect for the purpose of interaction.

internal respiration: Exchange of respiratory gases between the blood and cells in the tissues.

internal/deep: Within or near the center of the body.

interstitial fluid: Fluid in the tissue spaces between the cells.

interventricular septum: The partition that separates the right and left ventricles.

intracellular fluid: Fluid within the cells.

intravascular: Within the blood vessels.

intravenous (IV) line: A catheter inserted in a vein to administer fluids and simply referred to as an IV.

intravenous (IV): Of, pertaining to, or within, a vein.

intrinsic pathway: Coagulation pathway involving coagulation factors circulating within the bloodstream.

invasion of privacy: Violation of one's right to be left alone.

ionized calcium (iCa^{2+}): Form of calcium used by the body for such critical functions as muscular contraction, cardiac function, transmission of nerve impulses, and blood clotting.

iontophoresis: Electrical stimulation from electrodes placed on the skin. Used in the production of sweat in the sweat chloride test.

isolation procedures: Isolation procedures separate patients with certain transmissible infections.

jaundice: Also called icterus; a condition characterized by increased bilirubin (a product of the breakdown of red blood cells) in the blood, leading to deposits of yellow bile pigment in the skin, mucous membranes, and sclera (whites of the eyes), giving the patient a yellow appearance.

Joint Commission on the Accreditation of Healthcare Organizations (JCAHO): A voluntary, nongovernmental agency charged with (among other things) establishing standards for the operation of healthcare facilities and services.

K$^+$: Potassium.

keratinized: Having become hardened.

kidneys: Organs that form and excrete urine.

kinesics: The study of nonverbal communication.

kinesic slip: When the verbal and nonverbal messages do not match.

LAN: Local area network.

lancet: A sterile, disposable, sharp-pointed or bladed instrument that either punctures or makes an incision in the skin to obtain capillary blood specimens for testing.

large intestine: Part of the digestive system where undigested food is stored, formed into feces, and eliminated; also where normal intestinal bacteria act on food residue to produce vitamin K and some of the B-complex vitamins.

larynx: The enlarged upper end of the trachea that houses the vocal cords, the ends of which mark the division between the upper and lower respiratory tract.

lateral: Toward the side.

leukocytes: White blood cells (WBCs); nucleus-containing blood cells whose main function is to combat infection and remove disintegrated tissue.

leukopenia: An abnormal decrease of WBCs in the circulating blood.

lipase: Digestive enzyme secreted by the pancreas.

lipemia: Increased lipid content in the blood.

lipemic: Term used to describe serum or plasma that appears milky (cloudy white) or turbid due to high lipid content.

LIS: Laboratory information system.

liter: The basic unit of volume in the metric system, which is equivalent to 1000 mL.

liver: Accessory organ of the digestive system that stores glycogen, detoxifies harmful substances, secretes bile, and breaks down protein.

L/M: Liters per minute, as in oxygen therapy.

Lookback: Program that requires all components of a unit of blood to be traceable back to the donor and that also requires notification to all blood recipients when a donor for a blood product they have received has turned positive for a transmissible disease.

Luer adapter: In the Luer-Lok system, a device for connecting the syringe to the needle; when locked into place it gives a secure fit.

lumbar (spinal) puncture: Procedure in which a physician inserts a special needle into the spinal cavity to extract spinal fluid.

lumen: The internal space of a blood vessel or tube.

lungs: Organs that house the bronchial branches and the alveoli where gas exchange takes place.

lymph: Lymphatic system fluid derived from excess tissue fluid and similar in composition to plasma; also, an abbreviation for lymphocyte.

lymph nodes: Structures of the lymphatic system that contain special tissue that traps and destroys bacteria and foreign matter and functions in the production of lymphocytes.

lymphatic system: A system of vessels, nodes, and ducts that collect and filter excess tissue fluid called lymph and return it to the venous system.

lymphocytes (lymphs): Normally the second-most numerous WBC and the most numerous agranulocyte. Two main types of lymphocytes are T lymphocytes and B lymphocytes.

lymphostasis: Obstruction or stoppage of normal lymph flow.

lysis: Rupturing, as in the bursting of red blood cell.

lyse: To kill or destroy, as in ruptured red blood cells.

malpractice: A type of negligence committed by a professional.

mastectomy: Breast excision, or removal.

material safety data sheets (MSDS): A written document containing general information as well as precautionary and emergency information for any product with a hazardous warning on the label.

MCOs: Managed care organizations.

medial: Toward the midline or middle.

median cubital vein: The preferred vein for venipuncture, located in the middle of the antecubital fossa.

median cutaneous nerve: A major motor and sensory nerve in the arm that lies along the path of the brachial artery and in the vicinity of the basilic vein.

Medicaid: A federal and state program that provides medical assistance for low-income Americans.

medical terminology: Special vocabulary of the health professions.

Medicare: Federally funded program that provides healthcare to people over the age of 65 and the disabled.

megakaryocyte: Large bone marrow cell from which platelets are derived.

melanin: Dark pigment that colors the skin and protects it from the sun. Also found in hair and eyes.

meninges: Three layers of connective tissue that enclose the spinal cavity.

menu: A list of options from which the user may choose.

metabolism: The sum of all the physical and chemical reactions necessary to sustain life.

meter: The basic unit of linear measurement in the metric system; equal to 39.37 inches.

microbe: Short for microorganism; a microscopic organism or one that is not visible to the naked eye.

microcollection containers: Small plastic tubes used to collect the tiny amounts of blood obtained from capillary punctures; also called capillary tubes and microtubes and sometimes referred to as "bullets" because of their size and shape.

microhematocrit tubes: Disposable, narrow-bore plastic or plastic-clad glass capillary tubes that fill by capillary action.

midsagittal plane: Divides the body vertically into equal right and left portions.

midstream: Term applied to urine collection in which the specimen is collected in the middle of urination rather than at the beginning or end.

military time: Also called European time; based on a clock with 24 numbers instead of 12, eliminating the need to designate AM or PM.

mitosis: A type of cell duplication that involves DNA doubling and cell division.

mnemonic: Memory-aiding code or abbreviation used in LIS, for example.

monocytes (monos): Normally the largest WBCs and 1–7% of total WBCs, they are mononuclear phagocytic cells and one of the first lines of defense in the inflammatory process.

motor or efferent nerves: Nerves that carry impulses away from the CNS.

MR number: Medical record number used for patient ID.

MSDS: Material Safety Data Sheets.

multisample needle: A type of needle that allows multiple tubes to be collected with a single venipuncture.

murmurs: Abnormal heart sounds, often due to faulty valve action.

myocardial infarction (MI): Heart attack or necrosis (death) of heart muscle from lack of oxygen.

myocardial ischemia: Condition resulting from an insufficient supply of blood to meet the oxygen needs of the heart muscle.

myocardium: The middle muscle layer of the heart.

Na⁺: Sodium.

NAACLS: National Accrediting Agency for Clinical Laboratory Sciences.

nasopharyngeal (NP): Refers to the nasal cavity and pharynx.

National Fire Protection Association (NFPA): Federal agency that regulates disinfectant products and the disposal of hazardous waste among other responsibilities associated with developing and enforcing regulations that implement environmental laws enacted by Congress.

National Institute for Occupational Safety and Health (NIOSH): Federal agency responsible for conducting research and making recommendations for the prevention of work-related injury and illness.

needle phobia: Intense fear of needles.

Needlestick Safety and Prevention Act: Federal law that directed OSHA to revise the BBP standard in four key areas: revision of the exposure control plan, selecting engineering and work practice controls with employee input, modification of engineering control definitions, and new record-keeping requirements.

needle sheath: Needle cap or cover.

negligence: Failure to exercise due care.

nephron: The microscopic functional unit of the kidneys.

network: A group of computers that are all linked for the purpose of sharing resources.

neuron: Fundamental working unit of the nervous system.

neutropenic: Pertaining to an abnormally small number of neutrophil cells in the blood.

neutrophils: Normally the most numerous WBC in adults; averaging 65% of the total WBC count, with granules that are fine in texture and stain lavender; also called polys, PMNs, or segs.

newborn/neonatal screening: The routine testing of newborns for the presence of certain metabolic and genetic (inherited) disorders such as phenylketonuria.

NFPA: National Fire Protection Association.

NIDA: National Institute on Drug Abuse.

noninvasive: Not penetrating the skin.

NP: Nasopharyngeal.

NPO: Nothing by mouth (from Latin, *nulla per os*).

nosocomial infection: An infection acquired in a healthcare facility.

occlusion: Obstruction.

Occupational Safety and Health Administration: U.S. government agency that mandates and enforces safe working conditions for employees.

occult blood: Hidden blood. *see* **guaiac test.**

O&P: Ova and parasites; a test to detect the presence of intestinal parasites and their eggs in feces.

order of draw: A special sequence of tube collection that is intended to minimize additive carryover or cross-contamination problems.

OSHA: Occupational Safety and Health Administration.

osteochondritis: Inflammation of the bone and cartilage.

osteomyelitis: Inflammation of the bone marrow and adjacent bone.

output: Return of processed information or data to the user or to someone in another location.

ovum: Female gamete or sex cell.

oxalates: Anticoagulants that prevent clotting by precipitating calcium.

oxyhemoglobin: Oxygen combined with hemoglobin.

pacemaker: In the heart, the structure that generates the electrical impulse that initiates heart contraction; *see* **sinoatrial node.**

palmar: Concerning the palm of the hand.

palpate: Examine by feel or touch.

pancreas: An accessory organ to the digestive system that secretes hormones and produces digestive enzymes.

papillae (singular, papilla): Small elevations of the dermis that indent the bottom of the epidermis and give rise to the ridges and grooves that form the fingerprints.

papillary dermis: The dermal layer that adjoins the epidermis.

parenteral: Any route other than the digestive tract.

partial pressure (P): The pressure exerted by one gas in a mixture of gases.

partial pressure of carbon dioxide (PCO$_2$): A measure of the pressure exerted by dissolved CO$_2$ in the blood.

partial pressure of oxygen (PO$_2$): A measure of the pressure exerted by dissolved O$_2$ in the blood plasma.

password: A secret code that uniquely identifies a person and allows him or her to become a system user.

patency: State of being freely open, as in the normal condition of a vein.

pathogenic: Capable of causing disease.

pathogens: Microbes capable of causing disease.

patient ID: The process of verifying a patient's identity.

PCO$_2$: Partial pressure of carbon dioxide.

PDA: Personal digital assistants.

peak level: Drug level collected when the highest serum concentration of the drug is anticipated.

pelvic cavity: Body space that houses the reproductive organs.

percutaneous: Through the skin.

pericardial fluid: Fluid aspirated from the pericardial cavity that surrounds the heart.

pericardium: A thin, fluid-filled sac that surrounds the heart.

peripheral nervous system: All the nerves that connect the CNS to every part of the body.

peripherally inserted central catheter (PICC): A line inserted into the peripheral venous system (veins of the extremities) and threaded into the central venous system (main veins leading to the heart). It does not require surgical insertion and is typically placed in an antecubital vein just above or below the antecubital fossa.

peritoneal fluid: Fluid aspirated from the abdominal cavity.

permucosal: Through mucous membranes.

personal protective equipment (PPE): Protective clothing and other protective items worn by an individual.

petechiae: Tiny, nonraised red spots that appear on a patient's skin upon tourniquet application. They are minute drops of blood that escape the capillaries and come to the surface of the skin below the tourniquet most commonly as a result of capillary wall defects or platelet abnormalities.

pH: Abbreviation for potential hydrogen, a scale representing the relative acidity or alkalinity of a solution in which 7 is neutral, below 7 is acid, and above 7 is alkaline.

phagocytosis: Process in which a WBC surrounds, engulfs, and destroys a pathogen or foreign matter.

phalanges (singular, phalanx): Bones of the fingers or toes.

pharynx: A funnel-shaped passageway that receives food from the mouth and delivers it to the esophagus and air from the nose and carries it into the larynx.

phenylketonuria: Disorder that results from a defect in the enzyme that breaks down the amino acid phenylalanine, converting it into the amino acid tyrosine.

PHI: Protected health information.

phlebotomy: The process of blood-letting.

physiology: The function of an organism, or the science of the functions of living organisms.

PICC: Peripherally inserted central catheter.

pilocarpine: A sweat-stimulating drug used in the sweat chloride test.

pituitary gland: Endocrine gland under the control of the hypothalamus that secretes hormones that control other glands; sometimes called the master gland.

PKU: Phenylketonuria.

plaintiff: Injured party in the litigation process.

plantar surface: The sole or bottom surface of the foot.

plasma: The top layer of clear liquid used for testing; also, the fluid portion of the blood in the living body.

platelet adhesion: Platelets adhering (sticking) to an injured area.

platelet aggregation: Platelets sticking to one another.

platelet plug formation: Stage 2 of hemostasis in which platelets degranulate and stick to the site and each other and plug the site of injury.

platelets: Cellular elements that play a role in blood clotting; *see* **thrombocytes.**

pleura (pleural, pleurae): Layer of thin membrane that encases the lungs.

pleural cavity/space: A small space between the layers of the pleurae of the lungs.

pleural fluid: Fluid aspirated from the pleural cavity surrounding the lungs.

plunger: A rodlike device that fits tightly into the barrel of a syringe and creates a vacuum when pulled back in the process of filling the syringe.

PMN: Polymorphonuclear.

PNS: Peripheral nervous system.

PO₂: Partial pressure of oxygen.

POCT: Point-of-care testing

point-of-care testing: Alternate site testing (AST) or ancillary, bedside, or near-patient testing, often performed using portable or handheld instruments.

polycythemia: A disorder involving overproduction of red blood cells.

polymorphonuclear : Term used to describe a neutrophil whose nucleus is segmented (has multiple lobes).

posterior curvature: Medical term for the back of the heel.

posterior/dorsal: Refers to the back.

postprandial: After a meal.

potassium (K⁺): A mineral that is essential for normal muscle activity and the conduction of nerve impulses.

potassium oxalate: An anticoagulant commonly used with the antiglycolytic agent sodium fluoride.

PP: Postprandial.

PPD: Purified protein derivative; *see* **tuberculin test.**

PPOs: Preferred provider organizations.

PPS: Prospective payment system.

PPTs: Plasma preparation tubes.

preanalytical: Prior to analysis.

prefix: A word element that precedes a word root and modifies its meaning by adding information such as presence or absence, location, number, or size.

Pre-op/post-op: Before an operation or surgery (preoperative)/after an operation or surgery (postoperative).

primary care: Care by general physician who assumes ongoing responsibility for maintaining patients' health.

primary hemostasis: First two stages of the coagulation process that involve vasoconstriction and the formation of a platelet plug.

pronation: The condition of being prone or the act of turning the body or body part face down.

prone: Lying face down.

protective isolation: Type of isolation in which protective measures are taken to keep healthcare workers and others from transmitting infection to a patient who is highly susceptible to infection.

prothrombin test (PT): A test used to evaluate extrinsic pathway function and monitor coumarin therapy.

proxemics: The study of an individual's concept and use of space.

proximal: Nearest to the center of the body or point of attachment.

PSTs: Plasma separator tubes.

pulmonary circulation: Vascular pathway that carries blood from the heart to the lungs to remove carbon dioxide and returns oxygenated blood to the heart.

pulse: Rhythmic throbbing caused by the alternating contraction and expansion of an artery as a wave of blood passes through it.

pulse rate: Same as heart rate.

QA: Quality assurance.

QC: Quality control.

QI: Quality improvement.

QNS: Quantity not sufficient.

QSE: Quality system essentials.

quality indicators: Guides used as monitors of all areas of patient care.

radial artery: Artery located in the thumb side of the wrist that is the first choice and most common site used for arterial puncture.

RAM: Random-access memory.

reference laboratories: Large, independent laboratories that receive and test specimens from many different facilities.

reference ranges: Normal laboratory test values for healthy individuals.

reflux: Backflow of blood into a patient's vein from the collection tube during venipuncture.

requisition: The form on which test orders are entered and sent to the laboratory.

res ipsa loquitor: A Latin phrase meaning "the thing speaks for itself."

respondeat superior: Latin phrase meaning "let the master respond." In other words, employers must answer for damages their employees cause within the scope of their practice.

reservoir: The source of an infectious microorganism.

resheathing devices: Equipment such as shields that cover a needle after use.

reticulocytes (retics): Immature RBCs in the bloodstream that contain remnants of material from the nuclear phase.

reverse isolation: Same as protective isolation.

Rh blood group system: Blood group based on the presence or absence of an RBC antigen called the D antigen, also known as Rh factor.

Rh factor: Antigen called the D antigen that is the basis for the Rh blood group system.

Rh negative (Rh−): Rh blood type of an individual whose RBCs lack the D antigen.

Rh positive (Rh+): Rh blood type of an individual whose RBCs have the D antigen.

risk management: An internal process focused on identifying and minimizing situations that pose risk to patients and employees.

ROM: Read-only memory.

sagittal plane: Divides the body vertically into right and left portions.

saline lock: A catheter or cannula that is often placed in a vein in the lower arm above the wrist to provide access for administering medication or drawing blood and that can be left in place for up to 48 hours. It is periodically flushed with saline or heparin to prevent clotting.

salivary glands: Secrete saliva, which moistens food and contains enzymes that begin starch digestion.

sclerosed: Hardened.

sebaceous glands: Oil-secreting glands in the skin.

secondary care: Care by a physician (specialist) who can perform out-of-the-ordinary procedures in outpatient facilities.

secondary hemostasis: Stages 3 and 4 of the coagulation process, which involve fibrin clot formation and the ultimate dissolution of the clot after healing has occurred, respectively.

semilunar valves: Valves at the exits of the ventricles that are crescent shaped, like the moon (Latin, *luna*).

sensory or afferent (a'fer-ent) nerves: Nerves that carry impulses to the CNS.

septa (singular, septum): Partitions consisting mostly of myocardium that separate the right and left chambers of the heart.

septicemia: Microorganisms or their toxins in the blood.

serous fluid: Pale-yellow watery fluid found between the double-layered membranes that enclose the pleural, pericardial, and peritoneal cavities.

serum: Normally clear pale-yellow fluid that can be separated from a clotted blood specimen and has the same composition as plasma, except it does not contain fibrinogen.

sex cells: Gametes.

shaft: The long cylindrical portion of a needle.

sharps container: Special puncture-resistant, leak-proof, disposable container used to dispose of used needles, lancets, and other sharp objects.

short draw: An underfilled or partially filled tube.

short draw tubes: Tubes designed to partially fill without compromising test results.

silica: Glass particles used to enhance the coagulation process; a clot activator.

sinoatrial (SA) node: Structure that generates the electrical impulse that initiates heart contraction; also called the pacemaker.

skin antisepsis: Destruction of microorganisms on the skin.

small intestine: The longest part of the digestive tract where absorption of digested food, water, and minerals takes place.

sodium (Na⁺): An extracellular ion in the blood plasma that helps maintain fluid balance.

sodium citrate: An anticoagulant that prevents clotting by binding calcium and is used for coagulation tests because it does the best job of preserving the coagulation factors.

sodium fluoride: An additive that preserves glucose and inhibits the growth of bacteria.

sodium polyanethol sulfonate (SPS): An anticoagulant used in blood culture collection that also reduces the action of a protein called complement that destroys bacteria, slows down phagocytosis (ingestion of bacteria by leukocytes), and reduces the activity of certain antibiotics.

software: Programming or coded instruction required to control the hardware in processing of data.

solutes: Dissolved substances.

spermatozoa: Male gametes or sex cells.

sphygmomanometer: Blood pressure cuff; device used to measure blood pressure.

spinal cavity: Body space that houses the spinal cord.

sputum: Mucus or phlegm ejected from the trachea, bronchi, and lungs through deep coughing.

squamous: Scalelike.

SSTs: Serum separator tubes.

standard of care: The normal level of skill and care that a healthcare practitioner would be expected to practice to provide due care for patients.

standard precautions: Precautions to use in caring for all patients regardless of diagnosis or presumed infection status that are intended to minimize the risk of infection transmission from both recognized and unrecognized sources. They apply to blood, *all* body fluids (including all secretions and excretions except sweat, whether or not they contain visible blood), nonintact skin, and mucous membranes.

statute of limitations: A law setting the length of time after an alleged injury in which the injured person is permitted to file a lawsuit.

STAT/stat: Immediately (from Latin, *statim*, meaning immediately).

steady state: Stable condition required before obtaining blood gas specimens, in which there has been no exercise, suctioning, or respirator changes for at least 20–30 minutes.

stomach: Digestive tract organ that mixes food with digestive juices and moves it into the small intestine.

storage: Preserving information outside the CPU.

stratified: Arranged in layers.

stratum germinativum: Deepest layer of the epidermis; also called stratum basale.

subcutaneous: Beneath the skin.

subcutaneous layer: A layer of connective and adipose (fat) tissue that connects the skin to the surface muscles.

sudoriferous glands: Sweat-secreting glands in the skin.

suffix: A word ending that comes after a word root and either changes or adds to the meaning of the word root.

superior: Higher, above, or toward the head; also called cranial.

supination: The condition of being supine or the act of turning the body or body part face up.

supine: Lying on the back with the face up.

suprapubic: Term used to describe a urine specimen collected by inserting a needle directly into the urinary bladder and aspirating (withdrawing by suction) the urine directly from the bladder into a sterile syringe.

surfactant: Substance that coats the walls of the alveoli, lowering the surface tension and helping to keep them inflated.

susceptible host: An individual who has little resistance to an infectious agent.

sweat chloride test: Test that involves stimulating sweat production by electrical stimulation, then collecting the sweat and measuring the chloride content in it to diagnose cystic fibrosis.

syncope (sin' ko-pe): Medical term for fainting, the loss of consciousness and postural tone that results from insufficient blood flow to the brain.

synovial fluid: Viscid (sticky) colorless fluid found in joint cavities.

syringe system: A sterile safety needle, a disposable plastic syringe, and a syringe transfer device.

syringe transfer device: A special piece of equipment used to safely transfer blood from a syringe into ETS tubes.

systemic circulation: Vascular pathway that carries oxygenated blood from the heart, along with nutrients, to all the cells of the body and then returns the blood to the heart, carrying carbon dioxide and other waste products of cellular metabolism.

systole: Contracting phase of the cardiac cycle.

systolic pressure: Pressure in the arteries during contraction of the ventricles.

tachycardia: Fast heart rate; over 100 beats per minute.

TAT: Turnaround time.

TDM: Therapeutic drug monitoring.

terminal: A computer screen and keyboard.

tertiary care: Highly complex care and therapy services from practitioners in a hospital or overnight facility.

therapeutic drug monitoring (TDM): Testing of drug levels at specific intervals to help establish a drug dosage, maintain the dosage at a therapeutic (beneficial) level, or avoid drug toxicity.

third-party payer: An insurance company or government program that pays for healthcare services on behalf of a patient.

thixotropic gel: An inert (nonreacting) synthetic gel substance in some ETS tubes (e.g., SST, PST, and PPT) that prevents blood cells from continuing to metabolize substances in the serum or plasma by forming a physical barrier between the cells and serum or plasma when the specimen is centrifuged.

thoracic cavity: Body space above the diaphragm that houses the heart and lungs.

threshold values: The level of acceptable practice beyond which quality patient care cannot be assured.

thrombin: An enzyme that converts fibrinogen into the fibrin necessary for clot formation.

thrombocytes: Medical term for platelets, cellular elements that play a role in the coagulation process and are the smallest of the formed elements.

thrombocytopenia: Decreased platelets.

thrombocytosis: Increased platelets.

thrombophlebitis: Inflammation of a vein, particularly in the lower extremities, along with thrombus formation

thrombosed: Clotted; refers to a vessel that is affected by clotting.

tissue thromboplastin: A substance present in tissue fluid that activates the extrinsic coagulation pathway and can interfere with coagulation tests when picked up by the needle during venipuncture.

tort: A wrongful act, other than breach of contract, committed against one's person, property, reputation, or other legally protected right.

tourniquet: A device (typically a flat strip of stretchable material) applied to a limb prior to venipuncture to restrict venous flow, which distends the veins and makes them easier to find and pierce with a needle.

trace-element-free tubes: Tubes made of materials that are as free of trace element contamination as possible.

trachea: A tube that extends from the larynx into the upper part of the chest and carries air to the lungs.

transfusion reaction: An adverse reaction between donor cells and a recipient.

transmission-based precautions: Precautions used in addition to standard precautions for patients known or suspected to be infected or colonized with highly transmissible or epidemiologically significant pathogens.

transverse plane: Divides the body horizontally into equal upper and lower portions.

trough level: Drug level collected when the lowest serum concentration of the drug is expected, usually immediately prior to administration of the next scheduled dose.

trypsin: Digestive enzyme.

tube additive: Any substance placed within a tube other than the tube stopper or the coating of the tube.

tube holder: A clear, plastic disposable cylinder with a small threaded opening at one end where the needle is screwed into it and a large opening at the other end where an ETS collection tube is placed.

tuberculin (TB) test: Tuberculosis test; also called PPD test; *see* **PPD**.

tunica adventitia: The outer layer of a blood vessel, made up of connective tissue, and thicker in arteries than veins; also called the tunica externa.

tunica intima: The inner layer or lining of a blood vessel; made up of a single layer of endothelial cells, a basement membrane, a connective tissue layer, and an elastic internal membrane; also called the tunica interna.

tunica media: The middle layer of a blood vessel, made up of smooth muscle tissue and some elastic fibers and much thicker in arteries than in veins.

twenty-four hour urine: Pooled urine specimen collected over a period of 24-hours, usually beginning in the morning.

UA: Urinalysis

UBS drive: Universal Serial Bus device used for storing information.

ulnar artery: Artery located on the medial aspect or little finger side of the wrist.

unique plural endings: Plural forms of medical terms that follow the rules of the Greek or Latin languages from which they originated.

universal precautions (UP): Precautions established by the CDC and adopted by OSHA to prevent patient to personnel transmission of infection from body fluids. Under UP, blood and certain body fluids of *all* individuals were considered potentially infectious.

ureters: Ducts (tubes) that carry urine from the kidneys to the urinary bladder.

urethra: Ducts (tubes) through which urine is voided from the urinary bladder.

urinalysis (UA): Laboratory test that typically includes macroscopic, physical, chemical, and microscopic analysis of a urine specimen.

urinary bladder: A muscular sac that serves as a reservoir for urine.

urinary tract infection (UTI): Ailment caused by the presence of microorganisms in one or more structures of the urinary system.

uterus: Muscular organ in the female pelvis where a fetus develops during pregnancy.

UTI: Urinary tract infection.

vacuum: Negative pressure, or artificially created absence of air.

VAD: Vascular access device.

vasopressin: Antidiuretic hormone (ADH).

vasoconstriction: Stage 1 of hemostasis in which a damaged vessel constricts (narrows) to decrease the flow of blood to an injured area.

vasovagal syncope: Sudden faintness or loss of consciousness due to a nervous system response to abrupt pain, stress or trauma.

vector transmission: Transmission of an infectious agent by an insect, arthropod, or animal.

vehicle transmission: Transmission of an infectious agent through contaminated food, water, drugs, or transfusion of blood.

veins: Blood vessels that return blood to the heart.

vena cava (plural, vena cavae): Either of two veins, the superior vena cava and inferior vena, that return blood to the heart and are the largest veins in the body.

venostasis: Trapping of blood in an extremity by compression of veins.

venous stasis: Stagnation of the normal blood flow.

ventral: To the front of the body.

ventral cavities: Internal spaces located in the front.

ventricles: The lower pumping or delivering chambers on each side of the heart.

venules: The smallest veins at the junction of the capillaries.

viability: Ability to stay alive.

vicarious liability: Liability imposed by law on one person for acts committed by another.

virulence: Degree to which a microbe is capable of causing disease.

whole blood: Blood that is in the same form as when it circulated in the bloodstream.

whorls: Spiral pattern of the ridges and grooves that form the fingerprint.

winged infusion set: A $\frac{1}{2}$- to $\frac{3}{4}$-inch stainless steel needle permanently connected to a 5- to 12-inch length of tubing with either a Luer attachment for syringe use or a multisample Luer adapter for use with the evacuated tube; also called a butterfly needle.

word root: The part of a medical term that establishes its basic meaning and the foundation upon which the true meaning is built.

work practice controls: Practices that alter the manner in which a task is performed to reduce the likelihood of bloodborne pathogen exposure.

CHAPTER 1

Answers to Study & Review Questions

1. b	6. d	11. b
2. d	7. d	12. a
3. a	8. a	13. b
4. c	9. d	14. a
5. b	10. c	15. d

Answers to Case Studies

CASE STUDY 1-1: TELEPHONE ETIQUETTE AND IRATE CALLER

1. Sally let the phone ring too many times, lost the caller when transferring the call, and kept the line open, allowing her conversation to be heard.
2. Leaving the line open. This allows the caller to hear conversations, which could violate HIPAA regulations if they should involve protected health information.
3. Sally should have prepared herself ahead of time by having the receptionist show her how to put callers on hold and transfer calls.
4. It is the laboratory administrator's responsibility to offer employees training in telephone etiquette.

CHAPTER 2

Answers to Study & Review Questions

1. c	6. d	11. b
2. c	7. b	12. b
3. b	8. b	13. a
4. b	9. c	14. d
5. a	10. d	15. c

A-1

Answers to Case Studies

CASE STUDY 2-1: SCOPE OF DUTY

1. Although on the surface it seems like the proper thing to do, helping an inpatient walk to the bathroom is not in the phlebotomist's scope of duties and opens the phlebotomist up to liability issues as illustrated by this case. It would have been better to have nursing personnel, who are properly trained in this area, assist the patient.
2. The hospital may have liability for the injury because of the liquid spilled on the floor that caused the patient to slip.
3. Vicarious liability and respondeat superior could come into play if a lawsuit is filed on behalf of the patient. However, it is also possible for the phlebotomist to be seen as individually liable because helping the patient is not a normal duty of a phlebotomist.

CHAPTER 3

Answers to Study & Review Questions

1. c	5. a	9. b
2. d	6. b	10. a
3. a	7. c	11. d
4. a	8. c	12. d

Answers to Case Studies

CASE STUDY 3-1: AN ACCIDENT WAITING TO HAPPEN

1. The first thing the phlebotomist should do is wash the blood off of her arm, washing the scratch site thoroughly with soap and water for a minimum of 30 seconds.
2. The phlebotomist's actions that contributed to the accident included wearing heels and being in a hurry. It would have been better to wear appropriate shoes and change into heels just before going to lunch.
3. The phlebotomist should have had the scratch covered with a waterproof bandage.
4. The type of exposure she received can be classified as a parenteral exposure.

CHAPTER 4

Answers to Study & Review Questions

1. a	5. b	8. d
2. c	6. a	9. d
3. c	7. c	10. b
4. d		

Answers to Case Studies

CASE STUDY 4-1: LAB ORDERS

1. The blood culture specimens should be collected as soon as possible (ASAP). ASAP tests orders have priority over routine collections. Facility protocol must be followed for exact time limits for collection.
2. The patient is in the emergency room (ER).
3. FUO stands for "fever of unknown origin." FUO indicates that the patient may have septicemia (or microorganisms in the blood), which can be detected by blood cultures.

CASE STUDY 4-2: MISINTERPRETED INSTRUCTIONS

1. The student apparently did not notice the decimal point in the written instructions and filled the syringe with 1 mL of antigen.
2. The amount of antigen should have been written as 0.1 mL
3. The phlebotomist should not have left the student alone. If she had watched her throughout the process, she would have caught the error.
4. The patient received approximately 5 times as much antigen as the standard dose. If the patient has been exposed to TB, he or she could have a severe reaction.

CHAPTER 5

Answers to Study & Review Questions

1. b	5. d	8. a
2. d	6. b	9. d
3. c	7. c	10. b
4. c		

Answers to Case Studies

CASE STUDY 5-1: BODY SYSTEM STRUCTURES AND DISORDERS

1. The term for muscle pain is myalgia. Soreness of the tendons is most likely due to tendonitis (tendon inflammation).
2. The fluid-filled sac in the area of the elbow is called a bursa. Bursae help ease movement over and around areas subject to friction such as prominent joint parts or where tendons pass over bone. An inflamed bursa is called bursitis.
3. The student's leg muscles and tendons are probably stressed from the long weekend runs. Bursitis of the elbow most likely resulted from the long periods of lying on the floor resting on her elbows.

CASE STUDY 5-2: BODY SYSTEMS, DISORDERS, DIAGNOSTIC
TESTS, AND DIRECTIONAL TERMS

1. Glucose and insulin levels evaluate the endocrine system.
2. The patient may be a diabetic who is either in insulin shock or a diabetic coma.
3. The specimen was collected from the left arm, below the IV.

CHAPTER 6

Answers to Study & Review Questions

1. a	6. a	11. a
2. c	7. c	12. a
3. c	8. b	13. b
4. a	9. b	14. d
5. c	10. d	15. c

Answers to Case Studies

No case study.

CHAPTER 7

Answers to Study & Review Questions

1. d	5. b	8. c
2. a	6. a	9. b
3. d	7. d	10. b
4. c		

Answers to Case Studies

CASE STUDY 7-1: PROPER HANDLING OF
ANTICOAGULANT TUBES

1. Clots in EDTA specimens can be caused by inadequate mixing, a delay in mixing, or a delay in transferring a specimen collected in a syringe.
2. The clot in the CBC specimen was most likely caused by the delay in mixing it.
3. Yes. The problem with the second lavender top led to an even greater delay in mixing the specimen, which most likely contributed to the clotting problem
4. If Chi had mixed the first lavender top as soon as he removed it from the tube holder before putting it down, the problem with the second tube would not have had any effect on it.
5. Chi can prevent this from happening in the future by mixing all additive tubes as soon as they are removed from the tube holder.

CASE STUDY 7-2: ORDER OF DRAW

1. The green top for the stat electrolytes is compromised.
2. The specimen is compromised because it was drawn after the EDTA tube and may be contaminated by carryover of EDTA. Sodium or potassium levels (depending on the type of EDTA) may be increased by EDTA contamination.
3. If the situation were to arise in the future Jake could draw a few milliliters of blood into a plain discard tube to flush possible contamination from the needle before collecting the green top. If he didn't have a discard tube he could use an SST or another green top as the discard tube. Placing and removing a discard tube also helps remove residue on the outside of the needle. Jake should still indicate how the specimen was collected in case interference is suspected by lab personnel.

CHAPTER 8

Answers to Study & Review Questions

1. c	6. b	11. d
2. d	7. a	12. c
3. b	8. a	13. a
4. b	9. d	14. b
5. b	10. a	15. d

Answers to Case Studies

CASE STUDY 8-1: PATIENT IDENTIFICATION

1. Jenny didn't ask the patient to verbally state her name and date of birth.
2. Jenny assumed that because the woman was the only one left in the waiting room, she was the correct patient.
3. The patient may have been someone with a standing order that forgot to check in with the receptionist.
4. The real Jane Rogers can be drawn after a new requisition and labels have been created. The identity of the other patient may be discovered when a physician's office calls for results and there are none. The specimens on the unknown patient will have to be discarded, which is especially unfortunate because the patient was a difficult draw.

CASE STUDY 8-2: BLOOD DRAW REFUSAL

1. The phlebotomists did not obtain parental permission personally or check with the child's nurse to see if parental permission had been given for the blood draw.
2. The phlebotomists made the assumption that because permission to draw the child had been given previously, that it was all right to draw the child this time. They also made the assumption that the child was not telling the truth.
3. A lawsuit alleging assault and battery could be filed by the parents.

CHAPTER 9

Answers to Study & Review Questions

1. b	5. a	8. b
2. b	6. b	9. a
3. c	7. a	10. c
4. c		

Answers to Case Studies

CASE STUDY 9-1: PHYSIOLOGICAL VARIABLES, PROBLEM SITES, AND PATIENT COMPLICATIONS

1. Physiological variables associated with this collection site include the following: the patient is ill and may be dehydrated from vomiting, she is overweight, she has had a mastectomy on the left side, and she is normally a difficult draw. Charles will be limited to drawing from the right arm. He will most likely need to draw the specimen using a butterfly and the smallest tubes available. He should check the cephalic vein if he does not find a suitable antecubital vein. He may need to draw from a vein in the right hand, and he may need to warm the site to enhance blood flow. Because it is a physician office laboratory he should check with the patient's physician to see if it is advisable to offer the patient water because she is probably dehydrated. Dehydration would make it even more difficult to find a vein.

2. Because the patient appears ill, she should be asked to lie down to prevent her from fainting during specimen collection. An emesis basin or waste basket should be close at hand in case she vomits.

3. Charles should check the antecubital area of the left arm first, paying particular attention to the area of the cephalic vein if the median cubital vein is not palpable. If no suitable vein is found he should check for a hand vein followed by veins in the dorsal wrist (never the ventral or palmar area of the wrist) and the forearm.

4. If Charles is unable to find a proper venipuncture site he should consider capillary puncture. Both the CBC and glucose specimens can easily be collected by capillary puncture. The site will need to be warmed to enhance blood flow because the patient may be dehydrated.

CASE STUDY 9-2: TROUBLESHOOTING FAILED VENIPUNCTURE

1. Blood most likely spurted into the tube because although Sara thought the needle was in the vein, it may have been only partially in the vein with a tiny portion out of the skin. Therefore, the tube quickly lost vacuum.

2. The hissing sound and the fact that the tube no longer fills with blood even after repositioning the needle are clues that the tube has lost vacuum.

3. Sara must position the needle in the vein, making certain no part of the needle is out of the skin, and then replace the tube with a new one.

CHAPTER 10

Answers to Study & Review Questions

1. b	5. d	9. b
2. d	6. a	10. d
3. d	7. d	11. b
4. c	8. c	12. c

Answers to Case Studies

CASE STUDY 10-1: CAPILLARY PUNCTURE PROCEDURE

1. The phlebotomist tried to collect the specimen as it was running down the finger. A scooping or scraping motion during collection may have activated the platelets and caused them to clump. In addition, because the child was uncooperative, the specimen was not collected and mixed quickly, which may also have contributed to platelet clumping.

2. It appears that the phlebotomist started to collect the specimen without wiping away the first drop of blood. Consequently the hemolysis may have been caused by alcohol residue. Trying to collect the specimen as it ran down the finger may have resulted in scraping the blood from the skin, which can also cause hemolysis in the specimen.

3. Improper direction of puncture and presence of alcohol residue may have contributed to the blood running down the finger instead of forming drops, making it hard to collect the specimen. The phlebotomist's inexperience with children may have contributed to the child being uncooperative. In addition, if the phlebotomist had been more experienced with capillary puncture in children, he may have held the child's hand differently and prevented the child from pulling away.

CHAPTER 11

Answers to Study & Review Questions

1. a	5. c	9. d
2. b	6. c	10. c
3. a	7. c	11. b
4. b	8. c	12. b

Answers to Case Studies

CASE STUDY 11-1: PERFORMANCE OF A GLUCOSE TOLERANCE TEST

1. Mr. Smith should finish drinking the glucose drink within 5 minutes.

2. The timing for all of the GTT specimens begins when the patient finishes the glucose drink. The patient was given the drink at 0825. If he finishes it on time at 0830, the 1-hour specimen would be collected at 0930.

3. No. A level of 300 mg/dL at 30 minutes is abnormal according to the graph in Figure 11–12.
4. Normally, if a patient vomits within the first 30 minutes of a GTT, the test is discontinued and rescheduled. If the patient vomits after 45 minutes, the patient's physician should be consulted to determine if the test should be continued or not.

CHAPTER 12

Answers to Study & Review Questions

1. b	5. c	8. d
2. d	6. b	9. b
3. d	7. c	10. c
4. d		

Answers to Case Studies

CASE STUDY 12-1: ABG COLLECTION COMPLICATIONS

1. The phlebotomist should alert the patient's nurse to the problem.
2. A thrombus may be blocking blood flow and affecting the pulse.
3. The patient moving his arm very likely resulted in the phlebotomist missing the artery. In addition, the restless and agitated state of the patient may have contributed to an arteriospasm that made it harder to hit the artery.
4. The phlebotomist should have made an attempt to calm the patient. In addition, he should have been prepared for movement by the patient or he could have asked the patient's nurse to help steady the arm since the patient was restless and agitated.
5. Although the specimen appears dark in color, the phlebotomist can be fairly certain the specimen is arterial because it pulsed into the tube. It is probably dark in color because the patient has breathing difficulties.

CHAPTER 13

Answers to Study & Review Questions

1. d	5. c	8. d
2. c	6. d c	9. b
3. d	7. d	10. d
4. d		

Answers to Case Studies

CASE STUDY 13-1: 24-HOUR URINE SPECIMEN COLLECTION

1. No. The specimen is missing a critical portion of urine.
2. The phlebotomist should not accept the specimen without first consulting a supervisor. Whether or not the specimen will be accepted depends upon the type of test and

individual lab policy and may require consultation with the patient's physician. If it is determined that the specimen will be accepted, the phlebotomist should note the discrepancy in collection time and identify the person who authorized acceptance on the requisition or by computer entry.

3. Patients should be given verbal and written instructions in 24-hour urine collection procedures and verbal feedback should be obtained to ensure that the patient has complete understanding of the procedure. Patients should be made aware of the importance of timing and reminded to set an alarm, if necessary.

CHAPTER 14

Answers to Study & Review Questions

1. d	6. c	11. c
2. d	7. b	12. a
3. b	8. d	13. d
4. d	9. c	14. d
5. a	10. d	

Answers to Case Studies

CASE STUDY 14-1: MISSING RESULTS

1. Nurse Susan may have used the label for Betty Smith on the specimens she collected on Mr. Jones.
2. The lab reports results according to the identification on the specimen, with the assumption that it is correctly labeled.
3. Nurse Susan will have to follow hospital protocol, which typically involves reprinting a lab slip and recollecting the specimen.
4. The results on Mrs. Smith will have to be removed from all records and the reason why they are being removed must be documented according to laboratory protocol.

The following remarks or sentences are designed to assist the phlebotomist when conversing with a patient who speaks only Spanish. Before approaching the patient, these basic phrases should be said aloud several times to a person who could correct the pronunciation, if necessary. If these phrases are said incorrectly, the meanings could be changed enough to insult or bewilder the patient.

Hello	¡Hola!	(Ō-lah)
Good morning	Buenos días	(BWĀ-nos DĒ-ahs)
Good afternoon	Buenas tardes	(BWĀ-nahs TAHR-dās)
Good evening	Buenas noches	(BWĀ-nahs NO-chās)
I am from the laboratory	Soy del laboratorio	(soy dāl lah-bō-rah-tō-RĒ-ō)
My name is	Me llamo	(mā YAH-mō)
I am here to take a blood sample	Estoy aquí para tomarle una prueba de sangre	(ās-TOY ah-KĒ PAHR-ah tō-MAHR-lā UN-ah prū-bah dā SAHN-grā)
What is your name?	¿Cual es su nombre? OR ¿Como se llama?	(kwahl ās sū NŌM-brā?) (CŌ-mō sā YAH-mah?)
May I see your wristband?	¿Me permite ver su identificación?	(mā pār-MĒ-tā vār sū ē-dān-tē-fē-cah-sē-ŌN?)
Mr. or Sir	Señor	(sā-NYOR)
Mrs. or Madame	Señora	(sā-NYŌ-rah)
Ms. or Miss	Señorita	(sā-nyō-RĒ-tah)
Okay	Muy bien	(MŪ-ē- byān)
You are the person I need	Usted es la persona que necesito	(ūs-TED ās lah pār-SŌN-ah kā na-sā-SĒ-tō)

I am going to put a tourniquet on your arm	Le voy a poner un torniquete en el brazo	(lā voy ah pō-NĀR ūn tor-nē-KĀ-tā ān el BRAH-sō)
Please	Por favor	(por fah-VOR)
Close your hand	Cierra la mano	(SYĀ-rah lah MAH-nō)
Open your hand	Abra la mano	(AH-brah lah MAH-nō)
Straighten your arm	Enderezca el brazo	(en-dār-ĀZ-kah el BRAH-sō)
	OR Estire el brazo	(ās-TĒ-rā sū BRAH-sō)
Bend your arm	Doble el brazo	(DŌ-blā el BRAH-sō)
Relax	Relájese	(rā-lah HĀ-sā)
Sit here	Siéntese aquí	(syān-TĀ-sā ah-KĒ)
Your doctor ordered this	Su doctor ordeno esto	(sū dōc-TOR or DĀ-nō ĀS-tō)
You need to ask your doctor	Necesita preguntarle a su doctor	(nā-sā-SĒ-tah prā-gūn-TAHR-lā ah sū dōc-TOR)
Have you eaten?	¿Ha comido?	(ah cō-MĒ-dō)
It will hurt a little	Le dolerá un poco	(lā dō-lā-RAH ūn PŌ-kō)
I will get the nurse	Buscaré a la enfermera	(būs-cah-RĀ ah lah ām-fār-MĀ-rah)
Thank you	¡Gracias!	(GRAH-syahs)
Have a good day	Que le vaya bien	(kā lā VĪ-yah byān)
Someone will be back in a few minutes	Alguien regresará en un momento	(ahl-GWĒ-ān rā-grā-sah-RAH ān ūn mō-MĀN-tō
Make a fist	Haga un puño	(HAH-ga ūn pun yo)

TABLE C-1 Alphabetical Listing of Laboratory Tests

Test	Abbreviation	Sample Considerations	Dept.*	Clinical Correlation
Acid-fast bacillus culture (blood)	AFB	Green-top tube, isolator tube, or gel-barrier tube. Special cleaning for site and tube stopper	M	Isolate and identify myobacterium tuberculosis
Acid phosphatase	Acid p'tase	Gel-barrier tube. Centrifuge, separate, and freeze serum immediately. Transport frozen	C	Cancer of the prostate
Alanine transferase	ALT (SGPT)	Gel-barrier tube. Centrifuge for complete separate as soon as possible and refrigerate	C	Evaluate hepatic disease
Alcohol	ETOH	Gray (preferred) or gel-barrier tube. Use nonalcohol germicidal solution to cleanse skin; chain-of-custody required if for legal purposes	C	Intoxication
Aldosterone		Plain red top; gel-barrier tube unacceptable. Centrifuge, separate, and refrigerate serum. Draw "up-right" sample at least 1/2 hour after patient sits up	C	Overproduction of this hormone
Alkaline phosphatase	ALP	Gel-barrier tube. Centrifuge for complete separation as soon as possible. Fasting 8–12 hours is required	C	Liver function

*Test department codes: C = chemistry, CO = coagulation, H = hematology, I = immunohematology/blood bank, M = microbiology, S = serology/immunology

TABLE C-1 *(continued)*

Test	Abbreviation	Sample Considerations	Dept.*	Clinical Correlation
Alpha-fetoprotein	AFP	Gel-barrier tube. Avoid hemolysis; can be performed on amniotic fluid	C	Fetal abnormalities, adult hepatic carcinomas
Aluminum	Al	Royal blue tube; no additive. Avoid all sources of external contamination	C	Trace metal contamination, dialysis complication
Ammonia	NH3	Lavender-topped tube placed immediately on ice slurry. Centrifuge within 15 minutes without removing stopper; separate plasma and freeze in plastic vial	C	Evaluates liver function. High levels in the blood lead to a problem know as hepatic encephalopathy
Amylase		Gel-barrier tube. Centrifuge and refrigerate serum. Avoid hemolysis and lipemia	C	Acute pancreatitis
Antibody screen	Coombs' test, indirect	Collect whole blood (lavender); special ID procedure	I	Identifies any atypical antibodies present
Antinuclear antibodies (screen or titer)	ANA	Gel-barrier tube, refrigerated serum. Avoid hemolysis and lipemia	S	Systemic lupus erythematosus and other autoimmune connective tissue diseases
Anti-Rh antibody preparation		Special ID procedure	I	Administered to Rh-negative mothers to prevent Rh immunization
Antistreptolysin O test	ASO	Perform test immediately or refrigerate or freeze serum	S	Streptococcal infection
Antithrombin III activity	AT-III	Light blue top. Invert 3–4 times, centrifuge, separate, and immediately freeze plasma in plastic vial. Transport frozen	CO	Clotting factor deficiency
Aspartate aminotransferase	AST, GOT, SGOT	Gel-barrier tube. Centrifuge for complete separation and refrigerate	C	Acute and chronic liver disease
Basic metabolic panel	BMP	Gel-barrier tube, refrigerate unopened spun barrier tube. Separate within 45 minutes of venipuncture. Fasting 8–12 hours is required	C	A designated number of tests covering certain body systems

(continued)

TABLE C-1 *(continued)*

Test	Abbreviation	Sample Considerations	Dept.*	Clinical Correlation
Bilirubin, total and direct	Bili	Gel-barrier tube, spin and separate within 45 minutes. Wrap in foil to protect from light; refrigerate	C	Increased with types of jaundice (i.e., obstructive, hepatic, or hemolytic; hepatitis or cirrhosis)
Blood culture	BC	Whole blood inoculated into two blood culture bottles: one anaerobic and one aerobic from two different sites or yellow tube. Do not refrigerate	M	Isolate and identify potentially pathogenic organisms causing bacteremia or septicemia
Blood group & Rh type	ABO & Rh	Dedicated large lavender or pink top tube. Special ID procedure; hand label with special band	I	Detection of ABO and Rh antigens on the red blood cells. Detect atypical antibodies for prenatal screen or crossmatch
Calcitonin		Plain red, fasting specimen. Allow to clot 1–4 hours in an ice bath or refrigerator. Centrifuge in chilled holder or refrigerated centrifuge, separate, and freeze immediately in plastic vial	C	Evaluate suspected medullary carcinoma of the thyroid, characterized by hypersecretion of calcitonin
Carbon monoxide (carboxy-hemoglobin)	CO level	Fill lavender tube completely. Refrigerate immediately. Submit original, full unopened tube	C	Carboxyhemoglobin intoxication
Carcinogenic antigen	Ca 125	Serum gel tube. Refrigerate; freeze if testing is delayed.	C	Tumor marker primarily for ovarian carcinoma
Calcium, ionized	iCa²⁺	Gel-barrier tube. Centrifuge with cap on; do not pour over; refrigerate. Place a piece of tape over the top of tube and write "Do not open"	C	Bone cancer, nephritis, multiple myeloma
Carcinoembryonic antigen	CEA	Gel barrier tube; refrigerated serum	C	Monitoring of patients with diagnosed malignancies; malignant or benign liver disease; indicator of tumors
Carotene, beta		Gel-barrier tube. Transport in amber plastic tube with amber stopper, if available. Wrap in aluminum foil to protect from light. Freeze	C	Carotenemia

TABLE C-1 *(continued)*

Test	Abbreviation	Sample Considerations	Dept.*	Clinical Correlation
Chlamydia antibodies		Gel-barrier tube; refrigerated serum collected using aseptic technique. Centrifuge and separate serum from clot within 4 hours of collection	S	For trachoma, psittacosis, LGV, and pneumoniae
Cholesterol and HDL ratio	Chol HDL	Gel-barrier tube. Separate as soon as possible and refrigerate serum	C	Evaluates risk of coronary heart disease (CHD)
Chromium	Cr level	Royal blue—no additive; metal-free. Separate and refrigerate immediately	C	Associated with diabetes and aspartame toxicity
Cold agglutinins		Gel-barrier tube. Must be kept warm, incubate at 37°C and allow it to clot at 37°C before separation. Store and ship at room temperature	S	To diagnosis viral and atypical pneumonia caused by *Mycoplasma pneumoniae*
Complete blood count	CBC	Lavender top. Invert gently 6–8 times immediately after drawing; includes WBC, RBC, Hgb, Hct, indices, platelets, and diff	H	Blood diseases
Copper	Cu level	Royal blue—no additive; metal-free. Separate and transfer to a plastic transport tube immediately	C	Wilson's disease or nephritic syndrome
Cord blood		Refrigerated serum	I	Group and type infant's blood to detect the presence of incompatibilities, or mother for possible Rh immune globulin
Cortisol, timed		Gel-barrier tube; refrigerated serum. Clearly note time drawn	C	Cushing's syndrome
Creatine kinase	CK	Gel-barrier tube; refrigerated serum	C	Muscular dystrophy and trauma to skeletal muscle
Creatine kinase MB	CK-MB	Gel-barrier tube; refrigerated serum	C	Organ differentiation and to rule out myocardial infarction
Creatinine	Creat	Gel-barrier tube. Separate as soon as possible; refrigerate serum	C	Kidney function

(continued)

TABLE C-1 *(continued)*

Test	Abbreviation	Sample Considerations	Dept.*	Clinical Correlation
C-reactive protein	CRP	Gel-barrier tube; refrigerated serum	S	Chronic inflammation
Cryoglobulin		Gel-barrier tube. Draw and process at room temperature; separate from cells immediately	C	Associated with immunologic diseases (e.g., multiple myeloma or rheumatoid arthritis)
Cyclosporine		Whole blood or refrigerated serum from SST. Note: Use same type of specimen each time analyte is measured	C	Immunosuppressive drug for organ transplants
Culture		Collect the appropriate fluid or tissue using culture swab transport media. Indicate location of culture on the requisition	M	Identification of infective agent and appropriate antibiotic treatment
Cytomegalovirus antibody	CMV	Gel-barrier tube. Centrifuge ASAP; refrigerate serum	I	Screens donors and blood products for transplant programs
D-dimer	D-DI	1 mL frozen citrated plasma from a completely filled light blue tube. Separate and freeze plasma immediately in plastic vials. Transport frozen	CO	DIC and thrombotic episodes such as pulmonary emboli
Differential	Diff	Blood smear stained with Wright's stain	H	Classifying types of leukocytes, describing erythrocytes, and estimation of platelets
Direct antiglobulin test	DAT, Coombs test, direct	Dedicated lavender top. Special ID procedure	I	Detects antibodies attached to the patient's red blood cells
Disseminated intravascular coagulation panel	DIC panel	Light blue top, completely filled. Centrifuge, separate, and freeze plasma immediately in plastic vials. Transport frozen	CO	Distortion of the normal coagulation and fibrinolytic mechanisms

Test	Abbreviation	Sample Considerations	Dept.*	Clinical Correlation
Drug Monitoring	NA	Plain red; no gel barrier. Centrifuge and separate within 1 hour and transfer to plastic transfer tube	C	See individual drugs below
Amikacin	(Amikin)		C	Broad-spectrum antibiotic
Barbiturates	(Phenobarbital)		C	Anticonvulsant for seizures
Carbamazepine	(Tegretol)		C	Mood-stabilizing drug in bipolar affective disorder
Digoxin	(Lanoxin)		C	Heart stimulant
Gentamicin			C	Broad-spectrum antibiotic
Lithium			C	Manic-depression medication
Phenytoin	(Dilantin)		C	Treatment of epilepsy
Salicylates	(Aspirin)		C	Evaluation of therapy
Theophylline	(Aminophylline)		C	Asthma medication
Tobramycin			C	Broad-spectrum antibiotic
Valproic acid	(Depakote)		C	Seizures and symptomatic epilepsy
Vancomycin	(Vancocin)		C	Broad-spectrum antibiotic
Electrolytes	Na, K, Cl, CO_2, lytes	Gel barrier tube. Centrifuge within 30 minutes after drawing. Do not remove stopper. Avoid hemolysis and lipemia	C	Fluid balance, cardiotoxicity, heart failure, edema
Eosinophil	Eos	Lavender top. Invert gently 6–8 times immediately after drawing	H	Allergy studies
Epstein-Barr virus panel	EBV	Gel-barrier tube. Store serum at 2–8°C	S	Mononucleosis
Erythrocyte sedimentation rate	ESR	Lavender top. Invert gently 6–8 times immediately after drawing	H	Indication of degree of inflammation
Factor assays		Light blue top. Invert 3–4 times; centrifuge, separate, and freeze plasma immediately in plastic vials. 1 mL aliquot for each factor	CO	To detect factor deficiency
Febrile agglutinin Panel		Gel-barrier tube, random serum specimen. Avoid gross hemolysis and lipemia	S	Screens for *Salmonella*, *Tularemia*, *Rickettsia*, and *Brucella* antibodies

Test	Abbreviation	Sample Considerations	Dept.*	Clinical Correlation
Ferritin		Gel-barrier tube; refrigerated serum	C	Hemachromatosis, iron deficiency
Fibrinogen		Completely filled light blue top. Invert 3–4 times; centrifuge 15 minutes, separate, and freeze immediately. Place in plastic vial and transport frozen	CO	To investigate suspected bleeding disorders
Fibrin split products/fibrin degradation product	FSP/FDP	1 light blue top, completely filled. Inverted 6 times; immediately centrifuge for 15 minutes, separate and freeze. Transport frozen	CO	DIC and thrombotic episodes, valuable early diagnostic sign of increased rate of fibrin deposition
Fluorescent treponemal antibody absorption	FTA-ABS	Gel-barrier tube; refrigerated serum	S	Syphilis
Gamma-glutamyl transpeptidase	GGT	Gel-barrier tube; refrigerated serum. Spin and separate as soon as possible.	C	Assists in the diagnosis of liver problems; specific for hepatobiliary problems
Gastrin		Gel-barrier tube. Separate serum from cells within 1 hour after collection; freeze serum. Overnight fasting is required	C	Stomach disorders
Glucose, fasting	FBS	Gel-barrier tube. Separate from cells within one hour or use gray-top tube	C	Diabetes, hypoglycemia
Glycosylated hemoglobin	Hgb A1c	Lavender tube	C	Monitoring diabetes mellitus
Glucose-6-phosphate dehydro genase	G-6-PD	Lavender tube. Do not freeze	C	Drug-induced anemias
Gonorrhea screen	GC	Taken from the urethra of male or endocervical canal from female	M	Sexually transmitted disease
Hematocrit	Hct	Lavender top. Invert gently 6–8 times immediately after drawing	H	Anemia
Hemoglobin	Hgb	Lavender top. Invert gently 6–8 times immediately after drawing	H	Anemia
Hemoglobin A1c (see glycosylated hemoglobin)				
Hemoglobin electrophoresis		Refrigerated lavender top. Invert gently 6–8 times immediately after drawing	C	Hemoglobinopathies and thalassemia
Hepatitis B surface antibody	HBsAb	Gel-barrier tube; refrigerated serum	S	Determination of previous infection and immunity by hepatitis B

Test	Abbreviation	Sample Considerations	Dept.*	Clinical Correlation
Hepatitis B surface antigen	HBsAg	Gel-barrier tube; refrigerated serum	S	Diagnosis of acute or some chronic stages of infection and carrier status of hepatitis B
Homocysteine	Hcy	EDTA plasma (preferred) or serum gel-barrier tube. Place on ice immediately. Centrifuge and separate within 1 hour of draw. Refrigerate specimen.	C	Elevated levels indicate increased risk of atherosclerosis
Human immunodeficiency virus antigen	HIV-1	Gel-barrier tube; refrigerated serum. Do not ship in glass tubes. Use code number in place of patient name to protect patient confidentiality	S	Screen for donated blood and plasma as an aid in the diagnosis of HIV-1 infection
Human leukocyte antigen-B 27	HLA-B27	Yellow-top (ACD) tubes; unopened tube required. Do not freeze or refrigerate; ethnic origin must be included	I	Tested for disease association, matching prior to organ transplantation, platelet transfusion, paternity and forensic evaluation
Human chorionic gonadotropin	HCG	Gel-barrier tube; refrigerated serum	C	Pregnancy, testicular cancer
Immunoglobulins	IgA IgG IgM	Gel-barrier tube; refrigerated serum	C	Measurement of proteins capable of becoming antibodies, chronic liver disease, myeloma
Indices	MCV, MCH, MCHC	Lavender top, invert gently 6–8 times immediately after drawing	H	Indicates mean cell hemoglobin (MCH), hemoglobin concentration (MCHC), and volume (MCV)
Iron and total iron binding capacity	TIBC & Fe	Gel-barrier tube; refrigerated serum. Separate from cells within 1 hour of collection. Fasting morning specimen is preferred	C	Assist in differential diagnosis of anemia
Lactic acid (blood lactate)	Lact	Draw whole blood from a stasis-free vein into a gray-top tube. Centrifuge and separate plasma within 15 minutes of collection	C	Measurement of anaerobic glycolysis due to strenuous exercise; increased lactic acid can occur in liver disease
Lactate dehydrogenase	LD	Gel-barrier tube. Avoid hemolysis—do not freeze or refrigerate	C	Cardiac injury and other muscle damage

Test	Abbreviation	Sample Considerations	Dept.*	Clinical Correlation
Lead	Pb	Royal blue EDTA or tan-top lead-free tube. Use of other evacuated tubes or transfer tubes may produce falsely elevated results due to contamination	C	Lead toxicity, which can lead to neurologic dysfunction and possible permanent brain damage
Lipase		Gel-barrier tube; refrigerated serum	C	Used to distinguish between abdominal pain and that owing to acute pancreatitis
Lipoproteins		Gel-barrier tube; refrigerated serum	C	
High-density lipoprotein	HDL	Must be fasting a minimum of 12 hours		Evaluates lipid disorders and coronary artery disease risk
Low-density lipoprotein	LDL	Must be fasting a minimum of 12 hours		Evaluates lipid disorders and coronary artery disease risk
Magnesium	Mg	Gel-barrier tube. Separate from cells within 45 minutes. Maintain specimen at room temperature	C	Mineral metabolism, kidney function
Mononucleosis screen	Mono-test	Gel-barrier tube; refrigerated serum	S	Infectious mononucleosis
Partial thromboplastin time (Activated PTT)	PTT/APTT	Completely filled blue top. Invert 3–4 times immediately after drawing. Do not centrifuge or freeze if the sample will not be tested within 24 hours	CO	Clotting factor deficiency, monitoring heparin therapy
Phosphorus	P, PO4	Gel-barrier tube. Separate from cells within 45 minutes. Maintain specimen at room temperature	C	Thyroid function, bone disorders, and kidney disease
Plasminogen		Blue top. Centrifuge, separate, and freeze plasma immediately in plastic vials. Transport frozen.	CO	Fibrin clot formation prevention
Platelet aggregation	Plt. agg	4–5 mL sodium citrate tubes. Invert 3–4 times. Do not centrifuge. Do not refrigerate. Notify the lab before collection. Specimen must be received within 1 hour of collection	H	Hemostasis and thrombus formation
Platelet count	Plt. ct	Lavender top. Invert gently 6–8 times immediately after drawing	H	Bleeding disorders

Test	Abbreviation	Sample Considerations	Dept.*	Clinical Correlation
Prostatic specific antigen, total & free	PSA	Gel-barrier tube. Separate and freeze serum immediately in a plastic vial. Transport frozen	C	Screen for the presence of prostate cancer, to monitor the progression of the disease and monitor the response to treatment for prostate cancer
Prothrombin time	PT	Completely filled blue top. Invert 3–4 times immediately after drawing. Do not centrifuge or freeze if the sample needs to be transported	CO	Clotting factor deficiency, monitoring warfarin therapy
Red cell count	RBC	Lavender top. Invert gently 6–8 times immediately after drawing	H	Anemia
Reticulocyte count	Retic	Lavender top. Invert gently 6–8 times immediately after drawing	H	Anemia
Rheumatoid factor	RF	Gel-barrier tube; refrigerated serum. Overnight fasting is preferred	S	Arthritic conditions
Rapid plasmin reagin	RPR	Gel-barrier tube; refrigerated serum. Hemolysis and lipemia may alter test results	S	Syphilis
Sedimentation rate, Westergren	ESR	Lavender top. Invert gently 6–8 times immediately after drawing	H	Abnormal protein linkage
Serum protein electrophoresis	SPEP or PEP	Gel-barrier tube; refrigerated serum	C	Abnormal protein detection
Sputum screen		True sputum, not saliva—early morning sample	M	Tuberculosis
Streptococcus screen	strep	Submit culturette	M	Strep throat
Sweat chloride or electrolytes (iontop horesis)		Collect sweat specimen by iontophoresis	C	Cystic fibrosis
Thyroid profile (comprehensive)	FTI, T_3, T_4, TSH	Gel-barrier tube or red top tube that must be separated to plastic transfer tube	C	Hyper- or hypothyroid conditions
Triglycerides		Gel-barrier tube; refrigerated serum. Strict fasting 12–14 hours is required (water only)	C	Used to evaluate risk of coronary heart disease
Vitamin B_{12} and folate		Gel-barrier tube. Centrifuge, separate, and refrigerate. Protect from light	C	Macrocytic anemia
Urea nitrogen	BUN	Serum gel tube. Centrifuge for complete separation and refrigerate	C	Kidney function

Test	Abbreviation	Sample Considerations	Dept.*	Clinical Correlation
Uric acid		Serum gel tube or red top tube that must be separated within 45 minutes. Maintain specimen at room temperature	C	Gout
White cell count	WBC	Lavender top. Invert gently 6–8 times immediately after drawing	H	Infection (viral or bacterial)
Zinc (serum)	Zn	Non additive royal blue. Separate serum within 45 minutes and transfer to plastic transport tube	C	Liver dysfunction
Zinc (RBC)	ZNRBC	Royal blue EDTA. Refrigerate immediately; hemolysis unacceptable	C	Screening test for lead poisoning and iron deficiency

THE METRIC SYSTEM

The metric system is the system of measurement used in the healthcare industry. The metric system derives its name from its fundamental unit of distance, the meter (M or m). In the metric system, the meter is the basic unit of linear measure, the gram (G or g) is the basic unit of weight, and the liter (L or l) is the basic unit of volume. The metric system is a decimal system (a system based on the number 10). In a decimal system, units larger or smaller than the basic units are arrived at by multiplying or dividing by 10 or powers of 10.

In the metric system, prefixes added to the basic units indicate larger or smaller units. Prefixes are the same whether or not the units are meters, grams, or liters. Table D-1 shows prefixes commonly used in the medical laboratory. Basic metric units (grams, meters, liters) can be converted to larger units by moving the decimal point to the left according to the appropriate multiple. The multiple is the value of the exponent. The exponent is a number that indicates how many times a number is multiplied by itself. For example, a kilogram is 1,000 or $10 \times 10 \times 10$ or 10^3 g. The multiple, determined by the exponent, is three.

Example: Convert 100 grams to kilograms

From Table D-1 we determine that 1 kg is equal to 1,000 or 10^3 g. The multiple is 3. Therefore, to convert 100 grams to kilograms, move the decimal point three places to the left:

$$100 \text{ g} = 100.0 = 0.1 \text{ kg}$$

To convert basic metric units to smaller units, move the decimal point to the right the appropriate multiple.

Example: Convert 100 g to mg

From Table D-1, we see that 1 mg is equal to 10^{-3} g. The multiple is a minus three. We therefore move the decimal point three spaces to the right:

$$100 \text{ g} = 100.000 = 100,000 \text{ mg}$$

Metric units other than basic units can be converted to larger units by moving the decimal point to the left according to the appropriate multiple, determined by subtracting

TABLE D-1	Commonly Used Measurement Prefixes				
				Unit of Measure	
Prefix	Multiple	Meter (m)	Gram (g)		Liter (l)
Kilo- (k)	1,000 (10^3)	km	kg		kL
Deo- (d)	1/10 (10^{-1})	dm	dg		dL
Centi- (c)	1/100 (10^{-2})	cm	cg		cL
Milli- (m)	1/1,000 (10^{-3})	mm	mg		mL
Micro- (μ)	1/1,000,000 (10^{-6})	μm	μg		μL

the value of the exponent of the desired unit from the value of the exponent of the existing unit.

Example: Convert 200 mg to kg

From Table D-1, we determine that 1 mg is 10^{-3} and 1 kg is 10^3. The desired unit is kilograms; therefore, subtract -3 from 3 to determine the multiple:

$$3 - (-3) = 3 + 3 = 6$$

We are going from a smaller unit to a larger unit, so the decimal point moves to the left six spaces.

$$200 \text{ mg} = 000200. = 0.0002 \text{ kg}$$

Metric units other than basic units can be converted to smaller units by moving the decimal point to the right according to the appropriate multiple, determined by subtracting the value of the exponent of the desired unit from the value of the exponent of the existing unit.

Example: Convert 25 cm to μm

From Table D-1, we determine that 1 cm is 10^{-2} and 1 μm is 10^{-6}. The desired unit is micrometers; therefore subtract -6 from -2 to determine the multiple:

$$-2 - (-6) = -2 + 6 = 4$$

We are going from a larger unit to a smaller unit, so the decimal point moves to the right four spaces.

$$25 \text{ cm} = 25.0000 = 250,000 \text{ μm}$$

It is often necessary to convert our English system of units to metric units. Table D-2 lists English units and their metric equivalents commonly encountered in the healthcare setting.

To convert from English units to metric units, multiply by the factor listed. Metric units can be converted back to English units by dividing by the same factor or multiplying by the factor in the metric conversion chart.

Example: Convert 200 lb to kg
1 pound is equal to 0.454 kg

Therefore, multiply 200 × 0.454 to arrive at 90.8 kg

TABLE D-2	English-Metric Equivalents		
	English		**Metric**
Distance	Yard (yd)	=	0.9 meters (m)
	Inch (in)	=	2.54 centimeters (cm)
Weight	Pound (lb)	=	0.454 kilograms (kg) or 454 grams (g)
	Ounce (oz)	=	28 grams (g)
Volume	Quart (qt)	=	0.95 liters (L)
	Fluid ounce (fl oz)	=	30 milliliters (mL)
	Tablespoon (tbsp)	=	15 millimeters (mL)
	Teaspoon (tsp)	=	5 milliliters (mL)

Table D-3 shows the common equivalents for converting metric units to English units. To convert metric units to English units, multiply by the factor listed. To convert English units back to metric, divide by the same factor or multiply by the factor in the English unit conversion chart.

Example: Convert 15 mL to tsp

1.0 mL is equal to ⅕ tsp

Therefore, multiply 15 × ⅕ to arrive at ¹⁵⁄₅

or 3 tsp (or 15 × 0.2 = 3.0 tsp)

MILITARY TIME

Most hospitals use military (or European) time, which is based on a clock with 24 numbers instead of 12 (Fig. D-1). Twenty-four-hour time eliminates the need for designating AM or PM. Each time is expressed by four digits. The first two digits represent hours, and the

TABLE D-3	Metric-English Equivalents		
	Metric		**English**
Distance	Meter (m)	=	3.3 feet/39.37 inches
	Centimeter (cm)	=	0.4 inches
	Millimeter (mm)	=	0.04 inches
Weight	Gram (g)	=	0.0022 pounds
	Kilogram (kg)	=	2.2 pounds
Volume	Liter (L)	=	1.06 quarts
	Milliliter (mL)	=	0.03 fluid ounces
	Milliliter (mL)	=	0.20 or 1/5 tsp

Note: A milliliter (mL) is approximately equal to a cubic centimeter (cc), and the two terms are often used interchangeably.

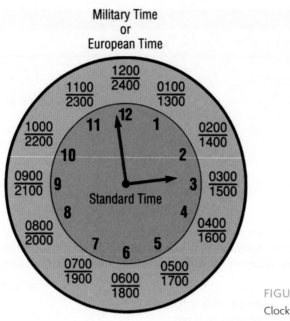

Military Time
or
European Time

Standard Time

FIGURE D-1

Clock showing 24-hour (military) time.

second two digits represent minutes. 1200 hours is noon and 2400 hours is midnight. One AM is 0100, 2 AM is 0200, and so on.

Noon is 1200; 1 PM is 1300

To convert regular (12-hour) time to 24-hour time, add 12 hours to the time from 1 PM on.

Example: 1:00 PM becomes 1:00 + 12 hours = 1300 hours
5:30 PM becomes 5:30 + 12 hours = 1730 hours

To convert 24-hour time to 12-hour time, subtract 12 hours after 1 PM.

Example: 1300 hours becomes 1300 − 12 hours = 1:00 PM.

TEMPERATURE MEASUREMENT

Two different temperature scales (Fig. D-2) are used in the healthcare setting. The Fahrenheit (F) scale is used to measure body temperature, whereas the Celsius (C), also known as the centigrade, scale is used to measure temperatures in the laboratory.

- Fahrenheit: The freezing point of water is 32°F, and the boiling point is 212°F. Normal body temperature expressed in Fahrenheit is 98.6°F.
- Celsius/centigrade: The freezing point of water is zero (0°C) and the boiling point is 100°C. Normal body temperature expressed in the Celsius scale is 37°C.

The following formulas can be used to convert from one temperature scale to the other:

Celsius temperature = ⅝ (°F − 32)
Fahrenheit temperature = ⅑°C + 32

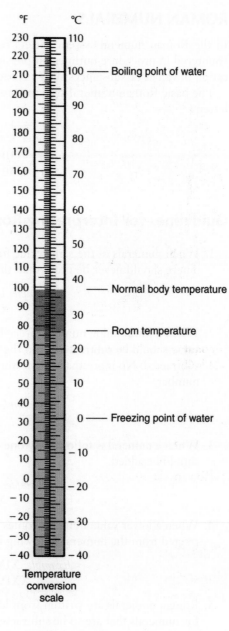

FIGURE D-2

Thermometer showing both Fahrenheit and Celsius degrees. (Memmler RL, Cohen BJ, Wood DL.)

ROMAN NUMERALS

In the Roman numeral system, letters represent numbers. Roman numerals may be encountered in procedure outlines, in physician's orders or prescriptions, and in the identification of values or substances such as coagulation factors.

The basic Roman numeral system consists of the following seven capital (or lowercase) letters:

$$
\begin{array}{llll}
I\ (i) &= 1 & C\ (c) &= 100 \\
V\ (v) &= 5 & D\ (d) &= 500 \\
X\ (x) &= 10 & M\ (m) &= 1{,}000 \\
L\ (l) &= 50 & &
\end{array}
$$

Guidelines for Interpreting Roman Numerals

1. When numerals of the same value follow in sequence, the values should be added. There should never be more than three of the same numeral in a sequence.

    Example: III = 1 + 1 + 1 = 3
    XX = 10 + 10 = 20

2. When a lower-value numeral precedes a numeral with a higher value, the lower value should be subtracted from the higher value. Numerals V, L, and D are never subtracted. No more than one lower value number should precede a higher value number.

    Example: IV = 5 − 1 = 4
    IX = 10 − 1 = 9

3. When a numeral is followed by one or more numerals of lower value, the values should be added.

    Example: XI = 10 + 1 = 11
    VII = 5 + 1 + 1 = 7

4. When a lower value numeral comes between two higher value numerals, it is subtracted from the numeral following it.

    Example: XIX = 10 + 10 − 1 = 19
    XXIV = 10 + 10 + 5 − 1 = 24

5. Roman numerals are written from left to right in order of decreasing value (except for numerals that are to be subtracted from subsequent numerals).

    Example: XXVII = 10 + 10 + 5 + 1 + 1 = 27
    MCMXCII = 1,000 + (1,000 − 100) + (100 − 10) + 1 + 1 = 1992

6. A line over a Roman numeral means multiply the numeral by 1,000.

    Example: $\overline{V}$ = V × 1,000 = 5,000

PERCENTAGE

Percent means per 100 and is represented by the symbol %. Two values are involved when a number is expressed as a percentage. They are the number itself, and 100.

Example: 10% means 10 per 100 or 10 parts in a total of 100 parts. To change a fraction to a percentage, multiply by 100 and add a percent sign to the result.

Example: Change ¾ to a percentage

$$^3/_4 \times {}^{100}/_1 = {}^{300}/_4 = 4\overline{)300}^{\,75} = 75\%$$

DILUTIONS

The concentration of laboratory reagents is often expressed as a percentage. For example, a solution of 70% isopropyl alcohol is used in skin cleansing before blood collection.

A 10% dilution of bleach (5.25% sodium hypochlorite) is used to disinfect countertops and other surfaces. A 10% dilution of bleach means that there are 10 parts of bleach in a solution containing a total of 100 parts. The above dilution can also be expressed as a ratio, showing the relationship between the part of the solution and the total solution. A 10% solution is also a 1:10 (1 to 10) solution or one part bleach in a total of 10 parts solution. A dilution of 10 parts in a total of 100 parts is the same as 1 part in a total of 100 parts, or a 1:10 dilution. A 10% dilution of bleach can be prepared by adding 10 mL bleach to 90 mL water, resulting in a total of 100 mL of bleach solution. The same percentage dilution would result from adding 1 mL bleach to 9 mL water, 20 mL bleach to 180 mL water, and so on.

BLOOD VOLUME

Blood volume in adults is generally stated as 5.0 quarts or 4.75 liters (L). Because people are not the same size, common sense tells us that they should not all have 5 quarts of blood. Actual blood volume is based on weight. Blood volume can be calculated for any size person from infant to adult, as long as the weight of the person is known. If the volume is calculated for adults and infants, it is important to realize that the value is not exact because the calculation is based on averages.

key • point   CLSI lists the following blood volumes for infants and children:

Premature infants	115 mL/kg
Newborns	80–100 mL/kg
Infants and children	75–100 mL/kg

Adult Blood Volume Calculation

Average adult blood volume is 70 mL per kg of weight.

Example: Calculate the amount of blood volume for a man who weighs 250 lb.

1. Change the weight in pounds to kilograms.
   Because 1 lb = 0.454 kg, you need to multiply 250 lb by 0.454 to arrive at 113.5 kg.
2. Next, multiply the number of kilograms by 70 because there are 70 mL of blood for each kg of weight.

$$113.5 \text{ kg} \times 70 \text{ mL/kg} = 7,945 \text{ mL}$$

3. Because blood volume is reported in liters rather than milliliters, divide the total number of mL by 1,000 (1 liter = 1000 mL).

$$\text{Blood volume} = 7,945 \text{ mL}/1,000 \text{ mL} = 7.945 \text{ L or } 7.9 \text{ L (rounded)}$$

Infant Blood Volume Calculation

ESTIMATING BLOOD VOLUME

When requested to collect blood specimens from infants, phlebotomists must be able to quickly estimate blood volume in their heads to avoid harming the patient. This can be accomplished by mentally dividing the patient's weight in pounds by 2 to convert them to kilograms and multiplying the kilograms by 100 to get estimated blood volume. This estimate will always be higher than the true value. (Ability to convert pounds to kilograms is also needed when deciding how much glucose beverage to give a child during a GTT).

It is very important to be able to calculate the blood volume of an infant, especially if that infant is in an intensive care unit where blood samples may be taken several times a day. A very small infant can become anemic if not monitored closely. Removal of more than 10% of an infant's blood volume in a short period of time can lead to serious consequences, such as iatrogenic anemia or cardiac arrest.

An average infant's blood volume is 100 mL per kg.

Example: Calculate the blood volume of a baby who weighs 5.5 lb.

1. Change the weight from pounds to kilograms using the same formula as for adults.

$$5.5 \text{ lb} \times 0.454 = 2.5 \text{ kg}$$

2. Multiply 2.5 kg by 100 for total blood volume in milliliters.

$$2.5 \text{ kg} \times 100 = 250 \text{ mL}$$

3. Change blood volume in mL/kg to liters.

$$250 \text{ mL}/1,000 \text{ mL} = 0.25 \text{ L}$$

WORK RESTRICTIONS FOR HEALTHCARE EMPLOYEES

Appendix E

TABLE E-1	Conditions Requiring Work Restrictions for Healthcare Employees
Condition	**Work Restriction**
Chicken pox (varicella)	Off work until 7 days after appearance of first eruption and lesions are dry and crusted
Hepatitis A	Off work until cleared by a physician
Hepatitis B	Off work until cleared by a physician
Herpes zoster	May work if no patient contact
Influenza	Work status determined by Employee Health Department depending on work area
Impetigo	Off work or no patient contact until crusts are gone
Measles	Off work until rash is gone (minimum 4 days)
Mononucleosis	Off work until cleared by a physician
MRSA (methicillin resistant *Staphylococcus aureus*)	May work, but no patient care until treatment is successful
Pink eye (acute conjunctivitis)	Off work until treatment is successful
Positive PPD test	May work depending upon evaluation and follow-up by Employee Health Department
Pregnancy	May work, but avoid contact with patients with rickettsial or viral infections, patients in isolation, and patients being treated with radioactive isotopes. Avoid areas with radioactive hazard symbol
Tuberculosis (active)	Off work until treated and AFB smears are negative for 2 weeks
Rubella (German measles)	Off work until rash is gone (minimum 5 days)
Salmonella	Varies depending on symptoms, treatment results, and Employee Health Department evaluation
Scabies	Off work until treated
Shigella	Varies depending on symptoms, treatment results, and Employee Health Department evaluation
Strep throat (group A)	Off work until 24 hours after antibiotic therapy is started and symptoms are gone
URI (upper respiratory infection)	Work status determined by Employee Health Department

INDEX

Page numbers in *italics* denote figures; those followed by a t denote tables.

BD Vacutainer® Venous Blood Collection
Tube Guide

For a full line of BD Vacutainer® Specimen Collection Products, visit www.bd.com/vacutainer.

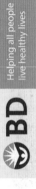

BD Vacutainer® Tubes with BD Hemogard™ Closure	BD Vacutainer® Tubes with Conventional Stopper	Additive	Inversions at Blood Collection*	Laboratory Use	Your Lab's Draw Volume/Remarks
Gold	Red/Black	• Clot activator and gel for serum separation	5	For serum determinations in chemistry. May be used for routine blood donor screening and diagnostic testing of serum for infectious disease.** Tube inversions ensure mixing of clot activator with blood. Blood clotting time: 30 minutes.	
Light Green	Green/Gray	• Lithium heparin and gel for plasma separation	8	BD Vacutainer® PST™ Tube for plasma determinations in chemistry. Tube inversions prevent clotting.	
Red	Red	• None (glass) • Clot activator (plastic)	0 5	For serum determinations in chemistry. May be used for routine blood donor screening and diagnostic testing of serum for infectious disease.** Tube inversions ensure mixing of clot activator with blood. Blood clotting time: 60 minutes.	
Orange	Gray/Yellow	• Thrombin	8	For stat serum determinations in chemistry. Tube inversions ensure complete clotting, which usually occurs in less than 5 minutes.	
Royal Blue		• Clot activator (plastic serum) • K_2EDTA (plastic)	8 8 0 5 8	For trace-element, toxicology, and nutritional-chemistry determinations. Special stopper formulation provides low levels of trace elements (see package insert).	
Green		• Sodium heparin • Lithium heparin	8 8	For plasma determinations in chemistry. Tube inversions prevent clotting.	
Gray		• Potassium oxalate/sodium fluoride • Sodium fluoride/Na_2 EDTA • Sodium fluoride (serum tube)	8 8 8	For glucose determinations. Oxalate and EDTA anticoagulants will give plasma samples. Sodium fluoride is the antiglycolytic agent. Tube inversions ensure proper mixing of additive and blood.	
Tan		• K_2EDTA (plastic)	8 8	For lead determinations. This tube is certified to contain less than .01 µg/mL(ppm) lead. Tube inversions prevent clotting.	
Yellow		• Sodium polyanethol sulfonate (SPS) • Acid citrate dextrose additives (ACD): **Solution A** - 22.0 g/L trisodium citrate, 8.0 g/L citric acid,	8 8	SPS for blood culture specimen collections in microbiology. Tube inversions prevent clotting. ACD for use in blood bank studies, HLA phenotyping, and DNA and paternity testing.	

Closure Color	Additive	Inversions*	Laboratory Use
	24.5 g/L dextrose **Solution B** - 13.2 g/L trisodium citrate, 4.8 g/L citric acid, 14.7 g/L dextrose	8	
Lavender	• Liquid K₂EDTA (glass) • Spray-coated K₂EDTA (plastic)	8 8	K₂EDTA and K₃EDTA for whole blood hematology determinations. K₂EDTA may be used for routine immunohematology testing and blood donor screening.*** Tube inversions prevent clotting.
White	• K₂EDTA with gel	8	For use in molecular diagnostic test methods (such as but not limited to polymerase chain reaction [PCR] and/or branched DNA [bDNA] amplification techniques).
Pink (New)	• Spray-coated K₂EDTA	8	For whole blood hematology determinations. May be used for routine immunohematology testing and blood donor screening.*** Designed with special cross-match label for patient information required by the AABB. Tube inversions prevent clotting.
Light Blue	• Buffered sodium citrate 0.105 M (=3.2%) glass, 0.109 M (=3.2%) plastic • Citrate, theophylline, adenosine, dipyridamole (CTAD)	3-4 3-4	For coagulation determinations. CTAD for selected platelet function assays and routine coagulation determination. Tube inversions prevent clotting.
Clear (New) Red/Gray	• None (plastic)	0	For use as a discard tube or secondary specimen collection tube.

Partial-draw Tubes (2 mL and 3 mL: 13 x 75 mm)   **Small-volume Pediatric Tubes** (2 mL: 10.25 x 47 mm, 3 mL: 10.25 x 64 mm)

Closure Color	Additive	Inversions*	Laboratory Use
Red	• None	0	For serum determinations in chemistry. May be used for routine blood donor screening, immunohematology testing,*** and diagnostic testing of serum for infectious disease.** Tube inversions ensure mixing of clot activator with blood. Blood clotting time: 60 minutes.
Green	• Sodium heparin • Lithium heparin	8 8	For plasma determinations in chemistry. Tube inversions prevent clotting.
Lavender	• Spray-coated K₂EDTA (plastic)	8 8	For whole blood hematology determinations. May be used for routine immunohematology testing and blood donor screening.*** Tube inversions prevent clotting.
Light Blue	• 0.105 M sodium citrate (=3.2%)	3-4	For coagulation determinations. Tube inversions prevent clotting.

* Invert gently; do not shake
** The performance characteristics of these tubes have not been established for infectious disease testing in general; therefore, users must validate the use of these tubes for their specific assay-instrument/reagent system combinations and specimen storage conditions.
*** The performance characteristics of these tubes have not been established for immunohematology testing in general; therefore, users must validate the use of these tubes for their specific assay-instrument/reagent system combinations and specimen storage conditions.

BD Diagnostics
Preanalytical Systems
1 Becton Drive
Franklin Lakes, NJ 07417 USA

BD Global Technical Services: 1.800.631.0174
vacutainer_techservice@bd.com
BD Customer Service: 1.888.237.2762
www.bd.com/vacutainer

Printed in USA   07/06   VS5229-8

BD, BD Logo and all other trademarks are property of Becton, Dickinson and Company © 2006 BD